OUTBREAK INVESTIGATION, PREVENTION, AND CONTROL IN HEALTH CARE SETTINGS

Critical Issues for Patient Safety

Second Edition

Kathleen Meehan Arias
MS, MT (ASCP), CIC

Arias Infection Control Consulting, LLC
Crownsville, Maryland

JONES AND BARTLETT PUBLISHERS
Sudbury, Massachusetts
BOSTON   TORONTO   LONDON   SINGAPORE

World Headquarters
Jones and Bartlett Publishers
40 Tall Pine Drive
Sudbury, MA 01776
978-443-5000
info@jbpub.com
www.jbpub.com

Jones and Bartlett Publishers Canada
6339 Ormindale Way
Mississauga, Ontario L5V 1J2
Canada

Jones and Bartlett Publishers International
Barb House, Barb Mews
London W6 7PA
United Kingdom

Jones and Bartlett's books and products are available through most bookstores and online booksellers. To contact Jones and Bartlett Publishers directly, call 800-832-0034, fax 978-443-8000, or visit our website www.jbpub.com.

Substantial discounts on bulk quantities of Jones and Bartlett's publications are available to corporations, professional associations, and other qualified organizations. For details and specific discount information, contact the special sales department at Jones and Bartlett via the above contact information or send an email to specialsales@jbpub.com.

This publication is designed to provide accurate and authoritative information in regard to the Subject Matter covered. It is sold with the understanding that the publisher is not engaged in rendering legal, accounting, or other professional service. If legal advice or other expert assistance is required, the service of a competent professional person should be sought.

Production Credits
Publisher: Michael Brown
Production Director: Amy Rose
Associate Editor: Katey Birtcher
Editorial Assistant: Catie Heverling
Senior Production Editor: Tracey Chapman
Production Assistant: Roya Millard
Marketing Manager: Sophie Fleck
Manufacturing and Inventory Control Supervisor: Amy Bacus
Composition: Achorn International
Cover Design: Scott Moden
Cover Image: © Daniela Illing/ShutterStock, Inc.
Printing and Binding: Malloy, Inc.
Cover Printing: Malloy, Inc.

Library of Congress Cataloging-in-Publication Data
Arias, Kathleen Meehan.
    Outbreak investigation, prevention, and control in health care settings: critical issues for patient safety / Kathleen Meehan Arias.
        p. ; cm.
    Rev. ed. of: Quick reference to outbreak investigation and control in health care facilities / Kathleen Meehan Arias. 2000.
    Includes bibliographical references.
    ISBN-13: 978-0-7637-5779-3 (pbk.)
    ISBN-10: 0-7637-5779-9 (pbk.)
    1. Health facilities—Sanitation—Handbooks, manuals, etc. 2. Nosocomial infections—Prevention—Handbooks, manuals, etc. 3. Cross infection—Prevention—Handbooks, manuals, etc. I. Arias, Kathleen Meehan. Quick reference to outbreak investigation and control in health care facilities. II. Title.
    [DNLM: 1. Health Facilities—Handbooks. 2. Infection Control—methods—Handbooks. 3. Disease Outbreaks—Handbooks. 4. Epidemiologic Methods—Handbooks. WX 39 A696o 2010]
    RA969.A736 2010
    614.4'4--dc22
                                                            2008029520

6048
Printed in the United States of America
13 12 11 10 09   10 9 8 7 6 5 4 3 2 1

For my wonderful husband, Bob.
For his patience, understanding, and support while I worked on the second edition of "the book."

I am indebted to the contributing authors (colleagues and friends who graciously shared their expertise) and to their families who were understanding of the time it takes to prepare a manuscript.

The author would like to thank Robert Arias, Patti Grant, and James Luby, MD, for reviewing sections of the manuscript and providing constructive criticism, and Shawn M. Phillips for sharing his mom.

Kathleen Meehan Arias

Contents

Preface to the Second Edition

Although optimists once imagined that serious infectious disease threats would by now be conquered, newly emerging (e.g., severe acute respiratory syndrome [SARS]), reemerging (e.g., West Nile virus), and even deliberately disseminated infectious diseases (e.g., anthrax bioterrorism) continue to appear throughout the world.

—Fauci AS, Touchette NA, Folkers GK. Emerging infectious diseases: a 10-year perspective from the National Institute of Allergy and Infectious Diseases. *Emerg Infect Dis*. 2005;11:519.

Since the 1970s, over 35 new human pathogens have been identified, and many known pathogens have emerged or reemerged. Many of these agents have caused outbreaks in healthcare settings. The ability of a previously unrecognized human pathogen to emerge and cause a pandemic was demonstrated by the severe acute respiratory syndrome (SARS) outbreak that began in late 2002 in the southern People's Republic of China and spread to over 25 countries on five continents before it was brought under control in July 2003.

Several major events have occurred since the first edition of this book was published. One was SARS, whose rapid global spread was facilitated by travelers on airplanes. Another was the intentional release of *Bacillus anthracis* spores through the United States postal system in September 2001. SARS caused clusters of respiratory disease in hospitals that resulted in deaths of healthcare workers. The anthrax cases that resulted from a bioterrorist event taxed the ability of healthcare facilities and public health agencies to respond quickly to identify and treat those who were infected, prevent further transmission, and care for the "worried-well". In the early 2000s a new hypervirulent strain of *C. difficile* caused widespread hospital outbreaks in Canada that were associated with severe morbidity and increased mortality. This more virulent strain is refractory to antibiotic treatment, has emerged in several countries, and has caused healthcare-associated outbreaks in the United States, United Kingdom, and Europe. The person-to-person transmission of the avian influenza virus, H5N1, was first documented in Asia in the early 2000s, and the potential exists for H5N1 to cause a pandemic in humans. Drug-resistant organisms, such as methicillin-resistant *Staphylococcus aureus* (MRSA) and multidrug-resistant strains of *Pseudomonas, Acinetobacter, Klebsiella*, and *Enterobacter* continue to evolve, spread globally, and cause outbreaks in healthcare settings worldwide.

All of these events highlight the need for infection surveillance, prevention, and control (ISPC) systems worldwide and a strong infrastructure to link and support these systems. Healthcare personnel and healthcare facilities play an integral role in interrupting the transmission of infectious agents and recognizing, preventing, and controlling outbreaks caused by infectious and noninfectious agents. The field of healthcare epidemiology was initially concerned with infection surveillance, prevention, and control in acute care hospitals. However, since the provision of health care continues to shift from the acute care hospital to a variety of ambulatory and long-term care settings, healthcare epidemiology has evolved beyond the hospital to include these settings and has expanded beyond infections to include the use of sound epidemiological principles in studying noninfectious outcomes of medical care. One factor that has greatly benefited infection surveillance, prevention, and control programs since 2000 is the growth of information technology (hardware, software, and Internet-based computer systems) to collect, store, analyze, report, and transmit data and information. The Internet is now widely used to gather and disseminate information on infectious diseases and outbreaks.

As with the first edition, this book was written for infection prevention and control (ICP) professionals, healthcare epidemiologists, clinical laboratory scientists, healthcare quality management personnel, public health personnel, students, and educators—those who are interested in using epidemiologic methods to monitor healthcare outcomes. This text has the following purposes:

1. Explain epidemiologic principles as they apply to the healthcare setting
2. Serve as a reference for published reports pertaining to the identification, investigation, prevention, and control of outbreaks in a variety of settings
3. Present practical guidelines for identifying, investigating, preventing, and controlling outbreaks caused by either infectious or noninfectious agents
4. Discuss the use of information technology (IT) in ISPC programs

The following changes and revisions have been made in this edition: The book title has been changed from *Quick Reference to Outbreak Investigation and Control in Health Care Facilities* to *Outbreak Investigation, Prevention, and Control in Health Care Settings: Critical Issues for Patient Safety*. The need to implement routine practices that can prevent outbreaks has become critical as pathogens develop multidrug resistance and the possibility of untreatable infections becomes a reality. Consequently, *prevention* has been added to the title, and infection prevention measures have been updated and expanded throughout the text. The word *facility* has been changed to *setting* because many healthcare facilities, especially hospitals, now encompass a wide variety of healthcare settings, such as outpatient offices, same-day (ambulatory) surgery, and rehabilitation and other long-term care services. The subtitle *Critical Issues for Patient Safety* has been added to focus on the essential role that ISPC play in providing a safe healthcare environment.

The title of Chapter 2 has been changed from "Surveillance Programs in Healthcare Facilities" to "Surveillance Programs, Public Health, and Emergency Preparedness." In response to events such as the SARS outbreak, anthrax bioterrorism, and the global spread of new and reemerging infections, information has been added on global surveillance programs, emergency preparedness, and the healthcare community's role in public health surveillance.

Chapter 9 (formerly "Conducting a Literature Search") has been renamed "Information Technology and Outbreak Investigation" and has been expanded to discuss the various roles that IT plays in detecting, investigating, preventing, and controlling outbreaks in the healthcare setting.

Chapter 11 has been renamed "The Role of the Laboratory in Outbreak Detection, Prevention, and Investigation" (formerly "The Role of the Laboratory in Outbreak Investigation"), and information on laboratory test methods and bioterrorism has been updated.

Information on outbreaks and pseudo-outbreaks that have occurred in acute, long-term, and ambulatory healthcare settings since the first edition has been added.

Updated information on emerging (new) and reemerging pathogens has been incorporated throughout the text.

The References and Suggested Reading and Resources sections at the end of each chapter have been updated and additional Web-based resources and links have been provided.

An increased emphasis has been placed on the integral role of the healthcare community in supporting the medical and public health infrastructures needed to effectively detect, investigate, prevent, and control outbreaks at the local, national, and international levels.

An Overview of the Content

Chapter 1 defines terms used in healthcare epidemiology, describes the different types of epidemiologic studies used in the healthcare setting, discusses the multifactorial nature of disease, and addresses the concepts of association and causation. Chapter 2 outlines the components of effective surveillance programs for a variety of healthcare settings—programs that are necessary to recognize a potential outbreak or occurrence of adverse events. Chapters 3 through 7 review reports of outbreaks and pseudo-outbreaks that have occurred in acute care, long-term care, and ambulatory care settings. By studying these reports, healthcare and public health personnel can expand their knowledge of the epidemiology of healthcare-associated outbreaks and identify effective interventions that can be used to interrupt and prevent outbreaks.

Chapter 8 presents practical guidelines for identifying, investigating, and controlling outbreaks in healthcare settings. Chapter 9 discusses the use of IT in outbreak detection, investigation, and control. Chapter 10 explains basic statistical terms and concepts used in outbreak investigation so the reader can recognize how and when to apply these methods to describe an outbreak, perform an epidemiologic study, analyze findings, and test a hypothesis on the likely cause of an outbreak. Chapter 11 outlines the integral role of the laboratory in the diagnosis and surveillance of infections and the detection and investigation of outbreaks. Chapter 12 gives practical information on collecting, organizing, and displaying epidemiologic data using tables, graphs, and charts.

The appendices (available for download at this text's Web site: http://www .jbpub.com/catalog/9780763757793/) contain a glossary of terms used in healthcare epidemiology, case definitions for infectious diseases, and infection prevention and control guidelines related to outbreak investigation, prevention, and control.

Contributors

Lorraine Messinger Harkavy, RN, MS
Consultant, Infection Control and Prevention
Potomac, Maryland

Deborah Y. Phillips, RN, BSN, MPH
Associate Director
Texas/Oklahoma AIDS Education and Training Center
Parkland Health and Hospital System
Dallas, Texas

CHAPTER 1

An Introduction to Epidemiology

Kathleen Meehan Arias

> Microbial threats continue to emerge, reemerge, and persist. Some microbes cause newly recognized diseases in humans; others are previously known pathogens that are infecting new or larger population groups or spreading into new geographic areas. . . . The emergence and spread of microbial threats are driven by a complex set of factors, the convergence of which can lead to consequences of disease much greater than any single factor might suggest.[1]

INTRODUCTION

Since the 1970s, over 35 new human pathogens have been identified, and many known pathogens have emerged or reemerged.[2,3] New and emergent pathogenic agents include bacteria such as *Borrelia burgdorferi*, *Campylobacter* sp, *Clostridium difficile*, *Ehrlichia chaffeensis*, *Escherichia coli* O157:H7, *Helicobacter pylori*, *Legionella pneumophila*, *Mycobacterium tuberculosis* (especially multidrug-resistant strains), methicillin-resistant *Staphylococcus aureus* (MRSA), *Streptococcus pyogenes* (group A strep), *Vibrio cholerae*, and *Vibrio vulnificus*; viruses such as adenovirus, avian influenza, the severe acute respiratory syndrome (SARS) coronavirus, Crimean-Congo hemorrhagic fever, chikungunya, dengue, Ebola, hantaviruses, hepatitis B, C, and E, the human immunodeficiency viruses, human parvovirus B19, influenza, Lassa, measles, monkeypox, norovirus, and rotavirus; prions such as those causing variant Creutzfeldt-Jakob disease and bovine spongiform encephalopathy or mad-cow disease; and other agents such as *Babesia*, *Cryptococcus*, *Cryptosporidium*, and *Pneumocystis carinii*. Many of these pathogens have caused outbreaks in healthcare settings. The ability of a previously unrecognized human pathogen to emerge and cause a pandemic was demonstrated by the SARS outbreak that began in late 2002 in the southern People's Republic of China and spread to more than 25 countries on five continents before it was brought under control in July 2003.[4]

This chapter provides the reader with information needed to investigate outbreaks in healthcare facilities and to understand that "complex set of factors, the convergence of which can lead to consequences of disease much greater than any single factor might suggest."[1(p1)]

DEFINITIONS USED IN HEALTHCARE EPIDEMIOLOGY

The term *epidemiology* is derived from three Greek words: *epi*, on or among, *demos*, people, and *logos*, the study of. Although many definitions can be found, the following is appropriate for use in the healthcare setting: "Epidemiology is the study of the distribution and determinants of health-related states and events in defined populations, and the application of this study to the control of health problems."[5]

In other words, epidemiology is used to describe what, who, where, when, and why disease and other health-related problems occur so that control measures can be identified and implemented. The information in this chapter focuses on the basic principles of epidemiology as they are applied to the surveillance, prevention, and control of healthcare-associated infections and other adverse events in healthcare facilities.

The terms defined in the following list are used in this text to describe the occurrence of disease The word *disease* is used throughout the text in a broad sense to include health-related conditions and events such as accidents, adverse drug reactions, and injuries. These definitions, as well as many others, can be found in the Glossary.

- Community acquired—A disease that results from exposure to physical, chemical, or biological agents in the community.
- Endemic—The usual or expected number of cases of disease within a specific geographic location or population.
- Epidemic—The occurrence of more cases of disease than expected in a given area or specific population over a specified period of time.
- Incidence—The number of new cases of disease in a particular population during a specified period of time.
- Nosocomial or healthcare-associated—A disease that results from exposure to physical, chemical, or biological agents in the healthcare setting.
- Pandemic—An epidemic that affects several countries or continents.
- Prevalence—The number of existing cases (both old and new) of disease in a particular population during a specified period of time.

A HISTORICAL PERSPECTIVE: SOME EPIDEMIOLOGIC TIDBITS

Epidemiologic principles have long been used to determine the suspected cause of diseases so that control measures can be identified and implemented to prevent their spread. We know from the Bible that lepers were isolated from society (c. 1400 BC) to prevent the spread of leprosy ("he shall dwell alone . . ." Leviticus 13:46). In the Mosaic code, the consumption of pork was forbidden ("The swine . . . is unclean to you." Leviticus 11:7), and this prohibition still exists today in some cultures. Around 400 BC, Hippocrates wrote his famous treatise, *On Airs, Waters, and Places*, in which he associated disease occurrence with environmental factors such as air, water, and places rather than with supernatural causes. In the Dark Ages (c. AD 500–1400), diseases were thought to be caused by miasmas or rising vapors, such as those from marshes, that were thought to infect the air. The word "quarantine" comes from 14th-century Italy where sailing vessels were detained for 40 days ("quaranta giorni") before travelers could disembark. This precaution was taken to prevent the spread of plague. This practice carries over to modern-day maritime regulations where a vessel, upon arrival from a foreign port, is required to display a square yellow flag until permission is granted to land.[6] The yellow signal flag represents the letter *Q* in the international code of flags that ships around the world use to communicate.

In the 1500s, Italian physician and poet Girolamo Fracastoro recognized that there were three modes of transmission (person-to-person, air, and objects), and in his 1546 work, *De Contagione et Contagiosis Morbis*, he suspected that minute agents caused disease.

The word *malaria* can be traced back to the 1700s and comes from the Italian *mala aria* or "bad air." This alludes to the former belief that malaria was spread by foul air from swamps. In the late 1700s, the British physician Edward Jenner observed that dairy workers who had contact with cows having cowpox did not succumb when exposed to smallpox. He discovered that individuals could be protected from smallpox if they were inoculated with cowpox—thus giving us the word *vaccine*, which is adopted from the Latin *vaccinus* for cow.

In 1846, Panum noticed that if measles were introduced to a population, there were fewer cases if some of the population previously had measles. He was the first person to scientifically explain herd immunity (i.e., the resistance of a population to invasion and spread of an infectious agent because many in the population are immune). In the 1840s Ignaz Phillipp Semmelweis noticed that there appeared to be more deaths from puerperal (childbed) fever in the first division of the Vienna Lying-In Hospital than in the second division. He reviewed the literature on the proposed causes of puerperal fever, observed practices, and carefully collected data on the numbers of deaths and possible risk factors, such as exposure to different types of medical personnel. After comparing mortality rates and risk factors between the two divisions, he formed the hypothesis that cadaveric material on the hands of medical students was somehow responsible for causing puerperal fever. Semmelweis then required students and physicians to wash their hands in chlorinated lime after performing autopsies prior to attending a patient. Semmelweis was able to demonstrate a dramatic decrease in maternal mortality rates after mandating hand disinfection.[7] Florence Nightingale began her reformation of the British army medical system by introducing sanitary practices, such as environmental cleanliness and safe food and water, during the Crimean War (1853–1855). After the war, she collaborated with the British statistician William Farr to study mortality rates in British hospitals. Using carefully collected epidemiologic data, they were able to show that many deaths were caused by communicable diseases, and they used this information to lobby for further improvements in hospital sanitation.[8]

In his well-known epidemiologic studies conducted in the 1850s, the anesthesiologist John Snow investigated the occurrence of cholera in the Golden Square area of London and deduced that the water supply coming from the Broad Street pump was associated with development of the disease.[9] Based on his findings, Snow reportedly removed the handle of the water pump, thus ending the cholera outbreak. John Snow is known as the "father" of field epidemiology because his studies classically illustrate the use of the epidemiologic principles used today to investigate and control outbreaks. It should be noted that Jenner, Panum, Semmelweis, Nightingale, and Snow used imagination, logic, and common sense to determine the most likely factors causing disease and to develop preventive measures—and all worked before the French chemist Louis Pasteur developed his germ theory in the late 1800s.

Any discussion of the evolution of epidemiology would be incomplete without mentioning Robert Koch (1843–1910) who won the Nobel Prize for his studies in microbiology. Among other things, Koch established techniques for growing microorganisms in pure culture and studied the relationship between *Mycobacterium tuberculosis* and tuberculosis (TB). He developed four postulates, now known as Koch's postulates, that he believed were necessary to prove that an organism was the cause of a disease:

1. The organism must be associated with all cases of a given disease.
2. The organism must be isolated in pure culture from persons with that disease.
3. When the pure culture is inoculated into a susceptible person or animal, it must cause the same disease.
4. The organism must then be isolated in pure culture from the person or animal infected by this inoculation.

Although Koch's postulates cannot be used to establish the etiologic relationship of some organisms, such as viruses and noncultivable agents, to the disease they are thought to cause, he created a scientific standard for establishing disease causation.[10]

THE MULTIFACTORIAL NATURE OF DISEASE

Etiologic Agents of Disease

The multifactorial nature of disease is now well recognized.[11] That is, a disease cannot be attributed to any one factor because there is a complex interrelationship between various agents, a host, and the environment—a concept known as the epidemiologic triangle.

Epidemiology was originally concerned with the study of infectious disease, and thus the epidemiologic triangle of agent, host, and the environment is the traditional model used to explain disease causation. Because the epidemiologic principles are now applied to the study of noninfectious conditions as well, the concept of the causative agent has been expanded beyond biological agents to include chemical and physical agents. Exhibit 1–1 provides examples of the various etiologic agents of disease.

Biological Agents

Despite advances in medicine, more people die annually worldwide from infectious diseases than from any other cause.[2] Many of the agents noted above as newly recognized or emerging since the 1970s have caused outbreaks in the community and in healthcare facilities. Several well-known pathogens have developed drug resistance and have caused serious epidemics: MRSA, vancomycin-resistant *Enterococcus* (VRE), and multidrug-resistant and extensively drug-resistant *Mycobacterium tuberculosis*.

Exhibit 1–1   Examples of Etiologic Agents of Disease

Biological Agents	*Examples*
Arthropods	*Sarcoptes* (mites); *Dermacentor, Amblyomma*, and *Ixodes* (ticks)
Bacteria	*Staphylococcus, Pseudomonas, Mycobacterium, Campylobacter, Clostridium, Ehrlichia*
Fungi	*Candida, Aspergillus, Cryptococcus, Histoplasmosis*
Metazoa	*Trichinella; Necator* and *Ancylostoma* (hookworm)
Prions	Creutzfeldt-Jakob Disease, bovine spongiform encephalopathy (mad cow disease)
Protozoa	*Plasmodium* (malaria), *Cryptosporidium, Giardia, Pneumocystis, Toxoplasma*
Rickettsiae	*Rickettsia*
Viruses	Hepatitis, human immunodeficiency virus, herpes, influenza, measles, norovirus, rotavirus

Chemical Agents	*Examples*
Food additives	Monosodium glutamate
Inorganic chemicals	Heavy metals
Occupational exposure	Industrial/laboratory reagents, silica, asbestos, latex
Organic chemicals	Aldehydes (e.g., gluteraldehyde), disinfectants
Pesticides	DDT, sterilants (e.g., ethylene oxide)
Pharmaceuticals	Antibiotics, analgesics, psychotropics

Physical Agents	*Examples*
Ionizing radiation	X-rays
Light	Ultraviolet, laser, lightning
Moving objects	Cars, bicycles, bullets
Noise	Music
Physical forces	Repetitive motion, lifting, falls
Thermal extremes	Heat, cold

Chemical Agents

Many chemical agents can cause adverse reactions in man. Personnel and patients in healthcare facilities have developed dermatitis and other allergic reactions following exposure to gluteraldehyde and latex, and patients have experienced hearing loss after therapy with gentamycin.

Physical Agents

Physical agents such as heat, cold, electricity, light, or ionizing radiation may cause injuries in the healthcare setting, For example, lasers have caused burns when they malfunctioned during surgery, and ultraviolet light has caused conjunctivitis in exposed personnel. Healthcare workers are also at risk for back injuries from lifting patients and from percutaneous injuries caused by needles and sharp instruments.

Host Factors Affecting Disease

Host factors are conditions that affect an individual's risk of exposure and resistance or susceptibility to disease. They include intrinsic factors such as age, sex, genetic composition, or race. Age is one of the most important host factors because it affects both risk of exposure and immunologic status. Factors that influence a person's risk of exposure to disease-causing agents include socioeconomic status, lifestyle behaviors, occupation, and marital status. Factors that influence a person's susceptibility or resistance to disease include immunologic and nutritional status, underlying disease, severity of illness, and psychological state.

Environmental Factors Affecting Disease

Environmental factors are extrinsic factors that affect either the agent or a person's opportunity for exposure to the agent. Factors that affect a person's risk of exposure to nosocomial events include hospitalization or residing in a long-term care facility. Crowding, sanitation, and living in a rural versus urban area are all environmental factors. In some instances, it is difficult to determine whether a particular factor should be classified as agent or environment. For instance, factors such as intravenous therapy, mechanical ventilation, surgery, and invasive diagnostic procedures all affect a patient's risk of exposure to both biological and physical agents; these procedures are also associated with the environment of health care.

Although the traditional epidemiologic triangle may not be appropriate for illustrating disease causation in many noninfectious conditions, it can facilitate understanding of the many interrelated factors that affect the occurrence of infectious diseases. This is an important concept that must be recognized when investigating outbreaks of disease.

STUDY METHODS USED IN EPIDEMIOLOGY: THE FIVE Ws— WHAT, WHO, WHERE, WHEN, AND WHY

Epidemiology is used to understand the causes of a disease (what) by studying its distribution (who, where, and when) and its determinants (why). This helps to characterize the natural history of a disease so that prevention and control measures can be identified. Note that a major purpose of epidemiology is to develop intervention and prevention programs rather than to find a cure.

Epidemiology is a population-based science. Many disciplines contribute to the knowledge of human health and disease—the basic sciences (such as microbiology and biochemistry), the clinical sciences (such as infectious diseases, pediatrics, and internal medicine), and population medicine (such as community medicine and public health)—and all are highly interrelated. The major difference between clinical medicine and population medicine is that the former focuses on an individual person, such as a patient with a respiratory disease, while the latter focuses on the community as a whole, such as an influenza outbreak. Epidemiology is a science of comparison and rates. The epidemiologist looks for groups with high or low rates of disease so that reasons for disease and freedom from disease can be postulated.

There are three types of epidemiologic studies: descriptive (or observational), analytic, and experimental. Descriptive and analytic studies are used to observe the natural course of events, such as an outbreak of food-borne illness or the course of the human immunodeficiency virus (HIV) epidemic; however, in an experimental study, the investigator studies the impact of varying some factor under his control (e.g., clinical trials of products or therapeutic agents).

Descriptive Epidemiology: Who, Where, and When

Descriptive studies are used to identify individuals and populations at greatest risk of acquiring a disease, to determine clues as to the etiology of disease, and to predict disease occurrence through knowledge of association of a disease with some risk factor. In descriptive epidemiology one studies the incidence (rates) and distribution (population at risk) of disease. Data are organized according to the variables of person, place, and time to identify factors that may be causally related to disease incidence.

Person

The major factors that affect a person's risk of developing a disease include:

- Age—Age is considered the most important factor among the personal variables because it affects one's potential for exposure (e.g., school children are exposed to childhood diseases and adults are exposed to occupational diseases), immune status (e.g., infants have poorly developed immune systems; the elderly have decreased resistance to many infections), and mental and physical condition (e.g., the elderly are generally more prone to falls than the young).
- Sex—Males have higher incidence rates for some diseases and conditions than females (e.g., HIV infection) while females have higher rates for others (e.g., breast cancer).
- Socioeconomic status—Variables such as social class, occupation, lifestyle, educational level, and family income affect nutritional status, travel, access to health care, and environmental living and working conditions— all of which influence a person's susceptibility or resistance to disease and risk of exposure to various agents and physical injury.
- Ethnic and racial groups—Cultural and religious differences can affect a person's risk of exposure to various agents, such as types of food eaten and methods of preparing it.[12]
- Genetic variables—Variables associated with genetic composition can affect susceptibility to some diseases, such as sickle cell, Tay-Sachs, and Kaposi's sarcoma.

Place

Depending on the event being studied, place may be characterized by birth-place, residence, school, hospital unit, place of employment, restaurant, and so on. One can use political boundaries such as country, state, city, county, or parish, or natural boundaries such as mountains, valleys, or watersheds. Some diseases are associated with the place where they were first recognized, such as Lyme disease with a town in Connecticut.

In the healthcare setting, surveillance data are usually collected and analyzed by the number of cases or the incidence rates in a specific place or area (e.g., the incidence of central line-associated bloodstream infections in an intensive care unit (ICU), intravenous therapy-related phlebitis on 3 West; or resident falls in the North Wing).

Many health departments use counties, census tracts, and ZIP codes to report statistics on injuries, illnesses, or communicable diseases (Table 1–1). Those responsible for infection control and other quality management programs in healthcare facilities should use this type of information to identify populations at risk for disease. Because exposure to many infectious diseases occurs both in the healthcare setting (through infected patients, residents, visitors, or personnel) and in the community (through infected relatives, friends, co-workers, classmates, etc.), outbreaks in healthcare facilities often reflect what is occurring locally. For example, community outbreaks of pertussis, chickenpox, rotavirus, TB, and influenza have caused simultaneous outbreaks in area hospitals and long-term care facilities.[13–16] In addition, community disease profiles should be used to conduct an assessment of the risk of healthcare workers' exposure to diseases such as TB.[17]

Table 1–1 Maryland Tuberculosis Incidence—New Cases and Rates per 100,000 Population by Geographic Area (2004–2007)

Jurisdiction	2004		2005		2006		2007	
High-Incidence Jurisdictions (6)	Cases	Rate	Cases	Rate	Cases	Rate	Cases	Rate
Montgomery	93	10.0	81	8.8	62	6.7	82	8.8
Baltimore City	58	9.1	68	10.6	35	5.5	47	7.4
Prince George's	72	8.6	57	6.7	72	8.5	66	7.9
Baltimore County	31	4.0	20	2.6	17	2.2	31	3.9
Anne Arundel	6	1.2	15	2.9	19	3.7	9	1.8
Howard	14	5.2	12	4.5	6	2.2	11	4.0
Remaining Counties (18)	40	2.5	30	1.8	42	2.6	24	1.5
Statewide	314	5.6	283	5.1	253	4.5	270	4.8

Source: Adapted from *Maryland Tuberculosis Incidence: New Cases and Rates per 100,000 Population by Geographic Area and Demographic Features* (1998–2007). Maryland Department of Health and Mental Hygiene, Office of Epidemiology and Disease Control Programs, Division of TB Control. http://edcp.org/tb/pdf/TB_Rate_Table.xls. Accessed February 22, 2008.

Time

Surveillance data are collected and analyzed over time for evidence of change in the incidence of an event (such as healthcare-associated infections or medication errors). These data are often shown on a graph with the number of cases or the incidence rate on the vertical axis (y-axis) and time on the horizontal axis (x-axis) (Figure 1–1). The time periods depicted on the x-axis may be hours, days, weeks, months, quarters, or years, depending on the event described.

Epidemic period. An epidemic is the occurrence of more cases of disease than expected in a given area or population over a specified period of time. For some diseases, a graph of an epidemic period, called an epidemic curve, can be used to provide insight into the time of exposure, the mode of transmission, and the agent causing the outbreak (Figure 1–2). Information on constructing and using epidemic curves can be found in Chapters 8 and 12.

Secular (long-term) trends. Surveillance data can be graphed over a period of years to show trends occurring over long periods of time. This information can be used to monitor the efficacy of infection prevention and control and performance improvement programs in healthcare facilities and in the public health sector. For example, Figure 1–3, a graph of the incidence of TB reported in the United States for the period 1982 through 2006 illustrates the increasing incidence that occurred in the late 1980s and early 1990s and the decline that followed through 2006.[18] According to the Centers for Disease Control and Prevention, factors that were associated with the resurgence of TB included the acquired immune deficiency syndrome (AIDS)/HIV epidemic; immigration of persons from countries where incidence rates are 10–30 times higher than in the United States; transmission of TB in settings such as hospitals, homeless

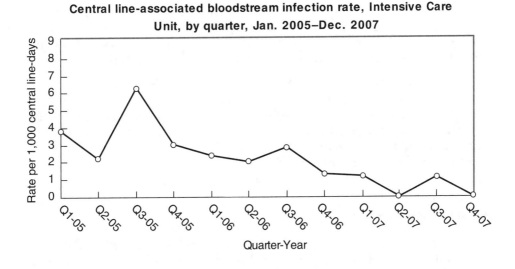

Figure 1–1 Surveillance Data Showing Infection Rates Over Time.

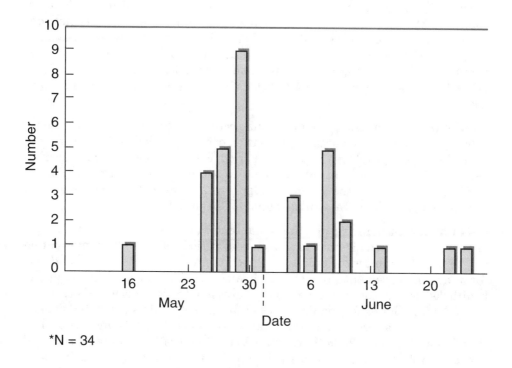

Figure 1-2 Epidemic Curve of a Measles Outbreak, Indiana, May–June, 2005.
Source: Centers for Disease Control and Prevention, Impact-Associated Measles Outbreak—Indiana, May–June 2005. *MMWR*. October 28, 2005; 54: 1073–1075. http://www.cdc.gov/mmwr/preview/mmwrhtml/mm5442a1.htm

shelters, and prisons; and declines in resources for TB control.[19] The downward trend that began in 1993 has been attributed to the implementation of stronger TB control programs that emphasize prompt identification of persons with TB, initiation of appropriate therapy, and completion of therapy.[20]

Seasonal occurrence. Some diseases have a characteristic seasonal pattern. For instance, in the United States the common cold caused by rhinovirus in adults occurs most frequently in the fall, and chickenpox occurs most frequently in winter and early spring. In temperate climates, outbreaks of influenza generally occur in winter. Information such as this can be used to recognize the possible causative agent of an outbreak of respiratory disease in a healthcare facility and to target the timing of influenza immunization campaigns.

Analytic Epidemiology: Why

When conducting an outbreak investigation, descriptive epidemiology is used to describe the outbreak or the cluster of events (i.e., the population involved, the time, and the place), and then rates can be calculated to identify the population with the highest rate of disease. The next step in the investiga-

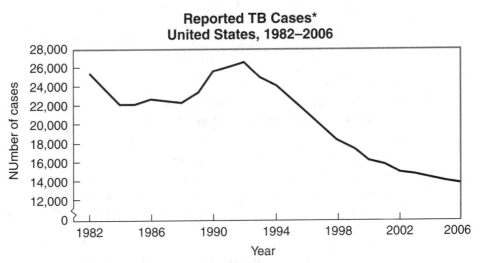

Figure 1–3 Graph Depicting Secular Trend of Tuberculosis from 1982 Through 2006 in the United States.
Source: Centers for Disease Control and Prevention. *Reported Tuberculosis in the United States 2006*. Atlanta, GA: U.S. Department of Health and Human Services, September 2007: 86. http://www.cdc.gov/tb/surv

tion is to use analytic methods to search for a probable cause by mathematically comparing risk factors (attack rates) between the population with the disease and the population without the disease. The statistical methods used are discussed in Chapter 10.

Two important concepts used in analytic epidemiology are *cause* and *association*. A cause is a factor that directly influences the occurrence of a disease. Reduction or elimination of the causative factor in a population will reduce or eliminate the occurrence of the disease in that population. An association is a statistical relationship between two or more variables.

It is commonly said that one cannot use statistics to prove that a particular factor caused an event. Therefore, when a population with a particular characteristic is more likely to develop a disease than a population without that characteristic, the characteristic is said to be associated with the occurrence of the disease.[21] In analytic epidemiology, the results of observational studies are analyzed to determine (1) if an association exists between a factor (exposure) and a disease and (2) the strength of that association if one does exist.

There are three types of statistical associations:

1. Artefactual, or spurious—A false association that occurs from chance alone or from some bias in the study method (this is also known as a type I error)

2. Indirect, or noncausal—An association that occurs between a factor and a disease only because both are related to some underlying condition

3. Causal—Factor *A* truly causes *B*. This occurs if, and only if, *A* occurs prior to *B*; a change in *A* correlates to a change in *B*; and this correlation is not the consequence of both *A* and *B* being correlated with some prior *C*.

Criteria for Judging Causality

The following criteria provide a basis for judging if an association is causal (i.e., the suspected factor is the likely cause of the event)[22]:

1. Strength of association—The prevalence of disease is higher in the exposed group than in the nonexposed group.

2. Dose-response relationship—There is a quantitative relationship between the factor and the frequency of disease. For example, those with the most exposure to the agent have the greatest frequency or severity of illness.

3. Consistency of association—The findings are reproducible; they have been confirmed by different investigators in different populations.

4. Chronological relationship—Exposure to the factor precedes the onset of disease. This criterion obviously must be met in order for a factor to be able to cause a disease.

5. Specificity of association—If the factor occurs, disease can be predicted.

6. Biologically plausible—The findings are coherent with existing information. They are acceptable in light of current knowledge.

Establishing Causal Relations

Two types of observational studies are used to determine causal relations: case-control and cohort. Case-control studies compare groups of people who have a disease (the cases) with groups from the same population who do not have the disease (the controls). Cohort studies compare groups of people based on their exposures to specific risk factors. In a cohort study the disease rate in the exposed group is compared with the disease rate in the unexposed group.

The case-control study. The case-control study is the most commonly used method for testing causal associations when investigating outbreaks in the healthcare setting. In a case-control study, cases are identified (i.e., persons identified as having a disease or condition) and compared with controls (i.e., persons from the same population who do not have the disease or condition). Case-control studies can be used to investigate outbreaks of either infectious or noninfectious events.[23,24] A statistical analysis is conducted to determine if the two groups differ in the proportion of persons who were exposed to a specific factor.

A case-control study is a retrospective method because it compares cases and controls to an exposure that has already occurred. For example, the microbiology laboratory in a hospital reports to the infection prevention and control department that it has isolated *Burkholderia cepacia* from the respiratory secretions of seven patients in the ICU in the past month. A review of microbiology reports for the previous 6 months reveals only one prior isolate of *B. cepacia*. Despite reinforcement of appropriate handwashing practices, the organism is isolated from the respiratory tract of two more patients in the ICU in the next 2 weeks. A case-control study could be designed to evaluate exposures among cases (those from whom *B. cepacia* is isolated) and controls (patients in the ICU at the same time as the cases but who do not have a positive culture for *B. cepacia*) in order to determine which risk factors (exposures) are associated with the occurrence of *B. cepacia*.

Information on designing, conducting, analyzing, and interpreting a case-control study can be found in Chapter 10.

The cohort study. In a cohort study, a defined group of individuals (a cohort) is studied to determine if specified exposures result in disease. Cohort studies may be conducted prospectively or retrospectively. A prospective cohort study begins with a group of subjects who are free of a given disease. The cohort is divided into groups, one of which is exposed to a potential risk factor and one of which is not. These are then followed over time (prospectively) to determine if there are differences in the rates at which disease develops in relation to the risk factor. The Framingham Heart Study, conducted by the National Heart, Lung, and Blood Institute in Massachusetts, is a well-known example of a long-term prospective study. Some of the subjects in this study have been followed for almost 40 years.[25]

By contrast, a retrospective cohort study can be used to analyze an outbreak in a small, well-defined population. For example, many of the 29 attendees of a luncheon at a long-term care facility are reported to have developed nausea, vomiting, and abdominal cramps within a 5-hour period following the luncheon. A few have diarrhea. A case definition for gastrointestinal illness should be developed and, using the methodology of a cohort study, the 29 attendees could be identified and questioned to determine whether or not they had become ill after attending the luncheon. An attack rate (the percentage of persons who became ill) could then be calculated. If the investigator found that 11 persons fit the case definition, this would be an attack rate of 38 % (11 ill out of 29 total attendees × 100). Since it is unusual for 38% of the attendees at a meal to develop these symptoms in such a short time period, it would be possible to develop a preliminary hypothesis that the attendees may have developed an acute food-borne illness following the consumption of a contaminated food or beverage at the luncheon. At this point, a retrospective cohort study could be designed to investigate possible associations between exposures to specific foods and the development of a gastrointestinal illness, as discussed in Chapter 10.

Experimental studies. Experimental studies are not used in the investigation of outbreaks, and they will not be covered in this text. However, infection prevention and control professionals, hospital epidemiologists, and quality management personnel frequently need to review published experimental studies before making decisions about the merits of a new device, product, or procedure. Therefore, they must be familiar with the principles, problems, and pitfalls in the design and interpretation of experimental studies. For information on conducting and interpreting experimental studies, refer to the Suggested

Reading list at the end of this chapter. In addition, many articles about critically reviewing the results of clinical trials have been published, and several of these are listed in the reference section.[26–29]

THE EPIDEMIOLOGY OF INFECTIOUS DISEASES

Because most outbreak investigations in healthcare facilities involve infectious diseases, this section will describe the spectrum of disease, explain the infectious disease process, and illustrate how these affect the surveillance, prevention, and control of infections.

The Infectious Disease Spectrum

By definition, a disease is an illness that is "characterized usually by at least two of these criteria: recognized etiologic agent(s), identifiable group of signs and symptoms, or consistent anatomical alterations."[30]

As illustrated in Figure 1–4, most diseases have a characteristic natural history, or progression, from onset to resolution unless medical intervention occurs. Although this concept applies to both infectious and noninfectious conditions, this discussion will focus on infectious diseases. Because not all infections result in disease (i.e., signs and symptoms), conducting an outbreak investigation requires familiarity with the natural history of a disease in order to identify persons who may be infected. If an outbreak is caused by an agent that frequently causes inapparent infection, many infected persons may be missed if an active search for cases is not conducted.

The infectious disease spectrum can be divided into three classes of infection: (1) infection is frequently inapparent, (2) infection results in clinical disease that is rarely fatal, and (3) infection results in severe disease that is usually fatal.

Frequently Inapparent Infection

Agents. Agents that often cause inapparent or subclinical infection include the hepatitis A, B, and C viruses, *M. tuberculosis*, polio virus, *N. gonorrhea* in females, *Chlamydia trachomatis*, HIV, many nontyphoid strains of Salmonella, and cytomegalovirus.

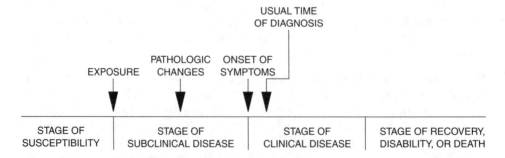

Figure 1–4 The Natural History of Disease.
Source: Centers for Disease Control and Prevention. *Principles of Epidemiology: An Introduction to Applied Epidemiology and Biostatistics.* 2nd ed. Atlanta, GA: U.S. Department of Health and Human Services, Centers for Disease Control and Prevention, Epidemiology Program Office; 1992:43.

Infection control/public health significance of inapparent infections.
Because they have no signs and symptoms, most persons with an inapparent
infection will not be identified, even though many may be able to spread the
infectious agent to others. Because only a small percentage of those infected (the
tip of the iceberg) develop clinical disease, only a few will seek medical attention.
Therefore, an even smaller percentage are likely to be hospitalized and/or
reported. Statistics on these types of infections are likely to be inaccurate because
the number of cases diagnosed and reported will be less than the true number.

If an outbreak is caused by an agent that rarely causes signs and symptoms,
it is necessary to actively search for cases by utilizing the appropriate diagnostic tests, such as serologic tests for the hepatitis viruses, stool cultures for *Salmonella*, and skin tests for *M. tuberculosis*, in order to identify infected
persons. If diagnostic tests are necessary, the laboratory should be consulted
in the early stages of an outbreak investigation to ensure that the correct tests
and specimen collection procedures are used, as discussed in Chapter 11.

Contact tracing (i.e., finding and treating the contacts of infectious persons)
is a public health method used to control the spread of these types of diseases. Contacts are persons who are exposed to an infectious individual in
such a way that infection is likely to occur. For instance, healthcare workers
with prolonged unprotected exposure to a patient subsequently found to be
infectious for *M. tuberculosis* would be identified as a contact and tested to
detect infection.

Carriers are persons who have no signs and symptoms but are infectious.
These cases are important from an infection control standpoint because they
may unwittingly spread their infection to others.

Because patients with inapparent infection may be infectious, healthcare
workers may transfer organisms from one patient to another, or to themselves,
if they do not properly follow standard precautions. It is important to remember that not everyone who has an inapparent infection is infectious. For example, most people who are infected with *M. tuberculosis* develop a latent
infection and will usually test positive by tuberculin skin test or blood assay,
but they are not infectious and cannot spread the infection to others.[17(p113)]

Infection Resulting in Rarely Fatal Clinical Disease

Agents. Agents that typically cause clinical disease in those who become
infected include the measles and chickenpox viruses and rhinovirus.

Infection control/public health significance. Most persons with measles
or chickenpox can be identified clinically. Nevertheless, diagnostic tests should
be used to confirm the diagnosis of measles because it is uncommonly seen in
the United States (due to a highly immunized population), and many clinicians are not familiar with its presentation.

Infection Resulting in Usually Fatal Severe Disease

Agents. Agents that cause severe infection that is invariably fatal if not
treated include the rabies virus, *Clostridium tetani,* and HIV. Infection
with HIV is unique in that it presents with a long subclinical phase in which

infection is inapparent and then develops into AIDS. Therefore HIV can be placed into two of the three classes in the infectious disease spectrum.

Infection control/public health significance. Statistics on incidence rates for these diseases are more accurate than the other two classes because these infections are more likely to be reported and can also be detected by surveillance systems that compile data from death certificates.

The Infectious Disease Process: The Chain of Infection

Certain conditions must be met in order for an infectious disease to be spread from person to person. This process, called the chain of infection, can occur only when all elements are present (Figure 1–5). For the infectious disease process to occur, an infectious agent must leave a reservoir through a portal of exit, be conveyed by an appropriate mode of transmission, and find a suitable portal of entry into a susceptible host. If an outbreak occurs, one must know or determine the likely chain of infection in order to identify effective control measures.

Infectious Agents

When an outbreak of unknown etiology occurs, it is important to remember that a variety of agents can produce similar clinical syndromes. For instance, an outbreak of diarrhea may be caused by a variety of biological agents, such as viruses, parasites, or bacteria; however, it could also be caused by a chemical agent such as a heavy metal or a toxin. Inherent characteristics of biological agents that affect their ability to cause disease are discussed in the following sections.

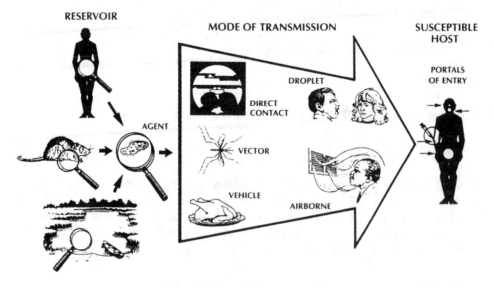

Figure 1–5 The Chain of Infection
Source: Centers for Disease Control and Prevention. *Principles of Epidemiology: An Introduction to Applied Epidemiology and Biostatistics*. 2nd ed. Atlanta, GA: U.S. Department of Health and Human Services, Centers for Disease Control and Prevention, Epidemiology Program Office; 1992:45.

Infectious dose. This is the number of organisms needed to cause infection; generally speaking, the larger the dose of infective microorganisms, the greater the chance that infection will result. For example, infection with *Coxiella burnetii*, the rickettsia that causes Q fever, can occur by inhaling only one organism. It is usually necessary to ingest 100–1000 *Salmonella* organisms to cause infection[31(p412)]; however, only a few *Shigella* (10–100 organisms) are needed for infection to occur.[31(p422)] In many food-borne outbreaks, persons who eat a large quantity of a contaminated food are more likely to develop symptoms than those who eat a small quantity because those who eat a greater amount are more likely to have ingested an infectious dose.

Invasiveness. This is the ability of an organism to enter the body and spread through tissue. Examples include the rabies virus, which has a predilection for the brain. Even if it enters the body through the leg, such as from a dog bite, the rabies virus can spread through tissue to reach the brain.

Infectivity. This is the ability of an agent to initiate and maintain infection. Examples include the chickenpox virus, exposure to which generally results in infection in a susceptible host.[32] By contrast, for *Treponema pallidum*, the causative agent of syphilis, only approximately 30% of exposures result in infection.[31(p451)]

Pathogenicity. This is the capacity of an agent to cause disease in a susceptible host. For example, the measles virus is highly pathogenic, and almost all persons who become infected will develop a rash, whereas *Enterococcus faecalis*, which is commonly found in the intestinal tract of man, rarely causes disease in a normal host and is considered to have low pathogenicity.

Virulence. This is the degree of pathogenicity of an infectious agent: the ability to cause severe disease or death. Virulence is a complex property that combines infectivity, invasiveness, and pathogenicity. For example, although measles is highly pathogenic (it easily causes disease in a susceptible person), it is not very virulent, because it rarely causes severe disease.[33] However, the rabies virus is both highly pathogenic (it causes disease in all who are infected) and extremely deadly, or virulent.[34]

Antigenic variation. This is the ability of an agent to change its antigenic components that are responsible for the specificity of immunity resulting from infection with that agent. For example, influenza A periodically modifies its antigenic structure.[35] This allows the virus to spread more easily through a population that does not have immunity to the new variant. For this reason, the influenza vaccine is modified yearly to protect against those strains of virus that are expected to be prevalent, and one must be immunized annually in order to obtain maximum protection.[35]

Viability in the free state. This is the ability of an organism to live outside of a host. For example, the hepatitis B virus (HBV) can survive for at least 7 days on inanimate surfaces at room temperature.[36] For this reason, environmental surfaces and fomites may very well be reservoirs for transmission in an outbreak of hepatitis B. Other organisms, such as HIV, *Neisseria meningitidis*, and *Neisseria gonorrhoeae*, are sensitive to air and will not survive for long on a dry surface, and the tubercle bacillus is readily killed by sunlight. Therefore, fomites are less important in the transmission of these organisms. (This explains why it is unlikely that one can catch a sexually transmitted disease from the often-maligned toilet seat.) Some organisms produce spores that may resist heat and drying—spores of *Bacillus anthracis* may remain infective for many years in contaminated soil and articles.

Host specificity. Some agents are species specific, and others will infect more than one species. For example, the measles virus, poliovirus, *Neisseria gonorrhoeae*, and *Treponema pallidum* infect only humans; other agents may infect many species. There are numerous serotypes of *Salmonella* that infect humans, other mammals, reptiles, and birds. In some cases, one can hypothesize a likely source of an outbreak if the organism and serotype are known. For instance, since humans are the reservoir for *Salmonella typhi*, one would look for a carrier or for a water or food source contaminated by human feces when investigating an outbreak caused by this organism. An outbreak caused by *Salmonella enteritidis*, however, would suggest a food-borne source because this organism infects both man and poultry, and outbreaks are commonly associated with consumption of raw or undercooked eggs.

Ability to develop resistance to antimicrobials. Some organisms develop resistance to multiple antibiotics while others remain fairly sensitive; predisposing factors and genetic predilection for developing resistance differs from genus to genus. For example: *Streptococcus pyogenes* (group A strep) has remained sensitive to penicillin, but *Streptococcus pneumoniae* has become increasingly resistant to penicillin and other antimicrobial agents. *Staphylococcus aureus* developed resistance to penicillin and to methicillin shortly after these antibiotics were introduced. MRSA, VRE, and antibiotic-resistant strains of gram-negative organisms, such as *Pseudomonas, Acinetobacter*, and the *Enterobacteriaceae* (especially *Klebsiella, Serratia, and Enterobacter*) are common causes of healthcare-associated infections in hospitals and long-term care facilities.

Immunogenicity. This is the ability of an agent to stimulate an immunogenic response. For example, infection with some agents will stimulate the production of antibodies that confer immunity. Some organisms, such as the measles, chickenpox, and HBV, promote a strong immunogenic response that generally results in long-term immunity to each specific disease. Organisms that stimulate a protective immune response are good candidates for vaccine development. Other agents, such as *Neisseria gonorrhoeae* and *Chlamydia trachomatis*, are poorly immunogenic, and reinfection can occur when a person is reexposed.

Reservoirs

The reservoir is the normal habitat in which an infectious agent lives, multiplies, and grows. Reservoirs for infectious agents exist in humans, animals, and the environment—any of these reservoirs may serve as the source of infection for a susceptible host. Viruses need a living reservoir (human, plant, or animal) to grow and multiply. Gram-positive bacteria such as *Staphylococcus* and *Streptococcus* grow well in a human reservoir but poorly in the environment. Gram-negative bacteria may have a human, animal, or environmental reservoir.

The terms *reservoir* and *source* are frequently used interchangeably; however, they may not be the same. A reservoir is the place where an organism normally lives and reproduces, and the source is the place from which an organism is transmitted to a host through some means of transmission. Sometimes the reservoir and source are the same (e.g., in an outbreak of chickenpox the reservoir and the source of the outbreak may be the same person), and sometimes they are different (e.g., water is a reservoir for *Pseudomonas aeruginosa* that may contaminate a bronchoscope that then becomes the source of an outbreak of respiratory tract infections). This difference may be important if one is investigating an outbreak and is trying to identify the source so control measures can be implemented. The inanimate environment, especially fluids, can become contaminated from a reservoir and can serve as the source of an outbreak in the healthcare setting (e.g., intravenous solutions contaminated with *Enterobacter*; hand lotion contaminated with *Serratia*; eggnog made with unpasteurized eggs harboring *Salmonella*).

Human reservoirs. There are three types of human reservoirs: carriers, colonized persons, and persons who are ill.

1. Carriers—Carriers are persons who are infected but who have no overt signs and symptoms, yet are able to transmit their infection to others. Carriers are potential sources of infection for others, especially because they usually do not know they are infectious and do not take precautions to prevent the spread of their infection to others. There are several types of carriers:

   - Those whose infection is inapparent throughout its course—Also known as subclinical infection, an example is hepatitis A infection, which in children is typically mild or inapparent, and jaundice is not a common manifestation. Hepatitis A spreads easily among children in the day care setting and on pediatric units because symptoms, if any, are so slight that little attention is paid to them. Outbreaks in these settings are frequently recognized only after parents or healthcare providers become infected and develop clinical disease.

   - Those who are in the incubatory stage—These are persons who are infected and are infectious but have not yet developed signs and symptoms. For example, a susceptible person who was exposed to chickenpox may have become infected and may be infectious 48 hours before the eruption of chickenpox[32]; because he does not know he is infectious, he does not limit contact with others and unwittingly spreads his infection to others.

   - Those who are in the convalescent phase—These are persons who continue to be infectious during and after return to health. Those who continue to harbor agents for a prolonged period of time are said to be chronic carriers. For example, approximately 10% of untreated persons infected with *Salmonella typhi* will continue to excrete bacilli for 3 months after onset of symptoms and 2–5% will become permanent carriers.[31(p504)]

2. Those who are colonized—These are persons who harbor an infectious agent but who do not have an infection. A person who is colonized with an infectious agent is a reservoir and may serve as the source of infection for that organism by transmitting it to another person, either by (1) direct contact, (2) by indirect contact with inanimate objects or environmental surfaces, or (3) by transferring the organism to another site on their own body. For example, approximately 20–30% of healthy persons carry *Staphylococcus aureus* (coagulase-positive staphylococci) in their anterior nares. These organisms can be transmitted to others or can be inoculated into a break in one's own skin. Autoinfection is thought to be responsible for at least one third of staphylococcal infections.[31(p430)] Many patients in hospitals and residents of long-term care facilities become colonized with antibiotic-resistant organisms, such as MRSA and VRE, and can serve as the source of infection for others if routine infection prevention measures such as hand hygiene and environmental cleanliness are not properly followed.

3. Those who are ill. These are persons who are infected and have signs and symptoms of disease. Because their illness is apparent and precautions can be taken to prevent transmission to others, acute clinical cases are probably less likely to spread their infection to others than those who are carriers or who are colonized. For example, if a resident in a long-term care facility develops diarrhea caused by *Clostridium difficile*, precautions such as hand hygiene and environmental disinfection can be implemented to prevent the transmission of the organism to other residents.

Animal reservoirs. As shown in Table 1–2, animals may serve as reservoirs for many agents that infect humans.[31,37–40] An animal may be a carrier, such as a chicken with *Salmonella,* or may be clinically infected, such as a cat with ringworm. Many food-borne outbreaks in the healthcare setting have been associated with animal reservoirs—most notably, outbreaks caused by *Salmonella* species from eggs, poultry, and other meats. Infectious agents may be transmitted directly from an animal to man (such as *Pasteurella multocida* transferred from the mouth of a cat to man by a cat bite), or they may be carried by an insect vector (such as *Borrelia burgdorferi*, the causative agent of Lyme disease, which is transmitted by a tick bite).

The author found no published accounts of outbreaks associated with animal-assisted activities or resident animals in healthcare facilities and few studies that evaluate the potential risk of transmission of zoonoses in the healthcare setting.[37,40] Personnel who work in facilities that have animal programs should be aware of the agents that can be transmitted from animals to patients or to residents and should ensure that appropriate precautions are taken by those in charge of the pets.[40,41] There is a report of an outbreak of *Malassezia pachydermatis* in an intensive care nursery that was associated with the colonization of healthcare workers' pet dogs at home[42] and an outbreak of surgical site infections caused by *Rhodococcus bronchialis* that was thought to be associated with a colonized nurse whose dogs were also colonized with *Rhodococcus*.[43]

Table 1–2   Diseases Transmitted from Animal Reservoirs to Humans (Zoonoses)

Disease	Causative Agent	Animal Reservoir(s)	Mode of Transmission
Anthrax	*Bacillus anthracis*	Herbivores, especially sheep and goats	Inhalation of spores from contaminated soil, wool, bones, or hides
Avian influenza	Influenza viruses	Swine, poultry	Close contact with animals
Brucellosis	*Brucella* species	Cattle, swine, sheep, goats, and dogs	Contact with blood, urine, and tissues (esp. placentas and aborted fetuses); ingestion of raw milk and dairy products
Hantavirus pulmonary syndrome	Hantaviruses	Rats, mice	Contact with urine and feces from infected rodents
Hookworm	*Ancylostoma* species	Cats, dogs	Contact with larva (from feces) in soil
Pasteurellosis	*Pasteurella multocida, P. haemolytica*	Cats, dogs	Animal bite
Plague	*Yersinia pestis*	Wild rodents (especially ground squirrels)	Bite of infected flea; contact with tissues of infected animals
Psittacosis	*Chlamydia psittaci*	Psittacine birds (parrots, parakeets); poultry	Inhalation of agent from desiccated feces, contaminated dust, or feathers
Ringworm	*Trichophyton* species, *Microsporum* species	Cats, dogs, cattle	Direct or indirect contact with infected animals
Rabies	Rabies virus	Skunks, raccoons, bats, dogs, coyotes, foxes, jackals, wolves,	Direct contact with saliva of infected animal; corneal transplants from infected person
Salmonellosis	Many *Salmonella* species	Poultry, swine, cattle, rodents, reptiles (esp. iguanas, turtles, and snakes), cats, dogs, hedgehogs	Ingestion of organisms in food; fecal-oral transmission
Toxocariasis	*Toxocara canis, T. cati*	Dogs, cats	Ingestion of Toxocara eggs from the environment

Table 1–2   *(Continued)*

Disease	Causative Agent	Animal Reservoir(s)	Mode of Transmission
Toxoplasmosis	*Toxoplasma gondii*	Cats and other felines are definitive hosts; sheep, swine, rodents, cattle, and birds may be intermediate hosts	Direct contact with feces; ingestion of raw or undercooked meat
Tularemia	*Francisella tularensis*	Rabbits, hares, muskrats, beavers, hard ticks	Direct contact with infected animal tissue (especially when skinning and processing meat of infected animals); ingestion of undercooked meat or contaminated water; tick bite

Environmental reservoirs. Water and soil are the primary environmental reservoirs for many agents that are pathogenic for man. *Pseudomonas, Legionellae, Cryptosporidium,* and some *Mycobacterium* species live and multiply in water.[40] Therefore, an aqueous source or reservoir should be considered when investigating an outbreak or cluster of infections caused by one of these organisms.[40] *Aspergillus, Histoplasma, Blastomyces, Cryptococcus,* and *Coccidioides* are fungi that live in the environment in soil or in decaying organic matter, and infection with these fungi occurs through inhalation. Outbreaks of *Aspergillus* in healthcare facilities are frequently associated with disruptions in the physical plant that occur during construction, demolition, and renovation.[40]

Portals of Exit

The portal of exit is the path by which an infectious agent leaves its host. The portals of exit and entry for an agent usually correspond to the site in which infection occurs in the body. Agents may leave their human or animal hosts through several portals:

- Respiratory tract—Diseases that are caused by agents released through the respiratory tract include the common cold, TB, influenza, chickenpox, measles, meningococcal disease, pneumococcal disease, infectious mononucleosis, diphtheria, mumps, rubella, and pertussis.[44]
- Genitourinary tract—Diseases of the genital tract that are spread through sexual contact include chlamydia, syphilis, gonorrhea, herpes, lymphogranuloma venereum, and granuloma inguinale.[44] HIV and HBV are blood-borne pathogens that may also be spread through semen and vaginal secretions.[44] Many types of organisms, both gram positive and

gram negative, can cause urinary tract infections, especially in a catheterized patient, and will be excreted in the urine. Cytomegalovirus is also shed in the urine and in cervical secretions.[44]

- Gastrointestinal tract—Agents that cause gastrointestinal infections and are excreted in feces include *Salmonella*, *Shigella*, *Clostridium difficile*, hepatitis A virus, *Vibrio cholerae*, poliovirus, *Campylobacter*, *Giardia lamblia*, *Yersinia enterocolitica*, norovirus, rotavirus, *Escherichia coli*, and the many viral agents that cause acute gastroenteritis.[44]

- Skin and mucous membranes—Organisms that are shed by the skin or mucous membranes include *Herpes simplex* from an oral, skin, or genital lesion; *Treponema pallidum* from a syphilitic lesion or rash; *Staphylococcus aureus* from a skin lesion or wound infection; and the many viral and bacterial agents that cause conjunctivitis.

- Blood—Organisms that are found in blood include HIV, HBV, hepatitis C virus, cytomegalovirus, *Treponema pallidum*, and *Plasmodium* species (malaria).[44]

- Transplacental route—Agents that may be transferred from mother to infant across the placenta include the rubella virus, cytomegalovirus, *Treponema pallidum*, HBV, HIV, and *Toxoplasma gondii*.[44]

Modes of Transmission

Because microorganisms cannot travel on their own, several modes of transmission facilitate the movement of an agent from its reservoir to a susceptible host. These may be classified as one of three modes of transmission: direct, indirect, and airborne.

Direct transmission. This implies immediate transmission of an infectious agent to an appropriate portal of entry (i.e., one through which infection can occur). Direct transmission can occur through touching, kissing, and sexual intercourse. Direct transmission can also occur through droplet spread. Droplets produced during coughing, talking, sneezing, spitting, or singing may contain infectious agents that can be carried for a short distance to reach the conjunctiva or mucous membranes of the nose or mouth of a susceptible host. Droplet spread is considered to be direct transmission because two people must be in close proximity for transmission to occur.[45] The meningococcus, pneumococcus, influenza virus, rhinovirus, and group A streptococcus are spread by the droplet route.

Indirect transmission. Transmission by the indirect route involves an intermediary (inanimate or animate) that carries the agent from the source to a susceptible host.[45] Agents can be vehicle borne, which occurs when an inanimate object (fomite) serves as a means of transmission. Vehicles in the healthcare setting include food, water, surgical instruments, medical devices and equipment, intravenous fluids, and blood and blood products. Some agents actively grow and multiply in the vehicle, and some can produce toxins in the vehicle. For example, *Pseudomonas* species readily grow and multiply in fluids; *S. aureus* produces an enterotoxin in contaminated foods; and other agents just passively hitch a ride, such as hepatitis A virus in a contaminated salad and

M. tuberculosis on a contaminated bronchoscope. In addition to inanimate vehicles, many agents that cause healthcare-associated infections and outbreaks in healthcare settings are frequently carried on the hands of healthcare workers who transfer the organisms to a person from an object or another person.

Indirect transmission can also be vector borne. Vectors are animate intermediaries that carry an infectious agent from host to host. Most vectors are arthropods such as flies, mosquitoes, fleas, lice, and ticks. Insects can transfer organisms by mechanical means (e.g., flies have been shown to carry pathogenic organisms on their feet) or they may be involved in the multiplication or life cycle development of the agent (e.g., *Plasmodium* species multiply in the *Anopheles* mosquito, which injects the organism into humans through a bite).

Airborne transmission. This occurs when microbial aerosols are suspended in air and reach the respiratory tract of a susceptible host.[17,45] Particles that are between 1 and 5 microns in size are easily inhaled and can bypass the defenses of the upper respiratory tract to be deposited in the alveoli where they grow and multiply. There are two types of aerosols:

- Small particles—Small particles can carry infective agents such as *Aspergillus conidia* from decaying matter and the Sin Nombre virus (a hantavirus) which is thought to be aerosolized from rodent excreta in soil.[39]
- Droplet nuclei—These are the dried residue of exhaled droplets; they can remain suspended for long periods of time and can be carried on air currents. Droplet nuclei can also be produced by medical procedures such as bronchoscopy and suctioning of the respiratory tract. Chickenpox, measles, and TB are spread by the airborne route in droplet nuclei.[45]

Portals of Entry

The portals of entry are similar to the portals of exit described above. Organisms require a specific portal of entry in order to cause infection. If they do not reach this specific portal of entry, they will not be able to establish an infection. For example, enteric pathogens are agents that are transmitted by direct or indirect contact with feces. They are spread by what is commonly called the fecal-oral route (i.e., they are excreted in the feces and enter the body through the mouth). Hepatitis A virus is spread through the fecal-oral route; it is excreted in the feces and is ingested by a host either through direct contact with feces (as may occur if one does not wash hands after changing a soiled diaper) or indirectly by eating or drinking contaminated food or water.

The skin is an excellent barrier against invasion from infectious agents. Only a few human pathogens, such as the larvae of hookworm and the cercariae of the schistosomes (blood flukes) can effectively penetrate intact skin. Organisms such as *Staphylococcus aureus* and group A *Streptococcus* can cause infection if they are introduced into a break in the skin; however, they are not able to initiate infection through intact skin. This is one reason why hand hygiene is such an important measure for preventing the transmission of infection. If transient organisms such as staphylococci can be removed from the hands before being introduced into a portal of entry, such as the nose or a wound, then they will not be able to cause an infection.

Salmonella and *Shigella* must be able to reach the intestinal lining in order to cause infection. For this to occur, these organisms generally must be ingested; however, they may also be iatrogenically introduced into the intestine. *Salmonella* has been transmitted in the healthcare setting by improperly disinfected endoscopes.

Mycobacterium tuberculosis is spread by the airborne route, and the tubercule bacilli must be able to reach the lung in order to initiate a pulmonary infection (i.e., the organism must be able to bypass the hairs, the cilia, and the mucus in the respiratory tract).[17] Generally, a person must inhale the organism for this to occur; however, the tubercule bacilli has also been nosocomially introduced into the lung via contaminated instruments, such as bronchoscopes. Extrapulmonary TB does occur and can affect any organ or tissue; however, the initial site of infection is almost always the respiratory tract with hematogenous spread to other parts of the body. Although the skin is an excellent barrier against *M. tuberculosis*, there are rare reports of primary cutaneous infection caused by direct innoculation.[46]

Susceptible Host

The susceptible host is the final link in the chain of infection. Several factors affect a host's ability to resist infection. These include inherent, or nonspecific, factors; acquired immunity; and secondary resistance factors.

Inherent factors—Inherent, or nonspecific, factors are those that we are born with, including:

- Natural barriers, such as skin, hairs in the nasal passages, mucous membranes, cilia of the respiratory tract, gastric acidity, and reflexes such as coughing, sneezing, and swallowing
- Special mechanisms such as the liver, spleen, and lymph nodes that can filter organisms from the bloodstream
- Hormonal activity such as estrogen that can protect premenopausal females from coronary artery disease

Acquired immunity refers to protective antibodies that are directed against a specific agent. There are two types—active immunity and passive immunity. Active immunity occurs when the host develops antibodies in response to an antigen and may be acquired naturally or artificially. It is acquired naturally when the host develops antibodies in response to an infection. For some diseases this immunity persists for the life of the host (e.g., measles and chickenpox). It is acquired artificially in response to a vaccine or toxoid; the duration of protection varies according to disease (e.g., active immunity induced by tetanus toxoid is not permanent, and booster doses are recommended every 10 years).47 Passive immunity results from borrowed antibodies and, like acquired immunity, may be acquired naturally or artificially.

Natural passive immunity is acquired through transfer of antibodies from mother to fetus; this immunity usually lasts from 6 to 9 months. Passive immunity is acquired artificially through injection of antiserum (e.g., hepatitis B or varicella-zoster immune globulin) or antitoxin; this protection usually lasts only 4 to 6 weeks.

Secondary resistance factors. Secondary resistance factors are those that affect the host's potential for exposure to an infectious agent. These include extrinsic and intrinsic factors. Extrinsic, or environmental, factors include lack of food, water, or rest; exposure to diagnostic or therapeutic procedures; temperature and humidity; and occupation and socioeconomic status. Examples of extrinsic factors that place the host at risk for healthcare-associated infection include devices such as ventilators and endotracheal tubes, which compromise the natural defenses in the respiratory tract; surgical procedures and intravascular catheters, which disrupt the skin barrier; urinary catheters, which allow organisms to enter the urinary tract; and chemotherapeutic agents, which are used to suppress the immune system in transplant patients. Intrinsic resistance factors include age, sex, genetic disposition, and diseases that impair the immune response. Examples of diseases that impair the immune response include neoplasias and HIV infection.

Identifying Effective Measures to Control or Prevent the Spread of Infection

If an agent can be identified—how it enters and exits a host and how it is transmitted—then appropriate prevention and control measures can be determined. These measures are aimed at one of the links in the chain of infection and are usually directed toward the reservoir or source, the mode of transmission, or the susceptibility of the host.

Measures Directed at the Reservoir or Source of an Agent

The nature of the reservoir is of paramount importance in determining the appropriate method of control. If domestic animals are the reservoir, measures include immunization (e.g., vaccinating dogs against rabies), testing of herds to identify infected animals (e.g., screening cows for bovine TB), and treatment or destruction of infected animals, such as the destruction of poultry to prevent the spread of avian influenza A to man. If wild animals are the reservoir, such as rodents for plague and hantavirus, control is more difficult but can be accomplished by limiting the entry of these animals into the living areas of man. When insects are the reservoir (e.g., mosquitoes for malaria), their entry into dwellings may be limited by screens or the insects may be eradicated with pesticides or repelled with chemicals. If the reservoir is man, obviously eradication of the host is not a viable option; however, if the infection is recognized, a person can be treated with an antimicrobial to eliminate the agent or can be isolated (i.e., restricted from exposing other persons, such as when a patient with infectious pulmonary TB is placed in an isolation room or is instructed to stay home until the period of communicability is over).

Measures Directed at Interrupting Transmission

Measures directed at interrupting transmission may be aimed at preventing the organism from entering or exiting the host or at limiting direct contact, indirect contact, or airborne dissemination. Examples include hand hygiene; standard precautions; protective barriers, such as gloves, gowns, respirators, and masks used by healthcare workers; aseptic technique; chemical repellents and window and door screens to protect against insects; isolation and quarantine; and dressings to cover wounds.

Contaminated vehicles can transmit infectious agents from one host to another. Food and water have the potential for affecting large numbers of people from one source and have been the vehicles for many outbreaks in the community and in healthcare facilities. Measures used to prevent this type of transmission include purification of drinking water; pasteurization of milk; irradiation of food; and safe handling and preparation of food, with an emphasis on hand hygiene, cleanliness of equipment, and proper refrigeration, cooking, and storage. Contaminated medication, equipment, instruments, and devices have served as vehicles in many outbreaks in the healthcare setting. Measures used to prevent or control these outbreaks include aseptic technique when handling medications and intravenous fluids, and proper cleaning, disinfection, and sterilization of instruments and medical devices.

Measures Directed at the Host

Measures directed at the host are aimed at reducing host susceptibility and include chemoprophylaxis and immunization. Examples in the healthcare setting include policies that require healthcare providers to show evidence of immunity to measles, mumps, rubella, and hepatitis B as a condition of employment (this may be required by law in some areas); blood-borne pathogens exposure management protocols that include hepatitis B vaccine (active immunization), hepatitis B immune globulin (passive immunization), and chemoprophylaxis for HIV; and TB control programs that include skin testing to identify infected persons so that chemoprophylaxis can be provided to prevent disease.

Sometimes there may be a shift in emphasis in the primary control measure used to prevent the spread of a disease—such has occurred for TB and measles. For TB the change was prompted by the development of effective antimicrobial agents; for measles the change occurred when an effective vaccine was produced. Before the discovery of effective chemotherapy, the primary control measure used to prevent transmission of TB was placement in a sanitarium or a specialized TB ward. Now the primary control method is prompt identification and treatment of infectious persons and follow-up of their contacts. Before the measles vaccine was widely implemented, the primary control method was isolation of an infected person; now immunization is the primary control method used.

SUMMARY

Microbes will continue to emerge, reemerge, and persist. To effectively prevent the spread of infectious agents and the occurrence of outbreaks, it is necessary to understand epidemiologic principles and the dynamic relationship between the host, microbial agents, and the environment. Additional information on epidemiology, infectious diseases, and infection prevention and control can be found in the Suggested Reading section at the end of this chapter.

REFERENCES

1. Smolinski MS, Hamburg MA, Lederberg J, eds. *Microbial Threats to Health: Emergence, Detection, and Response.* Washington, DC: National Academies Press; 2003. p.1 Executive Summary. http://www.nap.edu/catalog.php?record_id=10636. Accessed April 21, 2008.

2. Merrell DS, Falkow S. Frontal and stealth attack strategies in microbial pathogenesis. *Nature.* 2004;430:250–256.

3. Lederberg J, Shope R, Oaks S, eds. *Emerging Infections: Microbial Threats to Health in the United States.* Washington, DC: National Academy Press; 1992:36–41. http://www.nap.edu/catalog.php?record_id=2008. Accessed April 21, 2008.

4. Peiris JSM, Guan Y. Confronting SARS: a view from Hong Kong. *Philos Trans R Soc Lond B Biol Sci.* 2004;29:359:1075–1079. http://www.pubmedcentral.nih.gov/articlerender.fcgi?artid=1693390. Accessed July 28, 2008.

5. Last JM, ed. *Dictionary of Epidemiology.* 4th ed. New York, NY: Oxford University Press; 2001:61.

6. Maloney ES. *Chapman's Piloting, Seamanship and Small Boat Handling.* 62nd ed. New York, NY: Hearst Marine Books; 1996:55.

7. Miller PM. Semmelweis. *Infect Control.* 1982;3:405–409.

8. LaForce FM. The control of infections in hospitals: 1750 to 1950. In: Wenzel RP, ed. *Prevention and Control of Nosocomial Infections.* Baltimore, MD: Williams & Wilkins; 1987:1–12.

9. Snow J. *On the Mode of Communication of Cholera.* 2nd ed. London, England: Churchill; 1885. Reproduced in *Snow on Cholera.* New York, NY: Commonwealth Fund; 1936.

10. Fredericks DN, Relman DA. Sequence-based identification of microbial pathogens: a reconsideration of Koch's postulates. *Clin Microbiol Rev.* 1996;9:18–33.

11. The ecology of pathogenesis. In: Forum on Microbial Threats. Board on Global Health. Institute of Medicine of the National Academies. *Ending the War Metaphor: The Changing Agenda for Unraveling the Host-Microbe Relationship. Workshop Summary.* Washington, DC: National Academy Press; 2006:102–158. http://www.nap.edu. Accessed July 28, 2008.

12. Lee LA, Gerber AR, Lonsway DR. *Yersinia enterocolitica* O:3 infections in infants and children associated with the household preparation of chitterlings. *N Engl J Med.* 1990;322:984–987.

13. Christie CDC, Glover AM, Wilke MJ, et al. Containment of pertussis in the regional pediatric hospital during the Greater Cincinnati epidemic of 1993. *Infect Control Hosp Epidemiol.* 1995;16:556–563.

14. Faoagali J, Darcy D. Chickenpox outbreak among the staff of a large, urban adult hospital: costs of monitoring and control. *Am J Infect Control.* 1995;23:247–250.

15. Raad I, Sheretz R, Russell B, Reuman P. Uncontrolled nosocomial rotavirus transmission during a community outbreak. *Am J Infect Control.* 1990;18:24–28.

16. Agerton T, Valway S, Gore B, et al. Transmission of a highly drug-resistant strain (strain W1) of *Mycobacterium tuberculosis*: community outbreak and nosocomial transmission via a contaminated bronchoscope. *JAMA.* 1997;278:1073–1077.

17. Centers for Disease Control and Prevention. Guidelines for preventing the transmission of *Mycobacterium tuberculosis* in health-care settings, 2005. *MMWR*. 2005;54(RR17):1–141. http://www.cdc.gov/mmwr/preview/mmwrhtml/rr5417a1.htm?s_cid=rr5417a1_e. [errata http://www.cdc.gov/tb/pubs/mmwr/Errata09–25-06.pdf]. Accessed November 20, 2007.

18. *Reported Tuberculosis in the United States, 2006*. Atlanta, GA: U.S. Department of Health and Human Services, CDC; 2007. http://www.cdc.gov/tb/surv. Accessed November 19, 2007.

19. Cantwell MF, Snider DE, Cauthen GM, Onorato IM. Epidemiology of tuberculosis in the United States, 1985 through 1992. *JAMA*. 1994;272:535–539.

20. Centers for Disease Control and Prevention. Tuberculosis morbidity—United States, 1997. *MMWR*. 1998;47:253–257.

21. Centers for Disease Control and Prevention. *Principles of Epidemiology in Public Health Practice: An Introduction to Applied Epidemiology and Biostatistics*. 3rd ed. Atlanta, GA: US Department of Health and Human Services, Public Health Service, Centers for Disease Control and Prevention, Office of Workforce and Career Development; 2005. http://www2a .cdc.gov/TCEOnline/registration/detailpage.asp?res_id=1394. Accessed May 10, 2008.

22. Last JM, Tyler CW. Epidemiology. In: Last JM, Wallace RB, eds. *Maxcy-Rosenau-Last Public Health and Preventive Medicine*. 13th ed. Stamford, CT: Appleton & Lange; 1992:33.

23. Dwyer DM, Strickler H, Goodman RA, Armenian HK. Use of case-control studies in outbreak investigations. *Epidemiol Rev*. 1994;16:109–123.

24. Terdiman JP, Ostroff JW. Gastrointestinal bleeding in the hospitalized patient: a case-control study to assess risk factors, causes, and outcomes. *Am J Med*. 1998;104:349–354.

25. Post WS, Larson MG, Myers RH, et al. Heritability of left ventricular mass: the Framingham Heart Study. *Hypertens*. 1997;30:1025–1028.

26. Research Development Committee, Society for Research and Education in Primary Care Internal Medicine. Clinical research methods: an annotated bibliography. *Ann Intern Med*. 1983;99:419–424.

27. Carpenter LM. Is the study worth doing? *Lancet*. 1993;342:221–223.

28. Glynn JR. A question of attribution. *Lancet*. 1993;342:530–532.

29. Victoria CG. What's the denominator? *Lancet*. 1993;342:345–347.

30. *Stedman's Medical Dictionary*. 25th ed. Baltimore, MD: Williams & Wilkins; 1990:444

31. Benenson AS, ed. *Control of Communicable Diseases Manual*. 16th ed. Washington, DC: American Public Health Association; 1995.

32. Centers for Disease Control and Prevention. Varicella. In: Atkinson W, Hamborsky J, McIntyre L, Wolfe S, eds. *Epidemiology and Prevention of Vaccine-Preventable Diseases*. 10th ed. Washington, DC: Public Health Foundation; 2007. http://www.cdc.gov/vaccines/pubs/ pinkbook/default.htm. Accessed November 20, 2007.

33. Centers for Disease Control and Prevention. Measles. In: Atkinson W, Hamborsky J, McIntyre L, Wolfe S, eds. *Epidemiology and Prevention of Vaccine-Preventable Diseases*. 10th ed. Washington, DC: Public Health Foundation; 2007. http://www.cdc.gov/vaccines/pubs/ pinkbook/default.htm. Accessed November 20, 2007.

34. CDC. Human Rabies Prevention—United States, 1999. Recommendations of the Advisory Committee on Immunization Practices (ACIP). *MMWR*. 1999;48(RR-1):1–21. http://www .cdc.gov/mmwr/preview/mmwrhtml/00056176.htm. Accessed November 20, 2007.

35. Centers for Disease Control and Prevention. Influenza. In: Atkinson W, Hamborsky J, McIntyre L, Wolfe S, eds. *Epidemiology and Prevention of Vaccine-Preventable Diseases*. 10th ed. Washington, DC: Public Health Foundation; 2007. http://www.cdc.gov/vaccines/pubs/ pinkbook/default.htm. Accessed November 20, 2007.

36. Bond WW, Favero MS, Petersen NJ, Gravelle CR, Ebert JW, Maynard JE. Survival of hepatitis B after drying and storage for one week. *Lancet*. 1981;1:550–551.

37. Lefebvre SL, Waltner-Toews D, Peregrine AS, et al. Prevalence of zoonotic agents in dogs visiting hospitalized people in Ontario: implications for infection control. *J Hosp Infect*. 2006;62:458–466.

38. Plaut M, Zimmerman EM, Goldstein RA. Health hazards to humans associated with domestic pets. *Annu Rev Pub Health*. 1996;17:221–245.

39. Centers for Disease Control and Prevention. Hantavirus pulmonary syndrome—United States: updated recommendations for risk reduction. *MMWR*. 2002;51(RR09):1–12.

40. Sehulster L, Chinn LYW. Guidelines for environmental infection control in health-care facilities: recommendations of the CDC and the Healthcare Infection Control Practices Advisory Committee (HICPAC). *MMWR*. 2003;52:1–42.

41. Fredrickson M, Howie AR. Methods, standards, guidelines and considerations in selecting animals for animal-assisted therapy. Part B. Guidelines and standards for animal selection in animal-assisted activity and therapy programs. In: Fine AH, ed. *Academic Press Handbook on Animal Assisted Therapy: Theoretical Foundations and Guidelines for Practice*. San Diego, CA: Academic Press; 2000:99–114.

42. Chang HJ, Miller HL, Watkins N, et al. An epidemic of *Malassezia pachydermatis* in an intensive care nursery associated with colonization of healthcare workers' pet dogs. *N Engl J Med*. 1998;338:706–711.

43. Richet HM, Craven PC, Brown JM, et al. A cluster of *Rhodococcus* (*Gordona*) *bronchialis* sternal wound infections after coronary-artery bypass surgery. *N Engl J Med*. 1991;324:104–109.

44. Heyman DL, ed. *Control of Communicable Diseases Manual*. 18th ed. Washington, DC: American Public Health Association; 2004.

45. Siegel JD, Rhinehart E, Jackson M, Chiarello L, and the Healthcare Infection Control Practices Advisory Committee; *2007 Guideline for Isolation Precautions: Preventing Transmission of Infectious Agents in Healthcare Settings*. *http://www.cdc.gov/ncidod/dhqp/pdf/isolation2007.pdf*. Accessed November 19, 2007.

46. Genne D, Siegrist HH. Tuberculosis of the thumb following a needlestick injury. *Clin Infect Dis*. 1998;26:210–211.

47. Centers for Disease Control and Prevention. Recommended adult immunization schedule—United States, October 2006–September 2007. *MMWR*. 2006;55:Q1-Q4. http://www.cdc.gov/mmwr/pdf/wk/mm5540-Immunization.pdf. Accessed November 19, 2007.

SUGGESTED READING

Abramson JH. *Making Sense of Data: A Self-Instruction Manual on the Interpretation of Epidemiological Data*. 3rd ed. New York, NY: Oxford University Press; 2001.

American Academy of Pediatrics. *Red Book: 2008 Report of the Committee on Infectious Diseases*. Elk Grove, Village, IL: American Academy of Pediatrics; 2008.

APIC Text of Infection Control and Epidemiology. 2nd ed. Washington, DC: Association for Professionals in Infection Control and Epidemiology; 2005.

Centers for Disease Control and Prevention. *Principles of Epidemiology in Public Health Practice: An Introduction to Applied Epidemiology and Biostatistics*. 3rd ed. Atlanta, GA: US Department of Health and Human Services, Public Health Service, Centers for Disease Control and Prevention, Office of Workforce and Career Development; 2005. ttp://www2a.cdc.gov/TCEOnline/registration/detailpage.asp?res_id=1394. Accessed May 10, 2008.

Friedman GD. *Primer of Epidemiology*. 4th ed. New York, NY: McGraw Hill; 1994.

Heyman DL, ed. *Control of Communicable Diseases Manual*. 18th ed. Washington, DC: American Public Health Association; 2004

Jarvis WB, ed. *Bennett and Brachman's Hospital Infections*. 5th ed. Baltimore, MD: Lippincott Williams & Wilkins; 2007.

Last JM. *Public Health and Human Ecology*. 2nd ed. Stamford, CT: Appleton & Lange; 1997

Lederberg J, Shope R, Oaks S, ed. *Emerging Infections: Microbial Threats to Health in the United States*. Washington, DC: National Academy Press; 1992. http://www.nap.edu. Accessed November 19, 2007.

Lilienfeld DE, Stolley PD. *Foundations of Epidemiology*. 3rd ed. New York: Oxford University Press; 1994.

Mausner JS, Kramer S. *Epidemiology: An Introductory Text*. 2nd ed. Philadelphia, PA: WB Saunders; 1985.

Mayhall CG. *Hospital Epidemiology and Infection Control.* 3rd ed. Baltimore, MD: Lippincott, Williams & Wilkins; 2004.

Norman GR, Streiner DL. *Biostatistics: The Bare Essentials.* 3rd ed. Hamilton, Ontario: BC Decker; 2007.

Roueche B. *The Medical Detectives.* Vols. I, II. New York, NY: Washington Square Press; 1986.

Roueche B. *The Medical Detectives.* Reprint ed. New York, NY: Plume; 1991.

Sackett DL, Haynes RB, Guyatt GH, et al. *Clinical Epidemiology: A Basic Science for Clinical Medicine.* 2nd ed. Boston, MA: Little Brown; 1991.

Smolinski MS, Hamburg MA, Lederberg J, eds. Committee on Emerging Microbial Threats to Health in the 21st Century. *Microbial Threats to Health: Emergence, Detection, and Response.* Washington, DC: National Academies Press; 2003. http://www.nap.edu/catalog.php?record_id=10636. Accessed March 26, 2008.

Szklo M, Nieto FJ. *Epidemiology: Beyond the Basics.* 2nd ed. Sudbury, MA: Jones and Bartlett; 2006.

Wallace RB. *Public Health and Preventive Medicine (Maxcy-Rosenau-Last Public Health and Preventive Medicine).* 15th ed. Columbus, OH: McGraw-Hill; 2007.

Wenzel RP, ed. *Prevention and Control of Nosocomial Infections.* 4th ed. Baltimore: Lippincott Williams & Wilkins; 2002.

CHAPTER 2

Surveillance Programs, Public Health, and Emergency Preparedness

Kathleen Meehan Arias and Lorraine Messinger Harkavy

> Surveillance is undertaken to inform disease prevention and control measures.[1]
>
> —*World Health Organization*

INTRODUCTION

In February of 2003 an outbreak of a mysterious atypical pneumonia that caused much morbidity and mortality was first reported in the People's Republic of China. The disease rapidly spread to Hong Kong, Singapore, North Vietnam, and Canada, and nosocomial transmission between patients and healthcare providers occurred.[2] Within a few months, the illness, now known as the severe acute respiratory syndrome, or SARS, had spread to over 20 countries in Asia, North America, Europe, and South America.[3,4] News of SARS was quickly transmitted via the Internet,[4] and public health agencies worldwide rapidly developed and distributed guidelines to prevent disease transmission.

The rapid spread, recognition, and subsequent control of SARS demonstrates the need for both local and global disease surveillance systems. Both infection prevention and control personnel in healthcare facilities and public health personnel worldwide must monitor human health continually to detect outbreaks of disease, emerging infections, bioterrorist attacks, and potential pandemics so that control measures can quickly be implemented.

Surveillance is the foundation for an effective infection prevention and control program in the healthcare setting. A surveillance system is necessary to identify healthcare-associated infections (HAIs) and other adverse events so that prevention measures can be identified and implemented to minimize the risk for these events. An effective surveillance program is essential to recognize unusual infections and clusters or outbreaks of disease. In this chapter, the term *disease* is used to describe HAIs and other adverse events, such as falls, that are related to health care, and the term *patient* is used to describe patients in acute, subacute, long-term, and ambulatory care settings and residents in long-term care (LTC) facilities.

This chapter explains the reasons for implementing active infection surveillance programs, discusses the various components of an effective surveillance program for a healthcare setting, provides definitions for the identification of HAIs, outlines the steps in the surveillance process, and discusses how to use surveillance data to recognize problems such as potential outbreaks in order to identify and implement prevention and control measures. It also discusses regulations and other requirements affecting surveillance programs in health-care settings, national and global surveillance systems, and surveillance as it applies to emergency preparedness activities in healthcare settings.

This chapter will only briefly address surveillance in the home care setting. Readers who wish to obtain more information on infection surveillance, prevention, and control in home care are referred to the text by Rhinehart and Friedman.[5]

SURVEILLANCE PROGRAMS IN HEALTHCARE SETTINGS

In December 1970, the Hospital Infections Section of the US Centers for Disease Control and Prevention (CDC) first received reports of episodes of nosocomial bloodstream infections (BSIs) caused by *Enterobacter* species. "Between October 1970 and March 1, 1971, eight United States hospitals in seven states experienced 150 bacteremias caused by *Enterobacter cloacae* or gram-negative organisms of the *Erwinia* group. There were nine deaths; all were associated with intravenous (IV) fluid therapy. The *Enterobacter* bacteremias in all hospitals were substantially increased as compared to previous time periods. Four hospitals that isolated and identified *Erwinia* had not previously encountered infections with these organisms."[6(p1227)] The finding that two unusual organisms, *E. cloacae* and *Enterobacter agglomerans*, were causing BSIs at multiple hospitals pointed to the likelihood of a common source. The nationwide *Enterobacter* BSI outbreak that affected these hospitals was eventually traced to intrinsic contamination of the plastic cap liners of IV fluids from a single manufacturer. This outbreak of bacteremias associated with contaminated IV infusion fluids may not have been recognized had it not been for the ongoing infection surveillance programs that had been established in these hospitals. This outbreak, which was reported in the March 12, 1971, issue of *Morbidity and Mortality Weekly Report*, "would later be recognized as the largest and most lethal known outbreak of nosocomial infection associated with widespread distribution of a contaminated medical product in the United States. The report demonstrates the benefit of the emphasis that CDC had placed on nosocomial infection surveillance and control programs starting in the 1960s and illustrated the importance of being able to rapidly assemble data from multiple, widely scattered sites to resolve complex outbreaks."[6(p1227)] If the nosocomial infection surveillance programs had not existed in these hospitals, the detection of this outbreak would have been more difficult, and the outbreak likely would have resulted in additional deaths. This outbreak resulted in the development of the CDC's *Guidelines for Infection Control in Intravenous Therapy*,[7] which became the first in a series of CDC guidelines on the prevention of HAIs.

SURVEILLANCE: WHAT IS IT AND WHY DO IT?

Surveillance can be defined as "the ongoing, systematic collection, analysis, interpretation, and dissemination of data regarding a health-related event for use in public health action to reduce morbidity and mortality and to improve health."[8(p2)] Surveillance systems can be used to collect information about a variety of events. Although infection prevention and control professionals use surveillance to focus on healthcare- and community-associated infections, a surveillance system can also be used to detect medication errors, patient falls, sharps injuries in healthcare personnel, and an array of other quality care issues.

Surveillance can be used to measure either outcomes, which are the result of health care or performance (such as infections, decubitus ulcers, or patient falls), or processes, which are the actions that are taken to achieve an outcome (such as compliance with an established policy or protocol).[9–12] Two major goals of a surveillance program in a healthcare setting are to (1) improve the quality of health care; and (2) identify, implement, and evaluate strategies to prevent and control HAIs and other adverse events.

Four objectives of a surveillance program are to:

1. Provide baseline, or endemic, rates of disease
2. Identify increases in rates above the baseline, or expected, rates of disease
3. Identify risk factors for disease
4. Evaluate the effectiveness of prevention and control measures

Surveillance Programs in Hospitals

Surveillance programs in acute care hospitals are well-established in many countries. The Study on the Efficacy of Nosocomial Infection Control, or SENIC project, conducted by the CDC in the mid-1970s, was a landmark study that demonstrated the positive impact that infection control programs had on the reduction of HAI rates in hospitals.[13,14] SENIC found that hospitals could reduce their HAI rates by approximately 32% if they implemented an infection surveillance and control program that included certain critical components, such as appropriate surveillance activities, vigorous control efforts, and proper staffing.[13]

In 1970, the CDC established the National Nosocomial Infections Surveillance (NNIS) system to create a national database of hospital-associated infections and to improve surveillance methods in acute care hospitals.[15] In 2005, the CDC combined NNIS with two other national surveillance systems, the Dialysis Surveillance Network[16] and the National Surveillance System for Health Care Workers, to form the National Healthcare Safety Network (NHSN).[17] The healthcare facilities that participate in NHSN use standardized protocols and definitions for HAI[18] that are posted on the NHSN members page of the CDC Web site (http://www.cdc.gov/ncidod/dhqp/nhsn_members.html). Participating organizations submit their data to the CDC for analysis and aggregation into a national database. The aggregate NNIS/NHSN reports are periodically published in the *American Journal of Infection Control*[19] and are also available on the CDC's NHSN Web site. Data from NNIS/NHSN have been used to identify risk factors for nosocomial infection and measures that can be used to reduce these risks.[20] Some hospitals have used NNIS data to support the implementation of infection prevention and control measures and have been able to document a subsequent reduction in nosocomial infection rates.[21,22]

Additional examples of surveillance networks for HAIs include the following:

- Canadian Nosocomial Infection Surveillance Program—Established in 1994 to provide rates and trends of HAIs in Canadian healthcare facilities, to enable comparison of rates, and to provide data that can be used in the development of national guidelines related to HAIs. http://www.phac-aspc.gc.ca/nois-sinp/survprog_e.html. Accessed February 18, 2008.

- European Union's (EU) HELICS (Hospitals in Europe Link for Infection Control through Surveillance) network—An international network aimed at collecting, analyzing, and disseminating data on antibiotic resistance and the risks of HAIs in European hospitals. http://helics.univ-lyon1.fr/index.htm. Accessed February 18, 2008.

- Victorian Hospital-Acquired Infection Surveillance System in Australia—Established in 2002, it collects and analyses data on HAIs in acute care public hospitals in Victoria and reports individual hospital and aggregate data back to participants and the Department of Human Services. http://www.vicniss.org.au. Accessed February 18, 2008.

- European Centre for Disease Prevention and Control (ECDC)—Established by the European Parliament and Council in early 2004 to identify, assess, and communicate current and emerging threats to human health from communicable diseases. HAIs are included in the ECDC surveillance system that issued its first report in 2007.[23] http://ecdc.europa.eu/. Accessed February 18, 2008.

Surveillance Programs in Healthcare Settings Other Than Acute Care Hospitals

Many LTC facilities have HAI surveillance programs; however, these are generally not as well established as those in the acute care setting.[24–26] Little has been published about surveillance methods in the ambulatory care[16,27,28] and home care settings.[5,29–33] As of early 2008, the authors were unable to find a national surveillance system with a surveillance database for HAIs in long-term, home care, or ambulatory care settings other than hemodialysis.[16,18,34] In 2007, the NHSN included only hospitals and outpatient hemodialysis centers but will eventually expand to other healthcare settings, including long-term, ambulatory, and home care.[17] In 2006 the EU's HELICS conducted a survey to study the feasibility of developing a standardized approach to HAI surveillance in European nursing homes, and HELICS also plans to develop such a system.[35] In the United States, Stevenson et al. reported on a regional cohort of 17 LTC facilities in Idaho that used standard definitions and uniform case-finding methods and determined that a regional standardized approach to HAI surveillance in this setting is feasible.[36]

SURVEILLANCE METHODS

Each organization must develop a surveillance program that will meet the organization's needs, support its performance improvement initiatives, and fulfill regulatory and accreditation requirements. There is no one surveillance system that is appropriate for all types of settings and institutions. The Association for Professionals in Infection Control and Epidemiology (APIC) notes that "Although there is no single or 'right' method of surveillance design or implementation, sound epidemiologic principles must form the foundation of effective systems and be understood by key participants in the surveillance program and supported by senior management. . . . Each healthcare organization must tailor its surveillance systems to maximize resources by focusing on population characteristics, outcome priorities, and organizational objectives."[9(p427)]

Housewide (Comprehensive) Surveillance

Housewide (also known as comprehensive or total) surveillance was recommended by the CDC in the early 1970s and was the most common type of surveillance conducted in US hospitals throughout the 1970s. In housewide surveillance all patients are continuously monitored for HAIs at all body sites.[37,38] A major drawback of housewide surveillance is that it is labor intensive, especially if data are collected manually.[38] If housewide surveillance is conducted, an overall infection rate should not be calculated because such a rate is too insensitive to measure the influence of exposure to significant HAI risk factors such as urinary catheterization, mechanical ventilation, and surgical procedures. Instead of an overall rate, population-specific or event-related incidence rates, such as ventilator-associated pneumonia (VAP) in an intensive care unit (ICU), should be calculated.

From the early 1970s until the mid-1980s, hospitals in the NNIS system were required to perform housewide surveillance, and the denominator used to calculate infection rates was the number of patients discharged during the surveillance period. In 1986 NNIS changed its focus from a hospital-wide to a targeted approach and introduced four "surveillance components" in which hospitals could participate: housewide, adult and pediatric ICU, high-risk nursery, and surgical patient.[15,39] The purpose of the components was to fulfill the need for more precise measurement of HAIs and infection risk factors. In the mid-1990s the CDC dropped the hospital-wide component of the NNIS system.

Housewide surveillance is an ideal methodology because it can measure the occurrence and risk of HAIs and other monitored events in the entire patient population. However, many healthcare organizations do not have the trained personnel and other resources, such as computerization and technical support, needed to conduct comprehensive surveillance. In addition, many authorities believe that comprehensive infection surveillance is not an efficient use of resources provided an evidence-based infection prevention and control program is implemented housewide and personnel are held accountable for adhering to appropriate practices. Because of these reasons and the fact that the risk of developing an HAI varies by patient population and treatment and procedures provided, many experts recommend using targeted or focused surveillance programs.[39–41]

Targeted (Focused) Surveillance

In targeted surveillance (also known as focused, priority-directed, or surveillance by objective), selected events or populations are monitored.[37,39,42] A targeted surveillance program may focus on selected healthcare units (such as intensive care, hemodialysis, rehabilitation, pediatrics, or bone marrow transplant), specific procedures (such as surgery), infections associated with medical devices (such as VAP), or organisms of epidemiologic importance (such as methicillin-resistant *Staphylococcus aureus* [MRSA], *Clostridium difficile*, or *Mycobacterium tuberculosis*). Targeted surveillance programs generally focus on high-risk, high-volume, or high-cost HAIs that are potentially preventable.

Combining Housewide and Targeted Surveillance

Infection prevention and control personnel in many hospitals and other healthcare settings use a combination of housewide and targeted surveillance. For instance, a surveillance program can monitor central line-associated BSIs in a specific area while monitoring all patients and residents housewide for epidemiologically important organisms.

For additional information on surveillance methodologies, refer to one of several infection control texts that are listed in the Suggested Reading section at the end of this chapter (APIC text, Mayhall, or Wenzel) or to the CDC NHSN Web site (http://www.cdc.gov/ncidod/dhqp/nhsn.html).

GUIDELINES FOR DEVELOPING AND EVALUATING A SURVEILLANCE PROGRAM

Developing a Surveillance Program

A well-designed surveillance program should provide for the ongoing collection, management, analysis, and dissemination of data to control and prevent disease.

Regardless of the setting, those who are designing a surveillance program for a healthcare setting should establish a system that can prevent the most infections and other adverse events with the resources available. In 1984, Robert Haley, MD, recommended a priority-directed approach to surveillance that he termed "surveillance by objective."[42] Building on Dr. Haley's recommendations, the following guidelines can be used when designing a surveillance program today.

1. Target those outcomes that will be prevented (e.g., influenza, catheter-associated urinary tract infections, VAP, decubitus ulcers, medication errors, and sharps injuries) and those processes that will be improved (e.g., influenza immunization rates in healthcare providers and LTC facility residents, and personnel compliance with hand hygiene or aseptic technique when inserting vascular catheters), and develop specific indicators with objectives.

2. "Assign priorities to the specific objectives. Since there is never enough time or resources to do everything, one must rank the objectives."[42(p88)]

3. "Allocate time and resources commensurate with the assigned priorities."[42(p88)]

4. After completing the first three steps, design the surveillance, prevention, and control strategies so they can support the objectives.

5. After a defined period, evaluate the surveillance, prevention, and control program and revise it as needed.

Guidelines for developing and evaluating surveillance programs have been published by the CDC[8,18] and APIC.[9,43] Based on these references, a review of the literature,[5,11,12,15,18,24,25,37,38,41,43,44] and the authors' personal experience, the following steps should be taken (although not necessarily all in the order listed) when designing a surveillance system for the healthcare setting:

- Identify the surveillance methodology to be used.
- Assess and define the population(s) to be monitored, and select the events to be studied.
- Determine the time period for observation and the data collection.
- Select surveillance criteria for defining each event.
- Determine the data-gathering process.
- Identify how to calculate rates and analyze the data.
- Determine the personnel and other resources needed to implement and sustain the program.
- Design an interpretive surveillance report(s).
- Identify who will receive the report(s).
- Develop a written surveillance plan.
- Develop a mechanism for periodically evaluating the effectiveness of the surveillance program.

Identify the Surveillance Methodology to Be Used

When designing a surveillance program, an organization's management team must decide whether to conduct housewide surveillance (i.e., identify all HAIs in the entire population), targeted surveillance, or a combination of the two. Because government and accrediting agencies may require housewide surveillance, healthcare organizations should check external requirements before selecting the surveillance methodology. The authors recommend a combination housewide and targeted (or focused) approach to surveillance that fulfills internal performance needs and external agency requirements.

Assess and Define the Population and Select the Events to Be Monitored

Each organization must assess its patient, resident, and personnel populations and identify those who are at greatest risk for HAIs and other adverse health outcomes. The organization must then choose the indicators or events (outcomes, processes, and organisms) to be monitored. The surveillance events should be selected based on the characteristics of the population(s) to be studied, identified risk factors for infection, types of treatment provided and procedures performed, the level of care provided, relevant government and accrediting agency requirements, available resources, and performance improvement initiatives. An effective surveillance program will have a mixture of outcome and process monitors and will target organisms and diseases that have been demonstrated to cause healthcare-associated problems in the population being studied (or in similar populations as identified by a review of the literature). Some surveillance indicators should focus on personnel.

Acute care settings. In the acute care setting, the highest rates of HAIs occur in ICUs. ICU patients have been shown to be at high risk of infection due to their underlying disease and conditions, their compromised host status, and the invasive diagnostic and therapeutic treatments they receive.[45] Thus it is not surprising that many outbreaks reported in the literature occur in critical care unit patients, as discussed in Chapter 3. Those responsible for designing a surveillance program in a hospital should target their surveillance to defined populations (such as patients in a specific ICU or patients undergoing a specific surgical procedure) so that the number of patients in the population under study (i.e., the population at risk) can be identified. This is necessary if infection rates are to be calculated.[18]

Many infection prevention and control programs monitor device-associated infections, such as central line-associated BSI and VAP, because medical devices place a patient at risk for developing a nosocomial infection. Reports have shown that hospitals that have monitored device-related infection rates over time have been able to identify potential problem areas, implement practice changes to reduce the risk of infection, and reduce infection rates.[21,22,46] In addition, if a hospital uses NNIS/NHSN system methodology to define infections, collect data, and calculate rates, then it can use the published NNIS/NHSN rates for comparison with other hospitals.[19] Many hospital outbreaks have been associated with the improper use and care of ventilators, as discussed in Chapter 3. Because VAP can result in significant morbidity and mortality and increased patient costs and length of stay, many organizations conduct surveillance for VAP and use their surveillance data to identify and implement infection prevention and control measures.[46]

Patients who have surgery are at risk for developing surgical site infections (SSIs), and this risk is influenced by characteristics of the patient, the surgical procedure, personnel, and hospital.[47] Because it is neither necessary nor an efficient use of resources to monitor all surgical procedures all of the time (unless required by an external agency), most facilities select several high-risk, high-volume, or high-cost procedures that are performed at the facility. The CDC has published a list of operative procedures that are included in the NHSN.[18] Personnel who are responsible for developing a surveillance program in a hospital should consider monitoring one or more of these procedures, using the NHSN methodology, so that external comparative data are available (see caveats below). Much has been written about surveillance methods for SSIs. Because a complete discussion of this topic is beyond the scope of this chapter, the reader is referred to several references.[18,27,28,47–58]

Healthcare facilities should routinely conduct surveillance for epidemiologically significant organisms, such as *Clostridium difficile*;[59,60] respiratory syncytial virus (RSV);[61] rotavirus;[62] *M. tuberculosis*;[63,64] and multidrug-resistant organisms (MDROs)[65] such as MRSA,[66] vancomycin-resistant *Enterococcus, Acinetobacter* spp., *Stenotrophomonas* spp., *Pseudomonas aeruginosa, Enterobacter* spp., *Klebsiella pneumoniae, Burkholderia cepacia*, and *Ralstonia* spp., so that isolation precautions can be implemented as soon as possible to prevent transmission to other patients.[67] In addition, all healthcare organizations should routinely monitor laboratory reports for organisms of public health importance, such as *Salmonella* spp. or isolates of *Staphylococcus aureus* that have intermediate susceptibility to vancomycin (VISA) or are resistant to vancomycin (VRSA). All cases of *Salmonella* spp. should be reported to the local health department, and all cases of confirmed or presumptive VISA or VRSA should be reported immediately through local and state health departments to the CDC. Isolates of suspected VISA/VRSA should be saved for the CDC, and patients from whom VISA/VRSA is isolated should be placed on isolation precautions as specified by the CDC.[65,67] Each institution must choose which organisms to monitor based on the ages and the characteristics of the population served, the incidence or presence of an organism in the facility and in the community, and the institution's public health responsibilities (e.g., reporting reportable diseases). For example, pediatric units should monitor organisms that frequently cause nosocomial infections in children, such as RSV and rotavirus.

Healthcare providers and organizations play an integral role in recognizing community outbreaks. For instance, the staff of a community hospital detected a cluster of community-acquired Legionnaires' disease and reported this to the health department. This led to the recognition of an outbreak of legionellosis among the passengers of a cruise ship.[68]

Infection prevention and control personnel should also work with the employee health personnel to monitor and identify communicable infections in personnel, such as tuberculosis, chickenpox, and conjunctivitis, so that appropriate work restrictions can be implemented.

In addition to HAI surveillance in patients and in personnel, those responsible for performance improvement programs in hospitals should have a surveillance system for detecting noninfectious outcomes of care in patients, such as medication errors, and adverse events in personnel, such as sharps injuries. Personnel in both performance improvement and infection prevention and control programs should select several surveillance indicators that assess processes and activities that affect patient outcomes (such as biological monitoring of steam sterilizers and use of aseptic technique and barriers when inserting central lines) and the health of personnel (such as healthcare worker practices that result in sharps injuries and influenza immunization rates).

Ambulatory care settings. Few studies have been done on the risk factors for infection in the ambulatory care setting.[16,28,69–71] This is not surprising because the term *ambulatory care* encompasses a variety of settings. "Ambulatory care setting" as used in this chapter refers to a hospital-based or freestanding facility or office in which health care is provided and in which patients reside for less than 24 hours. Examples include emergency rooms, dialysis centers, physicians' offices, urgent care centers, ambulatory surgery centers, and clinics.

With the exception of patients in ambulatory surgery and dialysis centers, it is often difficult to identify specific populations at risk of developing a HAI that is related to health care provided in the ambulatory care setting.[28] When compared to the acute care and LTC settings, ambulatory care settings have a greater challenge regarding the surveillance of HAIs. Patients cared for in these locations are frequently seen for relatively brief periods, often over a few hours. The patients may not be well known to the provider, may be seen for only one encounter, and are frequently lost to follow-up once they leave the facility. Follow-up of these patients is usually left to the primary care provider, who may have a limited working relationship with other care providers.

Persons who are responsible for managing infection prevention and control programs in ambulatory care settings should be familiar with the numerous outbreaks that have occurred in these settings,[69,70] which are discussed in Chapter 5. Examples of frequently reported outbreaks in ambulatory care facilities include the following[69,70]:

- BSIs and hepatitis B infections associated with improper infection control practices in hemodialysis centers
- Tuberculosis associated with unrecognized cases of pulmonary disease or improper isolation precautions used for patients with known pulmonary tuberculosis
- Keratoconjunctivitis in ophthalmology clinics associated with poor infection prevention practices, such as lack of hand hygiene or improper disinfection of instruments.

In addition, bronchoscopy and gastrointestinal endoscopy procedures have been associated with many outbreaks in outpatient healthcare settings.[72] Infections associated with these procedures are difficult to detect unless they occur in clusters or are caused by an unusual or uncommon pathogen.

There is little published about effective surveillance methods for ambulatory care settings, with the exception of SSI surveillance in ambulatory surgery centers. Infection control professionals (ICPs) in ambulatory surgery centers should identify the operative procedures that are most commonly performed at the center and should use center-specific data and literature reviews to identify patients that have the highest risk for infectious and noninfectious complications.[27,47] If SSI surveillance is performed, high-volume and/or high-risk procedures should be monitored.

The NHSN includes a national surveillance system to study the incidence of bloodstream and vascular access-site infections, hospitalizations, and antimicrobial use in hemodialysis patients.[16,18] Hemodialysis centers should consider participating in this program. Information on the NHSN dialysis surveillance program can be obtained in the NHSN *Patient Safety Component Protocol*[18] and on the NHSN Web site (http://www.cdc.gov/ncidod/dhqp/nhsn.html). Hemodialysis centers should routinely perform quality assurance tests on hemodialysis water. Documentation of this testing and any actions taken based on the test results can serve as a process monitor.

Ophthalmology offices and clinics should conduct surveillance for patients who develop conjunctivitis following care in the office or clinic (an outcomes indicator). These settings should also select a few process indicators and implement a performance improvement initiative on the proper use of hand hygiene, multidose medications, or disinfection of equipment.

Personnel who are responsible for developing an infection surveillance, prevention, and control program in the ambulatory care setting should focus on both risk reduction and infection prevention activities (i.e., process indicators) and on outcomes measurements, such as infections. Process-oriented surveillance indicators for an ambulatory care setting such as a physician's office or a clinic could include compliance with reporting reportable diseases, compliance with sterility assurance protocols (i.e., biological, physical, and chemical monitoring) for all sterilizers used in the facility, and immunization rates for patients and personnel. Many studies have revealed glaring deficiencies in the processing of endoscopes, and numerous outbreaks have been associated with the use of contaminated bronchoscopes and gastrointestinal endoscopes.[72] Therefore, those who are designing a surveillance program for an endoscopy unit should develop process monitors, such as personnel compliance with specific cleaning and disinfection/sterilization protocols for endoscopes. In this setting, monitoring the processes used (i.e., attention to proper cleaning and disinfection practices) will more likely lead to improved patient care than monitoring an outcome such as infection, which is difficult to detect, especially in an ambulatory population that is frequently lost to follow-up. Ambulatory care facilities should also conduct surveillance for the occurrence of diseases of epidemiologic importance, such as salmonellosis, tuberculosis, and Legionnaires' disease, in their patient population and should report these diseases to the health department.

Long-Term Care Settings. Much has been published about endemic and epidemic nosocomial infections and risk factors for infection in the LTC setting.[25,73–85] However, infection surveillance methodology for the LTC setting has not been as well defined as it has been for the acute care setting, and many facilities probably lack an effective, ongoing surveillance program.[26,82] Surveillance programs in the LTC setting should be designed and implemented to promote the ongoing collection, analysis, and dissemination of information on infections in the setting. Surveillance data should be used to plan infection prevention and control activities, including educational programs.[81] Surveillance indicators should be based on those infections that commonly occur in the setting—especially on those that are potentially preventable—and on those processes shown to reduce the risk of HAIs in LTC facilities (e.g., annual influenza vaccination).[25] Guidelines for developing infection surveillance programs in LTC settings have been published by the APIC and the Society for Healthcare Epidemiology of America (SHEA),[25] Smith,[24,78] the Canadian Ministry of National Health and Welfare,[84] and Rosenbaum et al.[85] As in the acute care setting, targeted or focused surveillance programs are recommended because they are a more efficient use of infection prevention and control resources and they permit the calculation of site-specific rates (such as urinary tract infections).[25] Whenever designing a surveillance program, one has to ensure that it meets the requirements of regulatory and accrediting agencies.

The most commonly occurring outbreaks in the LTC setting are respiratory diseases (influenza and tuberculosis), gastrointestinal diseases, and scabies.[25] Colonization and infection with MRSA occurs frequently in many LTC settings. Therefore, surveillance programs must be capable of detecting these infections. Ahlbrecht et al. were able to demonstrate positive outcomes in a pilot study that involved infection surveillance and a team approach to infection prevention and control in a 220-bed community-based nursing home.[86] They also suggested some data elements in the minimum data set from the Health Care Financing Administration (now Centers for Medicare and Medicaid Services (CMS)) that may be useful in targeting surveillance in nursing home residents.

In addition to infection surveillance, LTC settings should have a program for monitoring noninfectious outcomes of care, such as falls, physical restraint use, and decubiti, and processes such as influenza immunization rates in residents and personnel.[12]

Selecting surveillance indicators. Table 2–1 lists suggested indicators and events for surveillance programs in a variety of healthcare settings and provides references, when available, that either explain or illustrate the use of these indicators or can provide criteria for developing an indicator.[11,18,30,32,33, 47–49,54–57,62,63,67,71,77,90–120]

Determine the Time Period for Data Collection

Surveillance data should be collected on an ongoing basis in order to identify trends, detect organisms and diseases of epidemiologic importance, and recognize clusters and outbreaks. There is no defined time period or number of events that must be measured; however, it is difficult to interpret rates for events that occur infrequently and for procedures that are rarely performed. In practice, many ICPs collect data on each indicator for a defined period, such as a month, quarter, or year, and analyze and assess the data to determine if they are useful for identifying potential problems and methods for improvement. If the indicator does not appear to be useful, its use should be discontinued. For example, if a facility selects noncentral line-related BSI rates as a HAI measure on a patient care unit and discovers that these infections rarely occur, then consideration should be given to discontinuing this particular measure.

Select Surveillance Criteria and Case Definitions

Criteria, or case definitions, are a key element of any surveillance system. To be able to accurately analyze surveillance data over time, consistent definitions must be used to determine the presence of a HAI or other health-related event or compliance to a policy. Criteria must be used the same way and applied consistently by all persons who collect or evaluate surveillance data to ensure the accuracy and reproducibility of the results. If data elements are not defined consistently, then it will not be possible to determine the presence and the true incidence of a disease or to determine if measures implemented to control a disease are effective.

Criteria allow all persons involved in the surveillance process (all those who collect, analyze, evaluate, and use the data) to have a common understanding

Table 2–1   Suggested Surveillance Indicators for Various Healthcare Settings

Indicator	Type(s) of Setting	Type of Indicator	Selected Reference(s)
Bloodstream infections associated with central lines	Acute, LTC, home	Outcome	11, 18, 30, 32, 46, 86, 120
Bloodstream infections in selected populations	Acute, LTC, home	Outcome	33, 87, 120
Local site infections and/or phlebitis associated with peripheral intravascular therapy	Acute, LTC, home	Outcome	88, 89
Ventilator-associated pneumonia	Acute, LTC	Outcome	11, 18, 86, 90
Catheter-associated urinary tract infections	Acute, LTC, home	Outcome	11, 18, 30, 33
Surgical site infections	Acute, amb surgery, home	Outcome	18, 30, 47–49, 54-57
Decubitus ulcers	LTC, acute	Outcome	77, 91–93
Conjunctivitis	Ophthalmology offices and clinics	Outcome	94
Influenza in residents and personnel	LTC	Outcome	90, 95
Sharps injuries in personnel	Acute, LTC, amb, home	Outcome	96–98
TST conversions in personnel	Acute, LTC, amb	Outcome	63, 99
TST conversions in residents	LTC	Outcome	63, 99
Newly diagnosed tuberculosis cases	Acute, LTC, amb	Outcome	63
Infection/colonization with MRSA or VRE	Acute, LTC	Outcome	65, 100
Respiratory syncytial virus (RSV) infection	Pediatric	Outcome	101
Rotavirus infection	Pediatric	Outcome	62
Clostridium difficile diarrhea	LTC, acute, home	Outcome	59, 102
Bloodstream infections, pyrogenic reactions, vascular access infections, MRSA, or VRE in hemodialysis patients	Hemodialysis centers	Outcome	16, 18
Resident or patient falls	LTC, acute	Outcome	103, 104
Medication errors	Acute, LTC	Outcome	105, 106
Occurrence of reportable diseases	Acute, LTC, amb	Outcome	Local, state, national regulations, 107

Continued

Table 2–1   *(Continued)*

Indicator	Type(s) of Setting	Type of Indicator	Selected Reference(s)
Influenza immunization rates in personnel, patients, and residents	LTC, acute, amb, home	Process	90, 108, 109
Personnel adherence to standard precautions or isolation precautions	Acute, LTC, amb	Process	67, 70
Personnel adherence to cleaning, disinfection, or sterilization protocols	Acute, LTC, amb	Process	110, 111, 113
Adherence to performance testing/ quality assurance program for sterilizers (e.g., appropriate use of biological indicator)	Wherever sterilizers are used	Process	111, 112
Proper functioning of isolation rooms used for tuberculosis and airborne isolation	Acute, LTC, amb	Process	63
Proper use of activated gluteraldehyde solutions	Wherever solutions are used	Process	According to instructions on product label
Adherence to infection prevention and control measures during construction and renovation	Acute, LTC	Process	90, 113
Hepatitis B immunization rates in personnel	Acute, LTC, amb	Process	114
Hepatitis B immunization rates in patients	Hemodialysis centers	Process	71
Adherence to reportable disease regulations	Acute, LTC, amb	Process	107, applicable regulations
Personnel adherence to appropriate hand hygiene practices	Acute, LTC, amb	Process	115–118

Note: LTC = long-term care; home = home care; amb = ambulatory care; MRSA = methicillin-resistant *Staphylococcus aureus,* VRE = vancomycin-resistant *Enterococcus*; TST = tuberculin skin test

of the events that are being monitored. To be acceptable to all of the users of the data, the criteria used in a surveillance program should reflect generally accepted definitions of the specific disease or event being studied. For example, if SSI surveillance is going to be performed, then the personnel from the infection prevention and control and the surgery departments must agree upon the criteria for defining the presence of an SSI.

Criteria frequently combine clinical findings with the results of laboratory and other diagnostic tests. In the United States the most widely used sets of definitions for HAIs in acute care hospitals are those developed by the CDC for the NNIS system. These definitions have been updated for use in the NHSN.[18] Definitions for surveillance of infections in LTC facilities were published by McGeer et al. in 1991.[119] The McGeer definitions were intended "for use in facilities that provide homes for elderly residents who require 24-hour personal care under professional nursing supervision."[119(p1)] The McGeer definitions focus on the clinical presentations of infections and minimize the need for confirmatory diagnostic and laboratory tests that are infrequently performed in the LTC setting.

Whenever possible, previously published, standardized definitions should be used. Ambulatory surgery facilities can use the NHSN criteria when conducting SSI surveillance,[19] and hemodialysis centers can use the NHSN definitions for healthcare events in these centers.[19]

The APIC-Healthcare Infection Control Practices Advisory Committe Surveillance Definitions for Home Health Care and Home Hospice Infections were published in 2008.[120]

Each organization must evaluate its population, case mix of patients, and the availability of diagnostic and laboratory facilities in order to determine which definitions are both appropriate and applicable to its setting. Factors that should be considered when evaluating surveillance criteria include the sophistication of the data collector, the applicability of the particular set of definitions to the population being surveyed, the availability and accuracy of laboratory and other diagnostic tests performed on the population, and the availability of laboratories that can provide needed feedback regarding specimen collection and analysis. Many organizations adapt available definitions for their use; however, changing the definitions makes it impossible for the organization to compare its performance to that of other institutions.

Some problems with current definitions. Many definitions of infections have serious drawbacks. ICPs have long recognized the difficulty of classifying some diseases, especially pneumonia and BSIs, when doing surveillance. Many investigators have proposed different definitions for classifying pneumonia, but there is little consensus on a practical definition for this disease.[121] Even though they have recently been revised, the CDC NHSN definitions for pneumonia and BSIs are difficult to use consistently. When evaluating a potential BSI, it is often difficult to determine if an organism isolated from a blood culture is a true infection or a contaminant. Those using definitions must realize that incidence rates may change when a definition is changed, and this must be recognized when analyzing surveillance data and must be noted when writing a surveillance report.

The characteristics of patients residing in licensed LTC facilities dramatically changed in the 1990s. The McGeer[119] definitions were written in 1989, before the widespread use of IV therapy and mechanical ventilators and the presence of patients with acquired immune deficiency syndrome in many LTC settings. Some LTC facilities, especially those that care for residents with significant acuity (such as those who are ventilator dependent or who have a central venous catheter), use the NNIS/NHSN definitions for use in their setting.[18]

Determine the Process for Gathering Data

The processes for gathering data will depend on the surveillance indicators that are chosen and available personnel and technical resources.[9,12,18,43]

Identify what data will be collected. Data collection should be limited to the essential information (i.e., data elements) needed to determine if the criteria for the disease or event being monitored are met. Although the variables to be collected will depend on the particular event being surveyed, when monitoring patient outcomes the following data points should be considered:

1. For HAIs:
   - Patient name, medical record or identification number, age, sex, location in the facility (unit, room number, bed number), physician name and service, date of admission, date of infection onset, type of infection, date of discharge, transfer, or death
   - Information needed to classify the specific HAI being monitored: relevant laboratory/diagnostic tests, date(s) done/results, cultures done (including date collected, body site cultured and result), antibiotic susceptibility pattern of significant isolates, signs/symptoms specific for the disease criteria
   - Risk factors for infection: host factors (such as underlying disease), surgical procedures (name of procedure, surgeon, American Society of Anesthesiologists [ASA] score, duration of procedure), presence of invasive devices (date of insertion, duration, location and types of vascular access devices; use and duration of urinary catheter or mechanical ventilator)

2. For noninfectious events:[12] Patient name; medical record or identification number; age; sex; location in the facility (unit, room number, bed number); physician name and service; date of admission; date, time, and location of the event; outcome of event; personnel involved (when relevant); date of discharge, transfer, or death; and risk factors for event (e.g., identified risk factors for falls include poor vision, preexisting neurologic deficits, and medications such as psychotropic drugs)

Identify when data will be collected. The approach to collecting surveillance data (i.e., concurrent and/or retrospective) depends on the event being studied and the available resources. The advantages of conducting concurrent surveillance (i.e., collecting data while the patient is still under the care of the facility) include the ability to observe findings that are not always recorded in the patient's record (such as the presence of drainage at a surgical incision site), to interview those caring for the patient (direct caregivers frequently provide insight into circumstances and factors that may influence patient outcomes), to detect clusters or potential outbreaks in a timely manner, to institute immediate control measures (such as isolation precautions), and to provide informal education about infection prevention and control to caregivers, patients, residents, or family members (this is especially important in LTC facilities that have high staff turnover rates). Some data, such as information on falls and other accidents, should be recorded at the time of the incident so that important information is not overlooked or forgotten. If data are collected concurrently, then patient length of stay will affect the frequency of data collection. Some experts recommend that routine infection surveillance be performed at least once a week in the LTC setting.[73]

The disadvantages of concurrent surveillance are the time involved in locating and reviewing charts on a busy unit and the incompleteness of the patient's medical record if test results are not yet available when the chart is reviewed. In some circumstances it may be more efficient to conduct retrospective or closed-record surveillance, especially if there is little or no opportunity for intervention. Retrospective chart review allows the surveyor to review laboratory and other diagnostic reports that may not be completed or placed in the medical record until after discharge.

Identify sources of data. After deciding what data elements are needed, the sources of the data should be identified. Sources may include the following[37,43]:

- Patient or resident records
- Daily microbiology reports provided by the laboratory
- Daily list of patients or residents admitted (including diagnosis) provided by the admissions department
- Monthly report of the number of patients admitted and discharged and the number of patient-days for each unit in the facility, as provided by the facility's administrative or financial department
- Interviews with caregivers
- Verbal and written reports from caregivers
- Kardex on the patient units
- Lists of patients on isolation precautions (this can sometimes be generated through the organization's computer information system)
- Antibiotic order reports generated by the pharmacy
- Chest radiograph results from the radiology department (these are often available through the hospital information system or through an audio system by telephone)
- Incident reports from the risk management department
- Observations of healthcare workers' practices
- Activity/procedure logs from the emergency room, operating room, respiratory therapy department, and outpatient offices or clinics
- Other personnel who regularly review records (such as quality management and utilization review)
- Employee health reports for needlesticks and other personnel injuries or exposures
- The medical records department for lists of patients who were coded with the same disease or condition.

ICPs should work with the organization's information services department to identify sources of data and how these data can be downloaded electronically to the infection prevention and control department.[122]

Identify who will collect the data. The persons who are responsible for collecting HAI surveillance data must be capable of interpreting clinical notes, collecting the data elements needed to evaluate the presence of nosocomial infection, and using a standardized data collection tool. The availability of surveillance personnel may affect the frequency and accuracy of data collection. If the person who is responsible for data collection leaves the position or is on extended leave of absence, then someone else should be trained and assigned responsibility for the data collection process. If data are not collected for short periods, it may not be of major consequence; however, if data collection is interrupted for long periods, significant events such as outbreaks or clusters may be missed.

For some HAI indicators, personnel in several departments may be given the responsibility for collecting data. For example, respiratory therapy personnel can often provide the number of ventilator-days in a specific patient care unit, and ICU personnel can collect and record each day the number of patients with a urinary catheter or a central line. (Note: *Central line* must be defined[19] so that data can be consistently collected each day regardless of who collects them.)

Design data collection tools. Standardized data collection tools must be designed and used to collect the necessary data elements for the surveillance indicators. Several types of data collection forms may be needed:

1. A case report form is usually used to collect surveillance data on each patient reviewed:
   - If a manual data collection and management system is used, this case report form should be designed so it is consistent with the order in the patient medical record so that information can be collected and recorded efficiently. This should minimize the need to search back and forth through the chart.
   - If a computer database is used, the case report form should be designed so its order is the same as the data entry screen on the computer. Whenever possible, both the computer database and the case report form should be set up so the information is consistent with the order in the patient medical record.
   - Case report forms may be paper based or electronic. A one-page data collection form should be used as much as possible.

2. A line-listing form or database should be used to record data on all cases that have a particular disease, such as all patients from whom MRSA has been isolated or all patients with an SSI following total hip arthroplasty, and to visualize data, such as factors that may be common to these patients.

3. A form should be used to record the number of patients on a specific unit who have a central line or urinary catheter or who are on mechanical ventilation.[11,18]

Examples of data collection forms can be found in several of the references.[12,18,78,84,95] Any of these forms can be used as prototypes upon which a facility-specific form can be modeled.

Using technology to collect, store, manage, and analyze surveillance data. Before data can be analyzed, they must be collected and organized. Data collection and consolidation can be accomplished using either a manual or electronic/computerized system. The basic premises are the same; however, the data can be more easily manipulated when a computer is used, so computers and computerized databases should be used whenever possible. Unfortunately, manual systems are frequently used even when computers may be readily available.

When manual data collection systems are used, the user should be able to take information from the individual or case forms in an orderly manner and enter it into an electronic database, such as Microsoft Excel, that is organized to correspond to the case form. Electronic line lists can then be generated to display data in a variety of ways (e.g., by organism, infection site, procedure, date of event, or service).

If they are not yet doing so, those responsible for coordinating infection surveillance, prevention, and control programs should learn to use computers to collect, store, manage, and analyze surveillance data. Basic software packages, such as Microsoft Office, contain word-processing, spreadsheet, database, and graphics programs that are useful for infection surveillance. Data collection forms can be designed using a word-processing program, and corresponding line listings can be developed using a word-processing, spreadsheet, or database program. Commercially available software programs designed to manage and display nosocomial infection surveillance data are available.[122] The use of information technology in the collection, management, and analysis of surveillance data is discussed in Chapter 9.

Data often are collected at the bedside or in clinical areas. Therefore, unless portable computers, personal digital assistants, or bedside terminals are used to collect the information, a paper form must still be used to record the data on site. The information then must be entered into a central computer program. Smyth et al. described the use of an automated data entry system employing optical scanning of a specially designed form to enter surveillance data into a computer database.[123] This method reduced both the time and errors associated with manual data entry. Although widely used for other purposes (such as grading examinations), optical scanning technology has rarely been used for entering surveillance data in healthcare facilities.

As discussed in Chapter 9, some facilities have developed comprehensive, hospital-wide software systems. These expert systems can merge and/or evaluate data in existing patient information databases to identify patients with a high probability of having a HAI. These patients can then be targeted for chart review, antibiotic management, or infection control intervention.[122,124]

Identify How to Calculate Rates and Analyze the Data

When designing a surveillance program, the types of measurements desired (usually rates and proportions) must be determined prior to conducting surveillance so that the appropriate data can be identified and consistently collected. Ratios, rates, and proportions are explained in detail in Chapter 10. The basic formula used to calculate rates, ratios, and proportions is:

rate, ratio, or proportion = $(x/y) \times 10^n$

where x (the numerator) is compared to y (the denominator) and 10^n is used to transform the result of the division into a uniform quantity. The value of n depends on the type of frequency measure being computed.

A rate is used in healthcare epidemiology to measure the frequency or occurrence of a disease or event in a specified population over time. The formula is:

$$\text{rate} = \frac{\text{number of cases or events occurring in a specified time period}}{\text{number of persons in the population at risk during the same time period}} \times 10^n$$

To calculate accurate rates of disease frequency, the appropriate numerators and denominators must be used. For instance, when calculating an incidence rate, persons who have the disease or condition being studied are called the "cases," and these become the numerator. The persons who are at risk of developing the disease or condition being studied are called the "population at risk," and these become the denominator.

Criteria or case definitions must be used to identify cases, as discussed earlier in this chapter. During the course of an outbreak investigation, the case definition may be expanded in order to identify all the persons who may be affected and later narrowed to include only those who have been diagnosed with the disease being studied, as explained in Chapter 8. However, when conducting routine surveillance, it is imperative that a single case definition for each disease or event be applied at all times, so that the surveyors can accurately track trends (rates) over time.

The selection of an appropriate denominator is one of the most important aspects of measuring disease frequency.[18,125] It is important to ensure that the number used closely represents the true population at risk. For example, incidence rates measure the frequency with which new cases or events occur in a defined population at risk during a specified period. The formula for calculating an incidence rate is:

$$\text{incidence rate} = \frac{\text{number of new cases or events that occur in a defined time period}}{\text{number of persons in population at risk during the same period}} \times 10^n$$

If one wishes to measure the incidence of primary bloodstream infections (PBSIs) in an ICU, the numerator would be the number of new PBSIs in the ICU during a defined period, and the denominator would be the number of patients discharged from the ICU during that period (because the number discharged would be a close approximation of the population at risk). However, because a patient's risk of developing a PBSI is known to increase as the time spent in the ICU increases, a more accurate measure of a patient's risk of developing a PBSI would be an incidence density rate. The incidence density is a type of incidence rate that incorporates time, such as patient-days, in the denominator. The formula is:

$$\text{incidence density} = \frac{\text{number of new cases that occur in a defined period}}{\substack{\text{the time each person in population at risk is observed,} \\ \text{totaled for all persons}}} \times 10^n$$

Using the above formula, one could calculate the incidence density rate of PBSI in the ICU as follows:

$$\text{ICU PBSI rate per 1000 patient-days} = \frac{\text{number of new cases of PBSI in the ICU in a defined period}}{\text{total number of patient-days in the ICU in the defined period}} \times 1000$$

where the denominator is the total number of days spent in the ICU by *all* patients who were in the ICU during the defined period, and $n = 3$ to show that rate per 1000 patient-days.

One can also calculate device-associated infection rates. One could calculate the number of BSIs that are associated with a central line in the above ICU population by using the steps shown in Exhibit 2–1.

Exhibit 2–1   How to Calculate a Device-Associated Infection Rate

Step 1. Decide on the time period for your analysis. It may be a month, a quarter, 6 months, a year, or some other period.

Step 2. Select the patient population for analysis (i.e., the type of intensive care unit or birth-weight category in a NICU).

Step 3. Select the infections to be used in the numerator. They must be site specific and must have occurred in the selected patient population. Their date of onset must be during the selected time period.

Step 4. Determine the number of device-days, which is used as the denominator of the rate. Device-days are the total number of days of exposure to the device (central line, umbilical catheter, ventilator, or urinary catheter) by all of the patients in the selected population during the selected time period.

Example: Five patients on the first day of the month had one or more central lines in place; five on day 2; two on day 3; five on day 4; three on day 5; four on day 6; and four on day 7. Adding the number of patients with central lines on days 1 through 7, we would have $5 + 5 + 2 + 5 + 3 + 4 + 4 = 28$ central line-days for the first week. If we continued for the entire month, the number of central line-days for the month is simply the sum of the daily counts.

Step 5. Calculate the device-associated infection rate (per 1000 device-days) using the following formula:

$$\text{Device-associated infection rate} = \frac{\text{Number of device-associated infections for an infection site}}{\text{Number device-days}} \times 1000$$

Example:

$$\text{Central line-associated BSI rate per 1000 central line-days} = \frac{\text{Number of central line-associated BSI}}{\text{Number of central line-days}} \times 1000$$

Source: Adapted from Edwards JR, Peterson KD, Andrus ML, et al. National Healthcare Safety Network (NHSN) Report, data summary for 2006, issued June 2007. *Am J Infect Control.* 2007;35: 290–301.
Author note: report is in public domain. http://download.journals.elsevierhealth.com/pdfs/journals/0196-6553/PIIS0196655307001472.pdf.

There are also many methods for calculating SSI rates.[49] One can calculate service-specific, surgeon-specific, or procedure-specific rates. In the examples below, $n = 2$, and the rate is expressed as a percentage:

$$\text{Cardiology service-specific rate (\%)} = \frac{\text{number SSIs in patients on cardiology service}}{\substack{\text{number patients on cardiology service} \\ \text{who had surgery}}} \times 100$$

$$\text{Surgeon-specific rate (\%)} = \frac{\text{number SSIs in patients operated on by Dr. A}}{\text{number patients operated on by Dr. A}} \times 100$$

$$\substack{\text{Procedure-specific} \\ \text{rate (\%)}} = \frac{\text{number SSIs after coronary artery bypass graft (CABG) surgery}}{\text{number CABG procedures done}} \times 100$$

Prevalence is a measure of the frequency of the occurrence of current (i.e., both existing and new) cases of a disease in a specified population during a defined time period. A prevalence rate is calculated using the formula:

$$\text{Prevalence rate} = \frac{\text{all new and existing cases during a specific time period}}{\text{population at risk during same time period}} \times 10^n$$

Incidence versus prevalence rates. A prevalence rate differs from an incidence rate in that a prevalence rate measures the occurrence of both new and existing cases of a disease while an incidence rate measures new cases only. For this reason, prevalence rates are generally higher than incidence rates. Some published studies report prevalence, not incidence, rates of infection. Therefore, one must be careful that the same types of rates are being compared when comparing rates in a facility to those in another facility or to rates published in the literature.

When developing a surveillance program, one must first identify which rates will be calculated and then identify which numerator and denominator will be used before any data are collected.[18]

Comparing rates: risk stratification, data collection, and making comparisons. Different populations have different risks for disease or injury. For instance, a new mother in a mother–baby unit is less likely to develop an HAI than a critically ill patient in an ICU. A healthcare worker who uses needles to give injections is more likely to sustain a needlestick than a clerk in the same facility. For this reason, a risk stratification method (a system of adjusting rates based on risk) must be incorporated into a surveillance program.[9,18,19,37,43,47,49]

Calculating incidence rates based on patient-days or device-days is one method of risk stratification, and this is used in the NHSN.[18,19] Surgical wound infection rates have long been calculated using risk adjustment systems.[49,18,19,126–128] The NNIS/NHSN uses a risk index based on wound classification, duration of the operation (time of incision to time of closure), and ASA score.[18]

Because a thorough discussion of risk stratification methods is beyond the scope of this chapter, for more information refer to the references noted above and to the review article by Gross.[129] It should be noted that risk adjustment systems must be used for measuring all outcomes of care, not only for HAIs.[130,131]

Data analysis should be limited to those personnel who are trained to consistently apply specific criteria for the event being monitored. Studies have shown that even when personnel are trained to identify the presence, type, and site of HAIs, there is variation in their ability to do so.[132,133] In addition, surveillance that is conducted prospectively (at least in part) has been shown to be more accurate than surveillance conducted by retrospective chart review.[134]

Factors that affect variations in data collection and analysis must be kept in mind when comparing rates over time in a healthcare setting and especially when comparing rates with other institutions.[135–139] Surveillance indicators that are used for comparing rates with external databases should meet the criteria delineated by SHEA and APIC.[135] For comparisons to be valid, those who are comparing their facility with another, or with a national database such as NHSN, must ensure that the same definitions for a HAI and the same methods for calculating rates are done in the facilities being compared.

Many hospitals use the NNIS/NHSN data for comparing HAI rates. To compare rates with NNIS/NHSN, an organization must use the NNIS/NHSN methodology for collecting data and for calculating and analyzing rates.[11,18] There is currently no similar national database for comparing or benchmarking nosocomial infection rates in the LTC setting; however, several government agencies are planning to develop one.[17,35] Stevenson et al. have published several reports of a regional data set of infection rates for LTC facilities that demonstrates the potential for developing a pooled data set for interfacility (among different facilities) comparison.[36,140] There are few national databases for comparing other types of events relating to health care. Although the use of benchmarking is attractive, and comparing rates to others can lead to improvement in the quality of care,[21,22] healthcare organizations must be aware of the problems inherent in comparing rates among facilities and the need for risk stratification, validation of the data collection process, and standardization of the methods used for analysis and interpretation of the findings.[135–144] These problems are being addressed in the United States and other countries where government agencies are requiring reporting of HAI rates and other healthcare quality data with the goal of improving healthcare quality.[145,146]

Develop an Interpretive Report

"Measurement, or surveillance, is an essential step in enabling an organization to learn about what it produces (outcomes) and how it produces it (process)."[147(p137)] Surveillance reports should be designed to provide accurate, interpretable information and to stimulate improvement of the process or the outcomes being measured. Methods for using visual displays (charts, graphs, and tables) to present the findings are discussed in Chapter 12.

The content, format, and level of detail of each report will depend on the intended audience. Reports should be designed to contain the following information: time frame of the study, numbers of cases or events detected, number in the population studied, the rates, the methodology that was used to collect the data and calculate the rates, the criteria that were used to define the numerator and denominator, any actions taken, the likely risk factors that influenced the occurrence of the events, and any recommendations for prevention and control measures.

Determine Who Should Receive the Report

Reports should be provided to those persons in the organization who can alter the outcomes or processes (i.e., those who can develop and implement strategies to reduce the risk factors). It is important to be expansive in determining who can alter the outcomes or processes of care. Although managers are most often thought of as those who can influence change, there are others on staff who also have this ability. Direct caregivers, such as nursing staff, physicians, and therapists, should also receive reports of surveillance findings. These personnel can make a substantial difference in preventing HAIs and improving adherence to proper infection prevention and control practices.

Those who produce the reports should periodically meet with those who receive the reports to discuss the findings, rates, any clusters detected, and any recommendations for improvement.

Develop a Written Surveillance Plan

A written surveillance plan should be developed and reviewed periodically, at least annually, to assess the usefulness of the program. The written plan should contain the following information:

- A brief description of the organization, population(s) served, and types of services provided
- The objectives of the surveillance program
- A brief description of the events and indicators monitored (both outcome and process)
- The methodology for data collection (housewide or targeted)
- The methodology for calculating and analyzing rates
- A description of the surveillance criteria used, such as NHSN[18] or McGeer[119]
- Delineation of who is responsible for collecting, managing, and analyzing data and preparing reports
- The types of reports provided and persons to whom they are provided
- The process for evaluating the program

Evaluating a Surveillance Program

Each surveillance program should be periodically assessed to evaluate its usefulness. Guidelines for evaluating surveillance systems have been published by the CDC.[8] A surveillance system is considered useful if it contributes to the prevention and control of adverse health events.

When assessing the usefulness of the program, one should begin with a review of the program's objectives. "Depending on the objectives of a particular surveillance system, the system might be considered useful if it satisfactorily addresses at least one of the following questions. Does the system:

- Detect diseases, injuries, or adverse or protective exposures of public importance in a timely way to permit accurate diagnosis or identification, prevention or treatment, and handling of contacts when appropriate?
- Provide estimates of the magnitude of morbidity and mortality related to the health-related event under surveillance, including the identification of factors associated with the event?
- Detect trends that signal changes in the occurrence of disease, injury, or adverse or protective exposure, including detection of epidemics (or outbreaks)?
- Permit assessment of the effect of prevention and control programs?
- Lead to improved clinical, behavioral, social, policy, or environmental practices?
- Stimulate research intended to lead to prevention or control?"[8(p14)]

REGULATIONS AND REQUIREMENTS AFFECTING SURVEILLANCE PROGRAMS IN HEALTHCARE SETTINGS

Many countries, including the United States and Canada, have state, regional or national requirements that healthcare facilities, such as hospitals and nursing homes, implement infection surveillance, prevention, and control measures or programs.[25,85,148–152] The CMS mandates the collection and analysis of data on outcomes and adverse events in facilities that receive Medicare and Medicaid payments. For example, the CMS Conditions of Participation for hospitals require a hospital to have a program for identifying, reporting, investigating, and controlling infections and communicable diseases in patients and personnel and to maintain a record of incidents and corrective actions related to infections.[152] CMS also requires LTC facilities to have an infection control program (CMS 42 CFR Part 83, Subpart B—Requirements for Long-Term Care Facilities).

In addition to government mandates, healthcare facilities are also subject to requirements of accrediting agencies, such as the Joint Commission and the Commission on Accreditation of Rehabilitation Facilities (CARF). The Joint Commission requires the healthcare organizations that it accredits (e.g., hospitals, LTC facilities, and ambulatory care facilities) to have infection surveillance, prevention, and control programs that include the ongoing review and analysis of data on HAIs.[153] The Joint Commission specifies that each healthcare organization must design and implement a surveillance program that is appropriate for its population and environment. Organizations that are accredited by CARF must have an infection prevention and control program that addresses infections acquired in the community, infections acquired in the facility, and trends.[154] Although the expectations of the various government, regulatory, and accrediting agencies regarding the methodology and type of data collected varies, there is consensus that a healthcare organization must collect data on HAIs, analyze the data to determine the significance of the findings, and implement programs and practices that will reduce the risk of HAIs.

Public health agencies worldwide have disease surveillance programs and requirements for reporting certain diseases and conditions to a local or national health department. All states and territories in the United States and many local municipalities mandate reporting of specific notifiable diseases by healthcare providers and laboratories.[155] Each year, the CDC publishes a list of nationally notifiable infectious diseases that should be reported to the National Notifiable Diseases Surveillance System[107]; however, state and local laws governing reporting vary for the diseases or conditions that must be reported by healthcare providers to the local health department.[155] The 2008 list of US nationally notifiable diseases is provided in Exhibit 2–2.

THE HEALTHCARE PROVIDER'S ROLE IN PUBLIC HEALTH SURVEILLANCE

Healthcare providers play a critical role in the identification, surveillance, and reporting of communicable diseases and in the early recognition of community outbreaks.[68] Even though it may not seem important to report one case of a notifiable disease, that case may be part of a larger outbreak that would not be recognized unless each healthcare provider reported each case diagnosed.

Outbreaks of infectious diseases are frequently first detected by healthcare providers when several patients present with the same symptoms within a short period of time. Healthcare providers and organizations should have a mechanism for routinely reporting suspected outbreaks of infectious and non-infectious diseases. For example, a few years ago a patient was admitted to a community hospital with dehydration and gastroenteritis. The patient told her attending physician that several of her friends, all of whom had attended the same wedding reception, were also ill and another had just been admitted to the same hospital with similar symptoms. The physician reported this to the infection control staff who interviewed both patients, confirmed the report, and called the local health department. The health department investigated the cases and uncovered an outbreak of *Salmonella enteritidis* food poisoning among the attendees of the wedding. The source of the *Salmonella* was eventually found to be a contaminated commercially packaged meat product. Contamination of the meat product may not have been recognized, and many more people may have become ill if this cluster of cases had not been promptly recognized, investigated, and reported.

GLOBAL SURVEILLANCE AND EMERGENCY PREPAREDNESS

In 2007 the World Health Organization (WHO) published its *World Health Report 2007, A Safer Future: Global Public Health Security in the*

Exhibit 2–2 Nationally Notifiable Infectious Diseases, United States, 2008

Acquired immunodeficiency
syndrome (AIDS)
Anthrax
Arboviral neuroinvasive and
nonneuroinvasive
diseases
- California serogroup
  virus disease
- Eastern equine
  encephalitis virus
  disease
- Powassan virus disease
- St. Louis encephalitis
  virus disease
- West Nile virus disease
- Western equine
  encephalitis virus
  disease
Botulism
Botulism, food-borne
Botulism, infant
Botulism, other (wound and
unspecified)
Brucellosis
Chancroid
Chlamydia trachomatis,
genital infections
Cholera
Coccidioidomycosis
Cryptosporidiosis
Cyclosporiasis
Diphtheria
Ehrlichiosis/Anaplasmosis
Ehrlichia chaffeensis
Ehrlichia ewingii Anaplasma
phagocytophilum
Undetermined
Giardiasis
Gonorrhea
Haemophilus influenzae,
invasive disease
Hansen disease (leprosy)
Hantavirus pulmonary
syndrome
Hemolytic uremic
syndrome, postdiarrheal

Hepatitis, viral, acute
- Hepatitis A, acute
- Hepatitis B, acute
- Hepatitis B virus,
  perinatal infection
- Hepatitis, C, acute
Hepatitis, viral, chronic
- Chronic hepatitis B
- Hepatitis C virus Infection
  (past or present)
HIV infection
HIV infection, adult
(> =13 years)
HIV infection, pediatric
(<13 years)
Influenza-associated
pediatric mortality
Legionellosis
Listeriosis
Lyme disease
Malaria
Measles
Meningococcal disease
Mumps
Novel influenza A virus
infections
Pertussis
Plague
Poliomyelitis, paralytic
Poliovirus infection,
nonparalytic
Psittacosis
Q fever
Rabies
- Rabies, animal
- Rabies, human
Rocky Mountain spotted
fever
Rubella
Rubella, congenital
syndrome
Salmonellosis
Severe acute respiratory
syndrome-associated
coronavirus (SARS-CoV)
disease

Shiga toxin-producing
Escherichia coli (STEC)
Shigellosis
Smallpox
Streptococcal disease,
invasive, group A
Streptococcal toxic-shock
syndrome
Streptococcus pneumoniae,
drug resistant, invasive
disease
Streptococcus pneumoniae,
invasive disease
non-drug-resistant, in
children less than
5 years of age
Syphilis
- Syphilis, primary
- Syphilis, secondary
- Syphilis, latent
- Syphilis, early latent
- Syphilis, late latent
- Syphilis, latent, unknown
  duration
- Neurosyphilis
- Syphilis, late,
  nonneurological
- Syphilitic stillbirth
- Syphilis, congenital
Tetanus
Toxic-shock syndrome (other
than streptococcal)
Trichinellosis (Trichinosis)
Tuberculosis
Tularemia
Typhoid fever
Vancomycin-intermediate
Staphylococcus aureus
(VISA)
Vancomycin-resistant
Staphylococcus aureus
(VRSA)
Varicella (morbidity)
Varicella (deaths only)
Vibriosis
Yellow fever

Source: Centers for Disease Control and Prevention. National Notifiable Diseases Surveillance
System. http://www.cdc.gov/ncphi/disss/nndss/phs/infdis.htm
Accessed February 16, 2008.

21st Century.[156] The report notes that 39 new diseases have emerged in the world since the 1970s. The need for a global surveillance system for infectious diseases is highlighted not only by the WHO report but also by the Forum on Microbial Threats[157] and events that have occurred since 2000: the rapid spread of SARS to several continents, a bioterrorist attack with *Bacillus anthracis*, the ongoing spread of avian influenza and the potential for an influenza pandemic, and the international spread of hypervirulent strains of *Clostridium difficile* and antimicrobial-resistant microorganisms.

In 2005 revised International Health Regulations, known as the IHR, were released to address issues that affect the health of people worldwide, such as infectious disease outbreaks, pandemics, and other events that may constitute a public health emergency of international concern.[158] The WHO is working to promote the IHR and the need for international efforts to identify and control emerging diseases; global collaboration in surveillance and outbreak alerts and response; and increased national and international resources for training, surveillance, laboratory capacity, response networks, and prevention efforts.

ICPs, healthcare epidemiologists, and healthcare providers play a critical role in detecting and reporting diseases and events of public health significance, such as emerging infections and potential outbreaks, so that prevention and control measures can be quickly implemented. They also play an important part in ensuring that their healthcare organizations have emergency plans in place to reduce the adverse impacts these events have on healthcare settings.[159] These plans should be developed by a multidisciplinary task force composed of personnel from the healthcare organization developing its plan and personnel from surrounding healthcare organizations, public health agencies, emergency responders, and other stakeholders. A discussion of emergency preparedness planning is beyond the scope of this text; however, there are many resources on the Internet for information on emergency preparedness planning. Public health agencies worldwide, such as the CDC, have developed and posted emergency preparedness plans on their Web sites.

SUMMARY

Routine surveillance programs should be implemented in healthcare settings to measure outcomes and processes related to health care. An effective surveillance program should be able to detect and quantify the occurrence of diseases of local and public health importance and of adverse events such as HAIs. Major objectives of a surveillance program are to improve the quality of health care and to identify clusters and outbreaks of disease so that measures can be implemented to prevent new cases from occurring. ICPs play a critical role in recognizing and preventing the spread of disease both in healthcare settings and in their community and in preparing and implementing their organization's response to public health emergencies.

REFERENCES

1. World Health Organization. Public health surveillance. http://www.who.int/immunization_monitoring/burden/routine_surveillance/en/. Accessed February 16, 2008.

2. Reynolds MG, Huy Anh B, Hoang Thu V, et al. Factors associated with nosocomial SARS-CoV transmission among healthcare workers in Hanoi, Vietnam; 2003. *BMC Public Health.* 2006;6:207. http://www.biomedcentral.com/1471-2458/6/207. Accessed February 17, 2008.

3. Outbreak of severe acute respiratory syndrome-worldwide; 2003. *MMWR.* 2003;52:226–228. [Erratum, *MMWR.* 2003;52:284].

4. ProMED-mail. Pneumonia—China (Guangdong). ProMed mail 2002; 11 February: 20030211.0369. http://www.promedmail.org. Accessed March 29, 2008.

5. Rhinehart E, Friedman MM. *Infection Control in Home Care and Hospice.* 2nd ed. Sudbury, MA: Jones and Bartlett Publishers; 2005.

6. Centers for Disease Control and Prevention. Nosocomial bacteremias associated with intravenous fluid therapy—USA. *MMWR.* 1997;46:1227–1233.

7. Goldmann DA, Maki DG, Rhame FS, Kaiser AB, Tenney JH, Bennett JV. Guidelines for infection control in intravenous therapy. *Ann Intern Med.* 1973;79:848–850.

8. Centers for Disease Control and Prevention. Updated guidelines for evaluating public health surveillance systems: recommendations from the guidelines working group. *MMWR.* 2001;50:1–35.

9. Lee TB, Montgomery OG, Marx J, Olmsted RN, Scheckler WE. Recommended practices for surveillance: Association for Professionals in Infection Control and Epidemiology (APIC), Inc. *Am J Infect Control.* 2007;35:427–440. http://www.apic.org/Content/NavigationMenu/PracticeGuidance/SurveillanceDefinitionsReportsandRecommendations/AJIC_Surveillance_2007.pdf. Accessed February 21, 2008.

10. Baker OG. Process surveillance: an epidemiologic challenge for all health care organizations. *Am J Infect Control.* 1997;25:96–101.

11. Lee TB. Surveillance in acute care and nonacute care settings: current issues and concepts. *Am J Infect Control.* 1997;25:121–124.

12. Massanari RM, Wilkerson K, Swartzendruber S. Designing surveillance for noninfectious outcomes of medical care. *Infect Control Hosp Epidemiol.* 1995;16:419–426.

13. Haley RW, Culver DH, White JW, et al. The efficacy of infection surveillance and control programs in preventing nosocomial infections in U.S. hospitals. *Am J Epidemiol.* 1985;121:182–205.

14. Centers for Disease Control and Prevention. Public health focus: surveillance, prevention and control of nosocomial infections. *MMWR.* 1992;41:783–787.

15. Emori TG, Culver DH, Horan TC, et al. National nosocomial infections surveillance system (NNIS): description of surveillance methods. *Am J Infect Control.* 1991;19:19–35.

16. Tokars JT, Miller ER, Stein G. A new national surveillance system for hemodialysis-associated infections: initial results. *Am J Infect Control.* 2002;30:288–295.

17. Tokars JI, Richards C, Andrus M, et al. The changing face of surveillance for health care-associated infections. *Clin Infect Dis.* 2004;39:1347–1352.

18. Centers for Disease Control and Prevention. *The National Healthcare Safety Network (NHSN) Manual. Patient Safety Component Protocol.* Division of Healthcare Quality Promotion, Atlanta, GA; 2008. http://www.cdc.gov/ncidod/dhqp/nhsn_members.html. Accessed February 9, 2008.

19. Edwards JR, Peterson KD, Andrus ML, et al. National Healthcare Safety Network (NHSN) Report. *Am J Infect Control.* 2007;35:290–301.

20. Gaynes RP, Culver DH, Emori TG, et al. The national nosocomial infections surveillance system: plans for the 1990s and beyond. *Am J Med.* 1991;91(Suppl 3B):3B-116S-3B-120S.

21. Gaynes RP, Solomon S. Improving hospital-acquired infection rates: the CDC experience. *J Qual Improve.* 1996;22:457–467.

22. Richards C, Emori TG, Peavey G, Gaynes R. Promoting quality through measurement of performance and response: prevention success stories. *Emerg Infect Dis.* 2001;7:299–301.

23. European Centre for Disease Prevention and Control. Annual epidemiological report on communicable diseases in Europe: report on the status of communicable diseases in the EU and EEA/EFTA countries. Stockholm; 7 June 2007. http://ecdc.europa.eu/pdf/ECDC_epi_report _2007.pdf. Accessed February 18, 2008.

24. Smith PW. Infection surveillance in long-term care facilities. *Infect Control Hosp Epidemiol.* 1991;12:55–58.

25. Smith P, Rusnack P. Infection prevention and control in the long-term-care facility. *Am J Infect Control.* 1997;25:488–512.

26. Goldrick BA. Infection control programs in long-term-care facilities: structure and process. *Infect Control Hosp Epidemiol.* 1999;20:764–769.

27. Manian FA. Surveillance of surgical site infections in alternative settings: exploring the current options. *Am J Infect Control.* 1997;25:102–105.

28. Nafziger DA, Lundstrom T, Chandra S, Massanari RM. Infection control in ambulatory care. *Infect Dis Clin North Am.* 1997;11:279–296.

29. Rhinehart E. Infection control in home care. *Emerg Infect Dis.* 2001;7:208–211.

30. Luehm D, Fauerbach L. Task force studies infection rates, surgical site management and Foley catheter infections. *Caring.* 1999;18:30–34.

31. Woomer N, Long C, Anderson CO, Greenberg EA. Benchmarking in home health care: a collaborative approach. *Caring.* 1999;18:22–28.

32. APIC Home Care Membership Section. Draft definitions for surveillance of infections in home health care. *Am J Infect Control.* 2000;28:449–453.

33. Rosenheimer L, Embry FC, Sanford J, Silver SR. Infection surveillance in home care: device-related incidence rates. *Am J Infect Control.* 1998;Jun26(3):359–363.

34. Manangan LP, Pearson M L, Tokars JL, Miller E, Jarvis WR. Feasibility of national surveillance of health-care-associated infections in home-care settings. *Emerg Infect Dis.* 2002;8: 233–236.

35. HELICS Improving Patient Safety in Europe. IPSE Annual Report, 2006. http://helics .univ-lyon1.fr/Documents/IPSE_Annual_Report_2006.pdf. Accessed February 18, 2008.

36. Stevenson KB, Moore J, Colwell H, Sleeper B. Standardized infection surveillance in long-term care: interfacility comparisons from a regional cohort of facilities. *Infect Control Hosp Epidemiol.* 2005;26:231–238.

37. Centers for Disease Control. *Outline for Healthcare-Associated Infections Surveillance. 2006.* Atlanta, GA: Centers for Disease Control; 2006. http://www.cdc.gov/ncidod/dhqp/pdf /nhsn/ OutlineForHAISurveillance.pdf. Accessed February 18, 2008.

38. Pottinger JM, Herwaldt LA, Perl TM. Basics of surveillance—an overview. *Infect Control Hosp Epidemiol.* 1997;18:513–527.

39. Scheckler WE. Surveillance, foundation for the future: a historical overview and evolution of methodologies. *Am J Infect Control.* 1997;25:106–111.

40. Tousey PM. Epidemiologic methods for selective surveillance. *Am J Infect Control.* 1987;15: 148–158.

41. Perl TM. Surveillance, reporting, and the use of computers. In: Wenzel RP, ed. *Prevention and Control of Nosocomial Infections.* 2nd ed. Baltimore, MD: Williams & Wilkins; 1993:139–176.

42. Haley RW. Surveillance by objective: a new priority-directed approach to the control of nosocomial infections. *Am J Infect Control.* 1985;13:78–89.

43. Arias KM. Surveillance. In: *APIC Text of Infection Control and Epidemiology.* 2nd ed. Washington, DC: Association for Professionals in Infection Control and Epidemiology; 2005; 3.1–3.18.

44. Gaynes RP, Horan TC. Surveillance of nosocomial infections. In: Mayhall CG, ed. *Hospital Epidemiology and Infection Control.* Baltimore, MD: Williams & Wilkins; 1996:1017–1031, App. A–App. C.

45. Wenzel RP, Thompson RL, Landry SM, et al. Hospital-acquired infections in intensive care unit patients: an overview with emphasis on epidemics. *Infect Control Hosp Epidemiol.* 1983;4:371–375.

46. Pronovost P, Needham D, Berenholtz S, et al. An intervention to decrease catheter-related bloodstream infections in the ICU. *N Engl J Med.* 2006;355:2725–2732.

47. Mangram AJ, Horan TC, Pearson ML, Silver LC, Jarvis WR, and the Hospital Infection Control Practices Advisory Committee. Guideline for the prevention of surgical site infection; 1999. *Infect Control Hosp Epidemiol.* 1999;20:247–280.

48. Platt R, Yokoe DS, Sands KE. Automated methods for surveillance of surgical site infections. *Emerg Infect Dis.* 2001;7:212–216.

49. Roy MC, Perl TM. Basics of surgical-site surveillance. *Infect Control Hosp Epidemiol.* 1997; 18:659–668.

50. Roberts FJ, Walsh A, Wing P, Dvorek M, Schweigel J. The influence of surveillance methods on surgical wound infection rates in a tertiary care spinal surgery service. *Spine.* 1998;23: 366–370.

51. Fields CL. Outcomes of a postdischarge surveillance system for surgical site infections at a Midwestern regional referral center hospital. *Am J Infect Control.* 1999;27:158–164.

52. Lee JT. Wound infection surveillance. *Infect Dis Clin North Am.* 1992;6:643–656.

53. Cardo DM, Falk PS, Mayhall CG. Validation of surgical wound surveillance. *Infect Control Hosp Epidemiol.* 1993;14:211–215.

54. Yokoe DS, Noskin GA, Cunningham SM, et al. Enhanced identification of postoperative infections among inpatients. *Emer Infect Dis.* 2004;10:1924–1930.

55. Miner AL, Sands KE, Yokoe DS, et al. Enhanced identification of postoperative infections among outpatients. *Emerg Infect Dis.* 2004;10:1931–1937.

56. Noy D, Creedy D. Postdischarge surveillance of surgical site infections: a multi-method approach to data collection. *Am J Infect Control.* 2002;30:417–424.

57. Petherick ES, Dalton JE, Moore PJ, Cullum N. Methods for identifying surgical wound infection after discharge from hospital: a systematic review. *BMC Infect Dis.* 2006;6:170. http://www.biomedcentral.com/1471–2334/6/170. Accessed February 19, 2008.

58. Schneeberger PM, Smits MHW, Zick REF, Wille JC. Surveillance as a starting point to reduce surgical-site infection rates in elective orthopaedic surgery. *J Hosp Infect.* 2002;51: 179–184.

59. Mylotte JM. Laboratory surveillance method for nosocomial *Clostridium difficile* diarrhea. *Am J Infect Control.* 1998;26:16–23.

60. McFarland LV, Beneda HW, Clarridge JE, Raugi GJ. Implications of the changing face of *Clostridium difficile* disease for health care practitioners. *Am J Infect Control.* 2007;35: 237–253.

61. Halasa NB, Williams JV, Wilson GJ, Walsh WF, Schaffner W, Wright PF. Medical and economic impact of a respiratory syncytial virus outbreak in a neonatal intensive care unit. *Pediatr Infect Dis J.* 2005;24(12):1040–1044.

62. Bernstein DI, Ward RL. Rotaviruses. In: Feigin RD, Cherry JD, eds. *Textbook of Pediatric Infectious Diseases.* 4th ed. Philadelphia, PA: WB Saunders Company; 1998:1901–1922.

63. Centers for Disease Control and Prevention. Guidelines for preventing the transmission of *Mycobacterium tuberculosis* in health-care settings; 2005. *MMWR.* 2005;54(RR-17):1–142. http://www.cdc.gov/ncidod/dhqp/index.html. Accessed February 15, 2008.

64. Tuberculosis Coalition for Technical Assistance. *International Standards for Tuberculosis Care (ISTC).* The Hague: Tuberculosis Coalition for Technical Assistance; 2006. http://www .nationaltbcenter.edu/international. Accessed February 15, 2008.

65. Siegel, JD, Rhinehart E, Jackson M, Chiarello L, and the Healthcare Infection Control Practices Advisory Committee. Management of multidrug-resistant organisms in healthcare settings; 2006. http://www.cdc.gov/ncidod/dhqp/index.html.

66. Klevens RM, Morison MA, Nadle J, et al. Invasive methicillin-resistant *Staphylococcus aureus* infections in the United States. *JAMA.* 2007;298(15):1763–1771.

67. Siegel JD, Rhinehart E, Jackson M, Chiarello L, and the Healthcare Infection Control Practices Advisory Committee; 2007. Guideline for isolation precautions: preventing transmission of infectious agents in healthcare settings; June 2007. http://www.cdc.gov/ncidod/dhqp/pdf/isolation2007.pdf. Accessed February 15, 2008.

68. Guerrero JC, Filippone C. A cluster of Legionnaire's disease in a community hospital—a clue to a larger epidemic. *Infect Control Hosp Epidemiol.* 1996;17:177–178.

69. Goodman RA, Solomon SL. Transmission of infectious diseases in outpatient health care settings. *JAMA.* 1991;265:2377–2380.

70. Herwaldt LA, Smith SD, Carter CD. Infection control in the outpatient setting. *Infect Control Hosp Epidemiol.* 1998;19:41–74.

71. Tokars JI, Miller ER, Alter MJ, Arduino MJ. *National Surveillance of Dialysis-Associated Diseases in the United States;* 1997. Atlanta, GA: National Center for Infectious Diseases, Centers for Disease Control and Prevention, Public Health Service, Department of Health and Human Services; 1999.

72. Kaczmarek RG, Moore RM, McCrohan J, et al. Multi-state investigation of the actual disinfection/sterilization of endoscopes in health care facilities. *Am J Med.* 1992;92:257–261.

73. Smith PW. Consensus conference on nosocomial infections in long-term care facilities. *Am J Infect Control.* 1987;15:97–100.

74. Jackson MM, Fierer J. Infections and infection risk in residents of long-term care facilities: a review of the literature; 1970–1984. *Am J Infect Control.* 1985;13:63–77.

75. Jacobson C, Strausbaugh LJ. Incidence and impact of infection in nursing home care unit. *Am J Infect Control.* 1990;18:151–159.

76. Vermaat JH, Rosebrugh E, Ford-Jones EL, Ciano J, Kobayashi J, Miller G. An epidemiologic study of nosocomial infections in a pediatric long-term care facility. *Am J Infect Control.* 1993;21:183–188.

77. Garibaldi RA, Brodine S, Matsumiya S. Infections among patients in nursing homes: policies, prevalence and problems. *N Engl J Med.* 1981;305:731–735.

78. Smith PW, ed. *Infection Control in Long-Term Care Facilities.* 2nd ed. Albany, NY: Delmar Publishers; 1994.

79. Jackson MM, Fierer J, Barrett-Connor E, et al. Intensive surveillance for infections in a three-year study of nursing home patients. *Am J Epidemiol.* 1992;135:685–696.

80. Darnowski SB, Gordon M, Simor AE. Two years of infection surveillance in a geriatric long-term care facility. *Am J Infect Control.* 1991;19:185–190.

81. Vlahov D, Tenney JH, Cervino KW, Shamer DK. Routine surveillance for infections in nursing homes: experience at two facilities. *Am J Infect Control.* 1987;15:47–53.

82. Goldrick BA. Infection control programs in skilled nursing long-term care facilities: an assessment; 1995. *Am J Infect Control.* 1999;27:4–9.

83. Nicolle LE, Garibaldi RA. Infection control in long-term care facilities. *Infect Control Hosp Epidemiol.* 1995;16:348–353.

84. Ministry of National Health and Welfare. *Canadian Infection Control Guidelines for Long Term Care Facilities.* Ottawa, Canada: Ministry of National Health and Welfare; 1994.

85. Rosenbaum P, Zeller J, Franck J, Pass MA. Long-term care. In: *APIC Text of Infection Control and Epidemiology.* 2nd ed. Washington, DC: Association for Professionals in Infection Control and Epidemiology. 2005;53.1–53.15.

86. Ahlbrecht H, Shearen C, Degelau J, Guay DRP. Team approach to infection prevention and control in the nursing home setting. *Am J Infect Control.* 1999;27:64–70.

87. Sheretz RJ. Surveillance for infections associated with vascular catheters. *Infect Control Hosp Epidemiol.* 1996;17:746–752.

88. Yokoe DS, Anderson J, Chambers R, et al. Simplified surveillance for nosocomial bloodstream infections. *Infect Control Hosp Epidemiol.* 1998;19:657–660.

89. Infusion Nurses Society. *The Infusion Nursing Standards of Practice.* Philadelphia, PA: Lippincott, Williams & Wilkins; 2006.

90. Tablan OC, Anderson LJ, Besser R, et al. and the Healthcare Infection Control Practices Advisory Committee. Guidelines for preventing health-care-associated pneumonia; 2003. http://www.cdc.gov/ncidod/dhqp/index.html. Accessed February 19, 2008.

91. Berlowitz DR, Halpern J. Evaluating and improving pressure ulcer care: the VA experience with administrative data. *Joint Comm J Qual Improv.* 1997;23:424–433.

92. Panel for the Prediction and Prevention of Pressure Ulcers in Adults. *Pressure Ulcers in Adults: Prediction and Prevention.* Clinical Practice Guideline, Number 3, Rockville, MD: AHCPR; 1992. AHCPR Publication No. 92–0047.

93. Wipke-Tevis DD, Williams DA, Rantz MJ, et al. Nursing home quality and pressure ulcer prevention and management practices. *J Am Geriatr Soc.* 2004;52(4):583–588.

94. Gottsch JD. Surveillance and control of epidemic keratoconjunctivitis. *Trans Am Ophthalmol Soc.* 1996;94:539–587.

95. Maryland Department of Health and Mental Hygiene (DHMH). *Guidelines for the Prevention and Control of Upper and Lower Acute Respiratory Illnesses (Including Influenza and Pneumonia) in Long Term Care Facilities; 2000.* Baltimore, MD: Maryland DHMH, Epidemiology and Disease Control Program; 2000. http://www.cha.state.md.us /edcp/guidelines/resp97 .html. Accessed February 21, 2008.

96. Patel N, Tignor GH. Device-specific sharps injury and usage rates: an analysis by hospital department. *Am J Infect Control.* 1997;25:77–84.

97. Centers for Disease Control and Prevention. Workbook for designing, implementing, and evaluating a sharps injury prevention program. http://www.cdc.gov/sharpssafety/index.html Accessed February 19, 2008.

98. World Health Organization. Sharps injuries: global burden of disease from sharps injuries to health-care workers. Geneva; 2003. http://www.who.int/quantifying_ehimpacts/publications/en/sharps.pdf. Accessed February 19, 2008.

99. Centers for Disease Control. Prevention and control of tuberculosis in facilities providing long-term care to the elderly: recommendations of the advisory committee for the elimination of tuberculosis. *MMWR.* 1990;39(RR-10).

100. Pittet D, Safran E, Harbarth S, et al. Automatic alerts for methicillin-resistant *Staphylococcus aureus* surveillance and control: role of a hospital information system. *Infect Control Hosp Epidemiol.* 1996;17:496–502.

101. Filippell MB, Rearick T. Respiratory syncytial virus. *Nurs Clin North Am.* 1993;28:651–671.

102. McDonald LC, Coignard B, Dunnerke E, et al. and the Ad Hoc *Clostridium difficile* Surveillance Working Group. Recommendations for surveillance of *Clostridium difficile*–associated disease. *Infect Control Hosp Epidemiol.* 2007; 28:140–145.

103. Mitchell A, Jones N. Striving to prevent falls in an acute care setting—action to enhance quality. *J Clin Nurs.* 1996;5:213–220.

104. Welton JM, Jarr S. Automating and improving the data quality of a nursing department quality management program at a university hospital. *Joint Comm J Qual Improv.* 1997;23:623–635.

105. Lesar TS, Briceland L, Stein DS. Factors related to errors in medication prescribing. *JAMA.* 1997;277:312–317.

106. Mohseni IE, Wong DH. Medication errors analysis is an opportunity to improve practice. *Am J Surg.* 1998;175:4–9.

107. Centers for Disease Control and Prevention. National notifiable diseases surveillance system. http://www.cdc.gov/ncphi/disss/nndss/nndsshis.htm. Accessed February 16, 2008.

108. Centers for Disease Control and Prevention. Prevention and control of influenza: recommendations of the Advisory Committee on Immunization Practices (ACIP); 2007. *MMWR.* 2007;56(RR-6):1–56. http://www.cdc.gov/mmwr/preview/mmwrhtml/rr5606a1.htm. Accessed February 21, 2008.

109. Bradley SF. Prevention of influenza in long-term-care facilities. Long-Term-Care Committee of the Society for Healthcare Epidemiology of America. *Infect Control Hosp Epidemiol.* 1999;20:629–637.

110. Rutala WA, and the APIC Guidelines Committee. APIC guideline for selection and use of disinfectants. *Am J Infect Control.* 1996;24:313–342.

111. Association of periOperative Registered Nurses. *2007 Standards and Recommended Practices.* Denver, CO: Association of periOperative Registered Nurses; 2007.

112. Association for the Advancement of Medical Instrumentation. *Comprehensive Guide to Steam Sterilization and Sterility Assurance in Health Care Facilities.* Arlington, VA: Association for the Advancement of Medical Instrumentation; 2006.

113. Sehulster LM, Chinn RYW, Arduino MJ, et al. Guidelines for environmental infection control in health-care facilities. Recommendations from CDC and the Healthcare Infection Control Practices Advisory Committee (HICPAC); 2003. *MMWR.* 2003;52(No RR-10):1–44. http://www.cdc.gov/ncidod/dhqp/gl_environinfection.html. Accessed February 19, 2008.

114. Doebbling BN, Ferguson KJ, Kohout FJ. Predictors of hepatitis B vaccine acceptance in health care workers. *Med Care.* 1996;34:58–72.

115. Larson E, Kretzer EK. Compliance with handwashing and barrier precautions. *J Hosp Infect.* 1995;30(Suppl):88–106.

116. Institute for Healthcare Improvement. How-to Guide: Improving Hand Hygiene—A Guide for Improving Practices among Health Care Workers. http://www.ihi.org. Accessed February 19, 2008.

117. Centers for Disease Control and Prevention. Guideline for hand hygiene in health-care settings: recommendations of the Healthcare Infection Control Practices Advisory Committee and the HICPAC/SHEA/APIC/IDSA Hand Hygiene Task Force. *MMWR.* 2002;51(RR16):1–45. http://www.cdc.gov/ncidod/dhqp/gl_handhygiene.html. Accessed February 19, 2008.

118. Centers for Disease Control and Prevention. Handwashing and glove use in a long-term care facility—Maryland; 1992. *MMWR.* 1993;42:672–675.

119. McGeer A, Campbell B, Emori TG, et al. Definitions of infection for surveillance in long-term care facilities. *Am J Infect Control.* 1991;19:1–7.

120. APIC-HICPAC. Surveillance definitions for home health care and home hospice infections. February 2008. http://www.apic.org/AM/Template.cfm?Section=Search&section=Surveillance_Definitions&template=/CM/ContentDisplay.cfm&ContentFileID=9898. Accessed May 10, 2008.

121. Goldmann D. Contemporary challenges for hospital epidemiology. *Am J Med.* 1991;91 (Suppl 3B):8S–15S.

122. Reagan DR. Microcomputers in hospital epidemiology. *Infect Control Hosp Epidemiol.* 1997;18:440–448.

123. Smyth ET, McIlvenny G, Barr JG, Dickson LM, Thompson IM. Automated entry of hospital infection surveillance data. *Infect Control Hosp Epidemiol.* 1997;18:486–491.

124. Carr JR, Fitzpatrick P, Izzo JL, et al. Changing the infection control paradigm from off-line to real time: the experience at Millard Fillmore Health System. *Infect Control Hosp Epidemiol.* 1997;18:255–259.

125. Victora CG. What's the denominator? *Lancet.* 1993;342:97–99.

126. Haley RW, Culver DH, Morgan WM, White JW, Emori TG, Hooton TM. Identifying patients at high risk of surgical wound infection: a simple multivariate index of patient susceptibility and wound contamination. *Am J Epidemiol.* 1985;121:206–215.

127. Haley RW. Nosocomial infections in surgical patients: developing valid measures of intrinsic patient risk. *Am J Med.* 1991;91(Suppl 3B):145S–151S.

128. Culver DH, Horan TC, Gaynes RP, et al. Surgical wound infection rates by wound class, operative procedure, and patient risk index. *Am J Med.* 1991;91(Suppl 3B):152S–157S.

129. Gross PA. Basics of stratifying for severity of illness. *Infect Control Hosp Epidemiol.* 1996;17:675–686.

130. Bailit JL, Dooley SL, Peaceman AN. Risk adjustment for interhospital comparison of primary cesarean rates. *Obstet Gynecol.* 1999;93:1025–1030.

131. Zinn JS, Aaronson WE, Rosko MD. The use of standardized indicators as quality improvement tools: an application in Pennsylvania nursing homes. *Am J Med Qual.* 1993;8:72–78.

132. Simonds DN, Horan TC, Kelley R, Jarvis WR. Detecting pediatric nosocomial infections: how do infection control and quality assurance personnel compare? *Am J Infect Control.* 1997;25: 202–208.

133. Larson E, Horan T, Cooper B, et al. Study of the definition of nosocomial infections (SDNI). *Am J Infect Control.* 1991;19:259–267.

134. Haley RW, Schaberg DR, McClish DK, et al. The accuracy of retrospective chart review in measuring nosocomial infection rates. *Am J Epidemiol.* 1980;111:516–533.

135. Scheckler WE, Brimhall D, Buck AS, et al. Requirements for infrastructure and essential activities of infection control and epidemiology in hospitals: a consensus panel report. *Am J Infect Control.* 1998;26:47–60. http://www.apic.org/AM/Template.cfm?Section=Guidelines& CONTENTID=1090&TEMPLATE=/CM/ContentDisplay.cfm. Accessed February 21, 2008.

136. Friedman C, Barnette M, Buck AS, et al. Requirements for infrastructure and essential activities of infection control and epidemiology in out-of-hospital settings: a consensus panel report. *Am J Infect Control.* 1999;27:418–430. http://www.apic.org/AM/Template.cfm?Section =Guidelines&CONTENTID=1082&TEMPLATE=/CM/ContentDisplay.cfm. Accessed February 21, 2008.

137. National Nosocomial Infection Surveillance System. Nosocomial infection rates for interhospital comparison: limitations and possible solutions. *Infect Control Hosp Epidemiol.* 1991;12:609–621.

138. The Quality Indicator Study Group. An approach to the evaluation of quality indicators of outcome of care in hospitalized patients, with a focus on nosocomial infection indicators. *Infect Control Hosp Epidemiol.* 1995;16:308–316.

139. Keita-Perse O, Gaynes RP. Severity of illness scoring systems to adjust nosocomial infection rates: a review and commentary. *Am J Infect Control.* 1996;24:429–434.

140. Stevenson KB. Regional data set of infection rates for long-term care facilities: description of a valuable benchmarking tool. *Am J Infect Control.* 1999;27:20–26.

141. Cleves MA, Weiner JP, Cohen W, et al. Assessing HCFA's Health Care Quality Improvement Program. *Joint Comm J Qual Improv.* 1997;23:550–560.

142. Hofer TP, Bernstein SJ, Hayward RA, DeMonner S. Validating quality indicators for hospital care. *Joint Comm J Qual Improv.* 1997;23:455–467.

143. Phillips CD, Zimmerman D, Bernabei R, Jonsson PV. Using the resident assessment instrument for quality enhancement in nursing homes. *Age Ageing.* 1997;26(Suppl 2):77–81.

144. Morris JN, Hawes C, Fries BE, et al. Designing the national resident assessment instrument for nursing homes. *Gerontologist.* 1990;30:293–307.

145. Steinbrook R. Public report cards—cardiac surgery and beyond. *N Engl J Med.* 2006;355: 1847–1849.

146. Leape LL. Reporting of adverse events. *N Engl J Med.* 2002;347:1633–1638.

147. Lovett LL, Massanari MM. Role of surveillance in emerging health systems: measurement is essential but not sufficient. *Am J Infect Control.* 1999;27:135–140.

148. Bobinski MA. Legal issues in hospital epidemiology and infection control. In: Mayhall CG, ed. *Hospital Epidemiology and Infection Control.* Baltimore, MD: Williams & Wilkins; 1996: 1138–1145.

149. Bartley J. Accrediting and regulatory agencies. In: *APIC Text of Infection Control and Epidemiology.* 2nd ed. Washington, DC: Association for Professionals in Infection Control and Epidemiology; 2005;10-1-10-12.

150. Occupational Safety and Health Administration. Directive - CPL 02-00-106 - CPL 2.106— enforcement procedures and scheduling for occupational exposure to tuberculosis. Occupational Safety and Health Administration; 1996. http://www.osha.gov/pls/oshaweb/owadisp .show_document?p_table=DIRECTIVES&p_id=1586. Accessed February 21, 2008.

151. Occupational Safety and Health Administration. Occupational exposure to bloodborne pathogens: final rule. *Federal Register.* December 6, 1991;56(235):64004–64182. http:// www.osha.gov/pls/oshaweb/owadisp.show_document?p_table=FEDERAL_REGISTER&p_id =13197. Accessed February 21, 2008.

152. Centers for Medicare and Medicaid Services, U.S. Department of Health and Human Services. Part 482—Conditions of Participation for Hospitals: 42CFR 482.42. October 1, 2002.

153. The Joint Commission. Surveillance, prevention, and control of infection. In: *2008 Comprehensive Accreditation Manual for Hospitals.* Chicago, IL: The Joint Commission; 2008.

154. Committee on Accreditation of Rehabilitation Facilities. *Medical Rehabilitation Standards Manual.* Tucson, AZ: CARF International; 2008.

155. Roush S, Birkhead G, Koo D, Cobb A, Fleming D. Mandatory reporting of diseases and conditions by health care professionals and laboratories. *JAMA.* 1999;282:164–170.

156. World Health Organization. *World Health Report 2007: A Safer Future: Global Public Health Security in the 21st Century.* Geneva: World Health Organization; 2007. http://www.who .int/whr/2007/whr07_en.pdf. Accessed February 18, 2008.

157. Lemon SM, Hamburg MA, Sparling PF, Choffnes ER, Mack A, and the Forum on Microbial Threats. *Global Infectious Disease Surveillance and Detection: Assessing the Challenges-Finding Solutions, Workshop Summary.* Washington, DC: National Academies Press; 2007. http://www.nap.edu/catalog.php?record_id=11996. Accessed February 17, 2008.

158. International health regulations (2005). Geneva, Switzerland: World Health Organization; 2006. http://www.who.int/csr/ihr. Accessed February 21, 2008.

159. Petrosillo N, Puro V, DiCarlo A, Ippolito G. The initial hospital response to an epidemic. *Arch Med Res.* 2005;36(6):706–712.

SUGGESTED READINGS AND RESOURCES

Readings

APIC Text of Infection Control and Epidemiology. 2nd ed. Washington, DC: Association for Professionals in Infection Control and Epidemiology; 2005.

CDC. Public health focus: surveillance, prevention, and control of nosocomial infections. *MMWR.* 1992;41:783–787.

Dato V, Wagner MM, Fapohunda A. How outbreaks are detected: a review of surveillance systems and outbreaks. *Pub Health Report.* 2004;119:464–471. http://www.publichealthreports.org/userfiles/119_5/119464.pdf. Accessed May 10, 2008.

Davis JR, Lederberg J, eds. Forum on emerging infections, board on global health. *Emerging Infectious Diseases from the Global to the Local Perspective: Workshop Summary.* Washington, DC: National Academies Press; 2001. http://books.nap.edu/catalog.php?record_id=10084. Accessed February 17, 2008.

Haley RW, Culver DH, White JW, et al. The efficacy of infection surveillance and control programs in preventing nosocomial infections in U.S. hospitals. *Am J Epidemiol.* 1985;121:182–205.

Jarvis WR, ed. *Bennett and Brachman's Hospital Infections.* 5th ed. Philadelphia, PA: Lippincott Williams & Wilkins; 2007.

Lee TB, Montgomery OG, Marx J, Olmsted RN, Scheckler WE. Recommended practices for surveillance: Association for Professionals in Infection Control and Epidemiology (APIC), Inc. *Am J Infect Control.* 2007;35:427–440. http://www.apic.org/Content/NavigationMenu/PracticeGuidance/SurveillanceDefinitionsReportsandRecommendations/AJIC_Surveillance_2007.pdf. Accessed February 21, 2008.

Massanari RM, Wilkerson K, Swartzendruber S. Designing surveillance for noninfectious outcomes of medical care. *Infect Control Hosp Epidemiol.* 1995;16:419–426.

Mayhall CG. *Hospital Epidemiology and Infection Control.* 3rd ed. Baltimore, MD: Lippincott, Williams & Wilkins; 2004.

Roy MC, Perl TM. Basics of surgical-site infection surveillance. *Infect Control Hosp Epidemiol.* 1997;18:659–668.

Smith PW, ed. *Infection Control in Long-Term Care Facilities.* 2nd ed. Albany, NY: Delmar Publishers; 1994.

Smith P, Rusnack P. Infection prevention and control in the long-term-care facility. *Am J Infect Control.* 1997;25:488–512.

Wenzel RP, ed. *Prevention and Control of Nosocomial Infections.* 4th ed. Baltimore: Lippincott Williams & Wilkins; 2002.

Resources

World Health Organization. International health regulations (2005). Geneva, Switzerland: World Health Organization; 2005. http://www.who.int/csr/ihr. Accessed May 10, 2008.

Surgical Care Improvement Project. http://www.medqic.org/dcs /ContentServer?cid=1122904930422 &pagename=Medqic%2FContent%2FParentShellTemplate&parentName=Topic&c=MQParents. Accessed February 19, 2008.

CDC National Healthcare Safety Network (NHSN). http://www.cdc.gov/ncidod/dhqp/nhsn.html. Accessed February 15, 2008.

Resources for information on emerging infections and emergency planning include the CDC's Emergency Preparedness and Response Web site (http://www.bt.cdc.gov/planning/), the online journal *Emerging Infectious Diseases* (http://www.cdc.gov/nciod/EID), the World Health Organization (http://www.who.int/en/), and the Agency for Healthcare Research and Quality, Public Health Emergency Preparedness (http://www.ahrq.gov/prep/). Accessed March 26, 2008.

CHAPTER 3

Outbreaks Reported in Acute Care Settings

Kathleen Meehan Arias

An ounce of prevention is worth a pound of cure.

—*Benjamin Franklin*

INTRODUCTION

Outbreaks of infectious diseases in hospitals have long been recognized. A study of the nosocomial transmission of epidemic louse-borne typhus fever was published in England in 1864[1] and "hospital fever" is one of the many names given to this disease. In the mid-1800s, Ignaz Semmelweis recommended hand washing to prevent the spread of puerperal fever, and Florence Nightingale promoted isolation of infected patients, a clean environment, and hygienic handling of food and water to prevent the spread of disease. Despite the advances of modern medicine, outbreaks continue to occur as a result of health care provided in a variety of settings.[2-9] The hospital outbreaks of typhus and puerperal fevers that occurred in the 1800s were replaced in the late 1900s by outbreaks of methicillin-resistant *Staphylococcus aureus* (MRSA) and vancomycin-resistant *Enterococcus* (VRE). However, the primary control measures used to prevent the spread of infectious agents remain the same: hand hygiene, isolation of infected persons, environmental cleanliness, and safe handling of food and water.

Personnel responsible for managing infection prevention and control and performance improvement programs in healthcare settings should study reports of outbreak investigations to expand their knowledge of the epidemiology of healthcare-associated infections (HAIs) and other iatrogenic events. By reviewing the findings of these investigations, it is possible to identify the following:

- Factors contributing to outbreaks, such as etiologic agents, common sources and reservoirs, and modes of transmission; devices, products, and other vehicles; and procedures, practices, and technical errors
- Measures for controlling or preventing a similar outbreak

If an outbreak is suspected in a healthcare setting, a literature search should be conducted to identify relevant articles, as discussed in Chapter 9.

The purpose of this chapter is to discuss outbreaks that have been reported in acute care facilities. It is not intended to be an exhaustive review of outbreaks that have occurred in hospitals. Rather, its purpose is to provide an overview of the wide variety of organisms, diseases, and conditions that have been responsible for epidemics in the acute care setting. Information on the agents, reservoirs, and modes of transmission is included, along with the control measures that were used to interrupt the outbreak. The outbreak reports discussed in this chapter were identified by conducting electronic literature searches of the PubMed databases from 1985 through March 2008, by reviewing the table of contents of selected journals and the references in relevant articles, and by performing targeted searches of the Internet. The reports of these outbreak investigations highlight the importance of maintaining an active surveillance program in all healthcare settings in order to identify an outbreak or a cluster of events so that control measures can be implemented as soon as possible.

Most of the outbreaks discussed in this text have been grouped into the settings in which they occurred. However, infection control professionals (ICPs) should be familiar with outbreaks that have been reported in all types of healthcare settings because procedures, practices, products, and devices may be used in more than one setting. The outbreaks discussed in this chapter occurred primarily in hospitals, although similar outbreaks may occur in other healthcare settings. Outbreaks caused by MRSA, VRE, *Mycobacterium tuberculosis*, *Sarcoptes scabiei*, *Clostridium difficile*, noroviruses, and the influenza virus occur in both acute care and long-term care settings and are discussed in Chapter 7 along with gastrointestinal and food-borne outbreaks. Although the terms *outbreak* and *epidemic* are most commonly used in reference to infectious diseases, they are also used to describe the sudden occurrence or increase of noninfectious diseases and conditions; therefore, examples of outbreaks caused by noninfectious agents are also included.

ENDEMIC VS. EPIDEMIC INFECTIONS

Most hospital-associated infections occur endemically; only a small proportion occur as part of an outbreak.[2] Results of one study showed that patients involved in epidemics accounted for 3.7% of all nosocomial infections detected over a 5-year period.[10] In another study it was estimated that true outbreaks involved approximately 2% of all patients who contracted a HAI.[3] Among infections reported to the Centers for Disease Control and Prevention (CDC) National Nosocomial Infections Surveillance system, approximately 5% occurred in epidemics.[5] Although these numbers are small, they are important because these infections (1) result in significant morbidity and mortality, (2) may cause disruption of services, (3) may be difficult to investigate and control, and (4) are potentially preventable.

ORGANISMS RESPONSIBLE FOR HOSPITAL-ASSOCIATED OUTBREAKS

The organisms responsible for the majority of endemic and epidemic infections in hospitals change over time. In the 1950s and 1960s, a pandemic of *S. aureus* caused major outbreaks in communities and hospitals. In the 1970s, gram-negative organisms, such as the Enterobacteriaceae and *Pseudomonas aeruginosa*, emerged as major nosocomial pathogens. Throughout the 1980s, MRSA became established in many hospitals, and in the late 1980s and early 1990s multidrug-resistant *Mycobacterium tuberculosis* (MDR-TB) caused multiple outbreaks in healthcare facilities, affecting both patients and personnel. A major concern in the 1990s was the evolution and nosocomial spread of antibiotic-resistant organisms such as the Enterobacteriaceae, MDR-TB, and VRE, and the anticipated emergence of vancomycin-resistant *S. aureus*.[11–13] In the early 2000s, novel virulent strains of *Clostridium difficile*, a well-known pathogen, caused hospital outbreaks that resulted in significant morbidity and mortality in several countries.[14] Antimicrobial-resistant organisms have continued to evolve and spread globally, and multidrug-resistant strains of *Pseudomonas*, *Acinetobacter*, *Klebsiella*, and *Enterobacter* have caused hospital-associated outbreaks worldwide.[15–17]

Infection prevention and control personnel and healthcare providers must be aware of both newly recognized infectious agents and reemerging pathogens that have the potential for causing endemic and epidemic HAI.[18–20] Since the 1970s over 35 new human pathogens have been identified, and many known pathogens have emerged or reemerged. New and reemerging pathogens that have caused outbreaks in hospitals include bacteria such as *Clostridium difficile*, *Legionella pneumophila*, *Mycobacterium tuberculosis* (especially multidrug- and extensively multidrug-resistant strains), MRSA, VRE, and *Streptococcus pyogenes* (group A streptococcus), and viruses such as adenovirus, Ebola, hepatitis B and C, norovirus, rotavirus, and the severe acute respiratory syndrome coronavirus.[14,18,20–23]

When the site of infection and the organism causing a suspected outbreak is known, it is possible to use the knowledge gained from published reports of outbreaks to develop hypotheses on the likely modes of transmission and potential sources and reservoirs. Four major modes of transmission are commonly involved in healthcare-associated outbreaks: contact, vehicle (common source), droplet spread, and airborne. Outbreaks caused by *S. aureus* are associated with human reservoirs, and this organism is transmitted directly by person-to-person contact, indirectly from patient to patient on the hands of personnel, or by a human disseminator, such as a nasal carrier. Organisms such as *Pseudomonas*, *Flavobacterium*, *Mycobacterium gordonae* and *M. chelonae*, and gram-negative bacteria such as *Klebsiella*, *Enterobacter*, and *Serratia* readily grow in fluids and are frequently associated with common-source outbreaks involving contaminated solutions. *Aspergillus* and *Legionella* are spread by airborne transmission. Epidemics caused by these two organisms usually involve environmental sources, such as cooling towers or contaminated potable water for *Legionella,* and construction or some disruption in the physical plant for *Aspergillus*. Many organisms have more than one mode of transmission and may have several potential sources or reservoirs in the healthcare setting, as shown in Table 3–1.[24–27]

Table 3–1   Organisms Associated with Outbreaks in the Healthcare Setting, Their Likely Modes of Transmission, and Potential Sources

Organism	Site of Infection	Likely Mode(s) of Transmission	Potential Sources/ Reservoirs
Clostridium difficile	Gastrointestinal	Contact/cross-infection via hands	Infected patients
		Vehicle/common source	Contaminated equipment
Enterococcus species	Genitourinary, Surgical wound	Contact/cross-infection via hands	Infected or colonized patients
		Vehicle/common source	Contaminated equipment
Group A streptococcus	Surgical wound	Contact	Infected personnel
	Pharyngitis	Vehicle/common source	Food contaminated by infected person
Hepatitis A	Hepatitis	Vehicle/common source	Food contaminated by infected person
		Contact/cross-infection via hands	Infected patients and personnel
Influenza	Respiratory	Droplet	Infected patients, personnel, and visitors
Legionella	Respiratory	Airborne	Contaminated water
		Vehicle/common source/contact of mucosal surfaces with water	Contaminated water
Mycobacterium species, not tuberculosis	Respiratory	Vehicle/common source	Contaminated bronchoscope
Mycobacterium tuberculosis	Respiratory	Airborne	Infected patients or personnel
		Vehicle/common source	Contaminated bronchoscope
Pseudomonas, Burkholderia, and Ralstonia species	Blood, Respiratory	Vehicle/common source	Contaminated fluids; devices and equipment with aqueous reservoirs
		Contact/cross-infection via hands	Infected and colonized patients

Table 3–1　*(Continued)*

Organism	Site of Infection	Likely Mode(s) of Transmission	Potential Sources/ Reservoirs
Salmonella species	Gastrointestinal	Vehicle/common source	Food contaminated by improper handling or by personnel carrier
		Contact/cross-infection via hands	Infected patients
Staphylococcus aureus	Surgical wound	Contact	Personnel carrier
	Skin, respiratory, blood	Contact/cross-infection via hands	Infected and colonized patients
	Gastrointestinal	Vehicle/common source	Food contaminated by infected person

OUTBREAKS ASSOCIATED WITH PRODUCTS, DEVICES, AND PROCEDURES (COMMON SOURCE OUTBREAKS)

Because some products, devices, and procedures are repeatedly associated with hospital epidemics, it is useful to study published reports of these outbreaks so that preventive measures can be identified and implemented. The Hospital Infections Program of the CDC conducted investigations of 125 healthcare-associated outbreaks occurring from January 1980 to July 1990 and reported the following.[4]

1. Products, procedures, or devices were involved in 46% of the outbreaks: 22% were product related, 13% were procedure related, and 11% were device related.

2. Bacterial pathogens caused 62% of the outbreaks, fungi caused 9%, viruses caused 8%, mycobacteria caused 4%, and toxins or other organisms caused 18%.

3. The proportion of outbreaks caused by products, devices, and procedures increased from 47% in the first half of the decade to 67% between 1986 and July 1990.

Outbreaks Associated with Products

Multiple outbreaks of infection and colonization, illnesses, or adverse reactions associated with the use of products have been reported.[28–65] Many of these outbreaks involved products that were intrinsically or extrinsically contaminated by microbial agents or their toxins; however, several outbreaks did not have an infectious etiology. ICPs in all healthcare settings should be familiar with the types of products associated with outbreaks because these products may be used not only in acute care facilities, but also in the long-term care and ambulatory care settings.[38,40,41,64,66]

Intrinsic Contamination of Products

As used here, the term *intrinsic* refers to contamination that occurs before a product's arrival at a healthcare facility, such as a product contaminated during manufacture. These products may cause widespread outbreaks in multiple facilities before they are recognized.[39,67-69] A variety of intrinsically contaminated products have caused outbreaks in hospitals: intravenous fluids, povidone-iodine solution, packed red blood cells, fresh-frozen plasma, intravenous immunoglobulin, gauze, skin lotion, polygeline plasma extender, powdered infant formula, saline solutions including prefilled saline syringes, alcohol-free mouthwash, fruit salads, a pediatric oxygen-delivery device, heparin solution, nebulized sulbutamol, ultrasound gel, lyophilized enteral nutrition, injectable steroids, and peritoneal dialysis fluid.[28-30,33,34,38,39,49,52,55,56,59-65,67-82] Examples of outbreaks caused by intrinsically contaminated products are shown in Table 3–2.

The use of pharmaceutical compounding has increased substantially in the past decade, and several outbreaks have been caused by contaminated products that were prepared at off-site compounding pharmacies.[74-76,83] Some of these contaminated medications resulted in meningitis and bloodstream infections and substantial morbidity and mortality.[83] Deficiencies that led to the contamination of the products included inadequate training of personnel, improper aseptic technique, incorrect autoclaving practices, and lack of end-product sterility testing.

If a product that is associated with a cluster of infections is believed to be intrinsically contaminated, hospital personnel should notify the manufacturer, the local health department, and the appropriate government agency. In the United States, if antiseptics, medications, or medical devices are believed to be intrinsically contaminated, the Food and Drug Administration (FDA) should be notified through the FDA MedWatch Adverse Event Reporting System (http://www.fda.gov/medwatch). In addition, healthcare providers using the item should immediately be notified of the suspected contamination and should be instructed to remove all of the implicated product from stock and save it for further study. Although healthcare facilities may not be able to prevent all infections associated with an intrinsically contaminated product, ICPs should be alert to clusters or increasing numbers of isolates of unusual organisms, because these may possibly be associated with contaminated products or medications. Active surveillance programs are necessary to recognize promptly any product-associated outbreaks so that measures can be taken to identify the implicated product and to prevent its continued use.[30]

Extrinsic Contamination of Products

Extrinsic contamination occurs during the use of a product. Extrinsically contaminated products associated with outbreaks include antimicrobial soap,

Table 3–2   Outbreaks Involving Intrinsically Contaminated Products

Outbreak	Year(s) Reported/ Reference No.	Product	Comments
Enterobacter cloacae and *Enterobacter agglomerans* septicemia	1976 (28, 29) 1978 (30)	Intravenous fluid	1971—Nationwide outbreak of septicemia (reference 29 is reprint of original report with a discussion of the outbreak)
Pseudomonas (currently *Burkholderia*) *cepacia* peritonitis and pseudobacteremia	1981 (33) 1992 (34)	Povidone iodine	1981—First report of nosocomial infections caused by intrinsically contaminated povidone iodine
Pseudomonas aeruginosa peritonitis and wound infection	1982 (38)	Poloxamer-iodine solution	Occurred in outpatients on chronic peritoneal dialysis
Hepatitis C infection	1994 (49)	Intravenous immunoglobulin	Worldwide outbreak; first recognized outbreak of blood-borne pathogens associated with immune globulin product licensed in the United States
Fever and hypotension after cardiac surgery	1995 (52)	Polygeline plasma extender	Product intrinsically contaminated by cell wall products of *Bacillus stearothermophilus*
Primary cutaneous Aspergillosis	1996 (55)	Contaminated gauze (one case prompted an investigation)	Gauze showed evidence of water exposure; contamination probably occurred prior to arrival at hospital
Cutaneous lesions caused by *Paecilomyces lilacinus*	1996 (56)	Skin lotion	Lesions occurred in immunocompromised patients; two patients died; product recalled
Burkholderia (currently *Ralstonia*) *pickettii* bacteremia	1997 (59)	Saline solution	Saline used to flush indwelling intravascular devices
Sterile peritonitis following continuous cycling peritoneal dialysis	1997 (60)	Peritoneal dialysis fluid	Nationwide outbreak resulted in recall of product; contaminated by endotoxin

Continued

Table 3–2   (*Continued*)

Outbreak	Year(s) Reported/ Reference No.	Product	Comments
Ralstonia pickettii respiratory tract colonization	1998 (62)	0.9% saline solution used for respiratory therapy	*R. pickettii* has been isolated from several products marketed as sterile
Pyrogenic reactions	1998 (63) 2000 (70)	Intravenous gentamicin	Associated with once-daily dosing of gentamicin received from one manufacturer; led to nationwide recall of product
Enterobacter cloacae bloodstream infections	1998 (64)	Prefilled saline syringes	Occurred in outpatient hematology/oncology service at a hospital
Burkholderia cepacia respiratory tract infection and colonization in intensive care units	1998 (65) 2000 (67)	Alcohol-free mouthwash	Product used for routine oral care of ventilated patients
Pseudomonas fluorescens and *Pseudomonas* sp. bloodstream infections	2005 (71)	Heparin/saline flush solution in preloaded syringe	Infections in four states led to nationwide recall of product from one manufacturer
Invasive *Enterobacter sakazakii* disease in infants	2006 (72)	Powdered infant formula	Multiple cases reported from North America, Europe, and the Middle East
Infection and colonization with *Ralstonia* species	2007 (73)	Pediatric oxygen-delivery device	*Ralstonia* spp. isolated from patients in 12 states led to national recall of device
Salmonella oranienburg infections	2007 (68)	Fruit salads served at healthcare facilities	Infections diagnosed in persons in 10 northeastern US states and one Canadian province; fruit salads were produced by one processing plant; source of contamination was not determined
Pseudomonas putida and *Stenotrophomonas maltophilia* infections	2008 (74)	Heparin catheter-lock solution	Solution purchased by hospital from a compounding pharmacy

benzalkonium chloride antiseptic, disinfectant solutions, saline solution, gauze dressings, gentian violet dye, albuterol, trypan blue solution, ultrasonography coupling gel, total parenteral nutrition (TPN) solution, radiopaque contrast medium, propofol, and dextrose solution.[31,35–37,40,41,45–48,50–53,58,61,84–88] Table 3–3 contains examples of outbreaks caused by in-use, or extrinsic, contamination of a product.

Some products, such as benzalkonium chloride solution, have been associated with multiple outbreaks and are no longer recommended for use in the healthcare setting because of the ease with which they can become contaminated.[66,89–91] In 1976 the CDC recommended the elimination of benzalkonium chloride solution as an antiseptic; however, a study reported in 1991 that many healthcare facilities were still using this product.[91] Personnel who are using benzalkonium chloride for skin antisepsis should be instructed to use an alternative product. Other products, such as the anesthetic agent propofol, have been associated with multiple outbreaks but are still widely used.[45–47] Healthcare personnel who use propofol should be made aware of the hazards associated with it and should be instructed to adhere to the manufacturer's instructions for preventing contamination.

Since many types of solutions have the potential to become contaminated during use, healthcare personnel should be educated on the proper handling of fluids and the use of aseptic technique. Even hand care products, such as lotions[92–94] and plain and antimicrobial soap,[58,95] can become contaminated during use and can serve as reservoirs for infectious agents.

Measures to prevent in-use contamination of products include the following:

- Education and competency testing of personnel on aseptic technique when preparing, handling, and administering fluids such as intravenous solutions and nutritional products
- Use of proper hand hygiene practices
- Protocols for proper use of multidose and single-dose vials and enforcement of these protocols
- Storage of medications and supplies in clean areas where they are protected against dust and water
- Adherence to proper protocols and quality assurance measures when compounding pharmaceuticals[83]

Noninfectious Adverse Events Related to Products

Clinicians also need to maintain surveillance for noninfectious adverse reactions due to procedures and therapeutic agents. Products that have resulted in clusters of illness, deaths, and injury in hospitals include disinfectants, intravenous additives, fiberboard infectious waste containers, transfusions with leukoreduced red blood cells, and contaminated heparin products as shown in Table 3–4.[32,39,54,57,77,82,96] If a therapeutic agent is associated with a cluster of adverse reactions, healthcare providers should notify the facility's pharmacy, the manufacturer, and the FDA (if the occurrence is in the United States).

Table 3–3   Outbreaks Involving Extrinsically Contaminated Products

Outbreak	Year(s) Reported/ Reference No.	Product	Comments; Reason for Extrinsic Contamination, When Applicable
Pseudobacteremia due to *Pseudomonas* (currently *Burkholderia*) *cepacia* and/or *Enterobacter* species	1976 (31)	Contaminated benzalkonium chloride antiseptic	Antiseptic used to prepare skin prior to venipuncture; several patients may have become bacteremic
Endotoxemia following computerized axial tomography	1980 (35)	Possible contamination of radiopaque contrast medium and glucagon	Source not determined but contaminated hot water bath had been used to warm contrast medium prior to infusion
Serratia marcescens bacteremia	1981 (36)	Heparinized saline irrigation fluid likely	Saline may have become contaminated when first mixed
Cutaneous Aspergillosis	1996 (37)	Outside packaging of dressing supplies	Outside of packages contaminated by spores and dust during construction in central inventory supply area
Mycobacterium chelonae surgical wound infections	1987 (40)	Gentian violet skin-marking solution	Gentian violet used to mark incision site prior to plastic surgery was contaminated with *M. chelonae*; occurred in a surgeon's office
Serratia marcescens septic arthritis	1987 (41)	Benzalkonium chloride antiseptic solution	Occurred in orthopedic surgeons' office among patients who had received injections of methylpred-nisolone; likely reservoir was canister of cotton balls soaking in benzalkonium chloride solution; *S. marcescens* was isolated from canister and office used multidose vials instead
Postoperative febrile episodes and bloodstream and surgical site infections	1990 (45) 1995 (46) 1997 (47)	Propofol	Multiple outbreaks have resulted from lack of aseptic technique; this lipid-based medication is easily contaminated

Table 3–3   *(Continued)*

Outbreak	Year(s) Reported/ Reference No.	Product	Comments; Reason for Extrinsic Contamination, When Applicable
Pseudomonas (currently *Ralstonia*) *pickettii* bacteremia	1991 (48)	Fentanyl citrate	Narcotic theft by employee who replaced fentanyl with contaminated distilled water
Burkholderia cepacia respiratory tract infection and colonization in mechanically ventilated patients	1995 (50) 1996 (51)	Albuterol multidose vial	Lack of aseptic technique by respiratory therapy and intensive care unit personnel; respiratory therapy personnel carried multidose vials in their pockets
Pseudomonas aeruginosa ventilator-associated respiratory tract infections and colonization	1995 (53)	Food coloring dye added to nasogastric tube feedings	*P. aeruginosa* isolated from 32 oz bottles of food coloring dye; multiple-use bottles were replaced by single-use vials
Neonatal infection and colonization with *Serratia marcescens*	1997 (58)	1% chlorxylenol antiseptic hand soap	Nursing staff used personal bottles of soap that became contaminated during use
Burkholderia cepacia septicemia in cardiac patients	1998 (61)	5% dextrose solution used to dilute heparin	One-liter bag of solution used to dilute heparin for multiple patients on cardiology ward
Pyoderma in neonates	2000 (84)	Ultrasound coupling gel	Common container of sonography gel was used and applied with a wooden spatula that was reused for multiple infants
Serratia marcescens bloodstream infections on a surgical ward	2006 (85)	Total parenteral nutrition (TPN) solution	Investigators observed incorrect use of single-dose and multidose vials and very low adherence to hand hygiene; single-dose vials used for multiple doses; TPN solution likely contaminated when nurses on unit added medications to the TPN bags

Table 3–4 Products Associated with Noninfectious Adverse Events

Outbreak	Year(s) Reported/ Reference	Product	Comments
Neonatal hyperbilirubinemia	1978 (32)	Phenolic disinfectant detergent	Hyperbilirubinemia developed in infants exposed to a phenol solution used for disinfecting nursery surfaces
Cluster of unusual illness and deaths in neonates	1986 (39)	Commercially available intravenous vitamin E preparation	Product was newly marketed; precise constituents in E-ferol that caused illness and death were not able to be determined
Needlestick injuries in hospital employees	1995 (54)	Fiberboard infectious waste containers	Hospital changed product; injuries occurred when needles pierced walls of new container
Illness and sudden deaths in adult patients	1997 (57)	Commercially available amino acid additive used for peripheral parenteral nutrition (PPN)	Additive caused precipitate in the PPN
Adverse ocular reactions ("red eye")	1998 (82) 2006 (96)	Leucocyte-reduced red blood cell product	Nationwide outbreak of red eye syndrome associated with transfusion of specific lots of leukoreduced red blood cell units led to recall of product
Acute allergic-type reactions among patients undergoing hemodialysis	2008 (77)	Intravenous heparin solution	Solution contaminated during manufacture with heparin-like product; led to nationwide recall

For additional information on outbreaks of hospital-associated infections related to contaminated substances, the reader is referred to the excellent review by Vonberg and Gastmeier.[97]

Outbreaks Associated with Devices

Devices used for therapeutic and diagnostic procedures have long been associated with outbreaks in the acute care and ambulatory care settings.[98–135]

When invasive devices are used, the risk of infection and of outbreaks increases. Outbreaks have been traced to contaminated endoscopes used for endoscopic retrograde cholangiopancreatography[98–101] and upper gastrointestinal procedures,[98,100,102–105] bronchoscopes,[98,106–112] automated endoscope washers,[100,105,108,109] respiratory therapy devices and equipment,[73,113,114] hemodynamic monitoring systems,[115–118] jet gun injectors,[119] reusable fingerstick blood-sampling devices,[120–121] urologic apparatus,[122–125] electronic thermometers,[126,127] hemodialysis equipment,[128] needleless valves used for intravascular access,[129,130] biopsy devices,[124,131] balloons used in manual ventilation,[132] and external ventricular catheters.[133] In addition, adverse reactions in patients have resulted from residual gluteraldehyde on devices that were not thoroughly rinsed after soaking in a gluteraldehyde solution.[134,135]

Table 3-5 lists examples of device-related outbreaks and the infection control and technical errors associated with their occurrence. The major reasons for these epidemics were (1) improper cleaning and disinfection procedures, (2) contamination of endoscopes by automatic washers/disinfectors, (3) improper handling of sterile fluids and equipment, and (4) lack of adherence to aseptic technique.

Measures used to prevent these types of outbreaks include the following:

- Careful attention to cleaning and disinfection protocols for endoscopes and bronchoscopes
- Careful maintenance and quality control of automated endoscope washing and disinfection machines
- Careful attention to cleaning and disinfection protocols for respiratory therapy equipment
- Proper use and dilution of disinfectant solutions
- Consistent use of disposable single-patient use equipment for hemodynamic monitoring and urodynamic testing
- Strict adherence to sterile technique when handling sterile supplies
- Correct use and cleaning of devices in accordance with manufacturers' instructions

Outbreaks Associated with Procedures

Many diagnostic and therapeutic procedures place a patient at risk for developing a HAI or other iatrogenic event, such as injury or allergic reaction. Most procedure-related infections are not associated with outbreaks and are usually thought to be a result of host factors such as impaired or disrupted host defenses, immunosuppression, colonization with healthcare-associated organisms, and underlying diseases. However, outbreaks have been associated with procedures such as gastrointestinal endoscopy,[98,100,102–105] bronchoscopy,[98,106–112] hemodialysis,[128,136–139] peritoneal dialysis,[140,141] hemodynamic pressure monitoring,[117–118] cystoscopy and transurethral resection of the prostate,[142,143] organ transplants,[144,145] pulsatile lavage for debridement,[146] ultrasonography,[147] and various surgical procedures.[148,149]

Table 3–5 Examples of Device-Related Outbreaks and Associated Infection Control or Technical Errors

Outbreak	Year Reported/ Reference No.	Device	Infection Control or Technical Error
Hepatitis B infection	1986 (119)	Jet gun injector	Nozzle tip contaminated with blood; was not properly disinfected
Mycobacterium tuberculosis	1989 (107)	Bronchoscope	Suction valve of bronchoscope not disinfected despite rigorous cleaning and disinfection
Pseudomonas aeruginosa infection and colonization post-UGI endoscopy	1991 (100)	UGI endoscope	Flawed automatic disinfector
Bloody diarrhea associated with endoscopy	1992 (134)	Endoscope	Residual gluteraldehyde in improperly rinsed endoscope
Proctitis following endorectal ultrasound examination	1993 (135)	Endoscope	Residual gluteraldehyde in improperly rinsed endoscope
Pseudomonas aeruginosa and Enterobacteriaceae bacteremia post-ERCP	1993 (99)	Endoscope	Flawed automatic disinfector
Pseudomonas cepacia respiratory tract colonization/ infection and bacteremia	1993 (113)	Reusable electronic ventilator probes	Improper disinfection solution used
Gram-negative bacteremia in cardiac surgery patients	1996 (115)	Hemodynamic pressure monitoring equipment	Pressure monitoring equipment left uncovered overnight in the operating room
Hepatitis C infection	1997 (104)	Colonoscope	Improper cleaning and disinfection of colonoscope
Multidrug-resistant *Mycobacterium tuberculosis*	1997 (110)	Bronchoscope	Inadequate cleaning and disinfection of bronchoscope
Multidrug-resistant *Pseudomonas aeruginosa* urinary tract infection and urosepsis	1997 (123)	Urodynamic transducer	Improperly processed transducer used for urodynamic testing

Table 3–5   (*Continued*)

Outbreak	Year Reported/ Reference No.	Device	Infection Control or Technical Error
Hepatitis B infection in a hospital and a nursing home	1997 (121)	Fingerstick blood sampling devices	Disposable component of device became contaminated with blood and was not routinely changed between patients
Bloodstream infections (BSIs) caused by multiple pathogens	1998 (128)	Hemodialysis equipment	Newly installed attachment used to drain spent priming saline became contaminated
Bacillus cereus systemic infections and colonization in a neonatal intensive care unit	2000 (132)	Balloons used in manual ventilation	The exteriors of the balloons were cleaned with detergent that did not reach the interior of balloon and was not sufficient to kill *B. cereus* spores; outbreak ended when balloons were sterilized by autoclaving
Pseudomonas aeruginosa urinary tract infections following urodynamic studies	2001 (125)	Pressure transducer cover for urodynamic system for measuring bladder pressure	The cover was labeled as a single-use device, but it was used on multiple patients
Burkholderia cepacia colonization and infection in two pediatric units	2003 (114)	Mechanical ventilator	Ventilator disinfection procedures not followed; poor separation of clean and dirty items
Increased incidence of catheter-related bloodstream infections	2006 (129) 2007 (130)	Positive pressure needleless valve used for intravascular access	Increased bloodstream infections noted after introduction of a new needleless valve intravenous access port reported by several investigators
Pseudomonas aeruginosa infections after transurethral resection of the prostate (TURP)	2007 (124)	Steel biopsy needle guide	Inadequate reprocessing procedures; device was disinfected with high-level disinfectant and then rinsed with tap water rather than sterilized as recommended by manufacturer

UGI = upper gastrointestinal; ERCP = endoscopic retrograde cholangiopancreatography

Gastrointestinal Endoscopy and Bronchoscopy

Numerous outbreaks and pseudo-outbreaks related to gastrointestinal endoscopy and bronchoscopy procedures have been reported in both the inpatient and outpatient settings.[9,98,150] Despite the fact that the risk of infection associated with these devices is well known, some personnel in endoscopy suites do not follow appropriate protocols for reprocessing scopes.[151–154] Because endoscopes are complex instruments that are difficult to clean and disinfect, staff responsible for processing them must be instructed to follow meticulously the proper protocols for cleaning, disinfecting, and sterilization of the endoscopes and their related parts. If automatic endoscope reprocessors are used, personnel must be instructed in their use.

A multisociety guideline for reprocessing gastrointestinal endoscopes was published in 2003 by the American Society for Gastrointestinal Endoscopy (ASGE) and the Society for Healthcare Epidemiology of America (SHEA).[153] The ASGE has published a variety of guidelines, including one on infection control during gastrointestinal endoscopy.[155] Culver et al. provide recommendations for bronchoscope reprocessing based on their review of outbreaks related to bronchoscopy.[156]

Measures to prevent infections and outbreaks related to endoscopy procedures include the following[153,155,156]:

- Implementation of an infection surveillance, prevention, and control program based on recognized standards and guidelines
- Establishment of an initial and ongoing training program for personnel who process endoscopes
- A mechanism to ensure that personnel adhere to protocols for cleaning and disinfection or sterilization of endoscopes and related accessories
- Following disinfection, use of either a sterile water rinse followed by forced-air drying or a tap water rinse followed by forced air drying and a 70% alcohol rinse
- Adherence to protocols for proper handling and storage of endoscopes after processing to prevent recontamination
- Rigorous adherence to established protocols and the manufacturer's instructions for the use of automatic endoscope reprocessors
- A quality assurance program to monitor the effectiveness of the disinfection and sterilization processes and the competency of the personnel who reprocess endoscopes and related accessories.

In 2001 and 2002, several hospitals in the United States and Europe reported HAIs related to bronchoscopy that were traced to a loose port on the bronchoscope.[111,112] The outbreaks resulted in a recall of several bronchoscope models.

Several outbreaks related to gastrointestinal endoscopy and bronchoscopy procedures are noted in Table 3-5. For additional information on outbreaks and pseudo-outbreaks associated with bronchoscopy, the reader is referred to the editorial by Weber and Rutala[150] and the review by Culver et al.[156]

Hemodialysis and Peritoneal Dialysis

HAIs are well-recognized complications of hemodialysis. Outbreaks in hemodialysis centers have occurred as a result of improper handling or inadequate cleaning and disinfection of reusable dialysers[136–138]; cross-contamination of blood tubing by ultrafiltrate waste[128]; sharing of staff, equipment, supplies, and medications between patients[139]; failure to isolate patients with chronic hepatitis B virus (HBV)[139]; and failure to vaccinate susceptible hemodialysis patients against HBV.[139]

Care must be taken to ensure that hemodialysis personnel are familiar with the proper use and disinfection of the equipment they are using. One outbreak of bloodstream infections occurred in two outpatient hemodialysis centers affiliated with a hospital; it was associated with a change in the setup of the hemodialysis system. The reservoir was a newly installed, commercially marketed attachment used to drain spent saline. The attachment became heavily contaminated with multiple gram-positive, gram-negative, and fungal pathogens and served as a portal of entry into the blood tubing.[128]

Outbreaks related to peritoneal dialysis have been associated with contaminated peritoneal dialysis machines[140,141] and the use of intrinsically contaminated povidone iodine solution.[28] Personnel responsible for cleaning, disinfecting, and handling equipment used for peritoneal dialysis must practice strict aseptic technique and carefully follow manufacturers' directions for the specific equipment they are using.

Outbreaks related to hemodialysis and peritoneal dialysis and measures to prevent transmission of infectious agents in the dialysis setting are further discussed in Chapter 5.

Outbreaks Associated with Surgery

Most surgical site infections are caused by endogenous or exogenous organisms that are introduced into the wound at the time of surgery. However, outbreaks associated with surgical procedures may be caused either by contaminated antiseptics,[157] dressings,[158–160] equipment,[115,148] medications or solutions,[40,88,161] or by organisms disseminated by a personnel carrier. These outbreaks are generally recognized when a cluster of surgical site infections caused by the same organism is detected. The type of organism causing the infections will often provide a clue to a source or reservoir. Outbreaks of postoperative infections caused by *S. aureus* or group A streptococci are invariably associated with a human carrier. Outbreaks caused by gram-negative organisms and fungi are frequently associated with an environmental source.[115]

In addition to surgery-related outbreaks caused by infectious agents, clusters of adverse events associated with exposure to chemicals have also been reported in surgical patients. In one report, six patients who had cardiac surgery developed postoperative bleeding, which was caused by residual detergent in reprocessed laparotomy sponges.[162] In another, an outbreak of corneal edema following cataract surgery was thought to be caused by inadequate rinsing of small-lumen surgical instruments that had been disinfected by soaking in gluteraldehyde.[163]

Although postoperative infections and complications following cataract surgery are uncommon, they can be devastating.[164–166] Outbreaks associated with cataract surgery are discussed in Chapter 5.

OUTBREAKS ASSOCIATED WITH *PSEUDOMONAS, RALSTONIA,* AND *BURKHOLDERIA* SPECIES

Outbreaks associated with *Ralstonia pickettii, Pseudomonas aeruginosa,* and *Burkholderia cepacia* are frequently related to therapeutic and diagnostic procedures and contaminated devices and solutions, as demonstrated in Tables 3–2, 3–3 and 3–5.[167–169] Whenever a cluster of colonizations or infections with one of these organisms is identified, a contaminated solution or aqueous reservoir should be suspected.

OUTBREAKS ASSOCIATED WITH HUMAN CARRIERS OR DISSEMINATORS

Human carriers and disseminators have been responsible for hospital outbreaks of *S. aureus, Streptococcus pyogenes* (group A beta-hemolytic streptococci [GAS]), *Candida* species, *Serratia marcescens, Pseudomonas aeruginosa,* hepatitis A, hepatitis B, hepatitis C, and *Salmonella.* Many organisms have more than one mode of transmission. Although hospital outbreaks caused by *S. aureus,* group A streptococcus, and hepatitis A are often associated with a human carrier, each of these organisms can be spread either by direct person-to-person contact or by food that is contaminated by a carrier. HBV may be directly transmitted from person to person by a carrier or indirectly via contaminated medications or equipment. *Salmonella* may be directly transmitted from person to person or via contaminated food.

Staphylococcus aureus

Although cross-infection on the hands of personnel is thought to be the primary mode of transmission of *S. aureus* in healthcare settings, some outbreaks have been associated with colonized or infected healthcare workers.[170,171] Healthcare workers commonly carry *S. aureus* in their nares and on their hands.[172] Outbreaks of surgical site infections caused by *S. aureus* have been associated with personnel carrying the organism on their skin and hair [173] and in their nares.[174,175] One outbreak of MRSA surgical site infections was associated with a healthcare worker with chronic sinusitis who was a carrier for prolonged periods.[175] One of his family members was also found to be a carrier of the epidemic strain. Staphylococcal outbreaks in nurseries[171,176,177] and intensive care units (ICU)[171,178] have also been associated with personnel carriers. In a review of 165 MRSA outbreaks, Vonberg et al. determined that there was strong evidence that healthcare workers were the source in 11 (6.6%) of the outbreaks.[171] In 8 of these outbreaks, the healthcare worker had a respiratory tract infection or skin infection; in only 3 (1.6%) was the healthcare worker source an asymptomatic carrier.

There is a phenomenon of airborne dispersal of *Staphylococcus aureus* that is called the "cloud" phenomenon; several outbreaks have been associated with healthcare workers who were considered to be airborne dispersers.[170,178] These outbreaks can occur despite personnel adherence to standard precautions and good hand hygiene and are difficult to control until the carrier is identified and effectively treated or removed from the setting.

Outbreaks caused by MRSA are discussed in Chapter 7. Since the control measures for preventing the transmission of MRSA are essentially the same as those for methicillin-sensitive *S. aureus,* the reader is referred to Chapter 7 for a review of control measures used to interrupt staphylococcal outbreaks.

S. aureus was the fourth most frequently identified bacterial agent causing food-borne outbreaks in the United States, as reported to the CDC between 1998 and 2002.[179] Dietary personnel who have a staphylococcal infection may contaminate food and be the source of a food-borne outbreak. Hospital personnel who have boils or skin lesions known or suspected to be infected with *S. aureus*—especially on the hands—should be restricted from patient care activities and from handling food until they have been treated and their infection has resolved. If investigators suspect a common source outbreak (i.e., a personnel carrier), they should examine personnel for evidence of skin breakdown or infection.

Group A Beta-Hemolytic Streptococcus

GAS can spread rapidly from person to person and can cause serious disease in a variety of healthcare settings.[180] Numerous outbreaks of healthcare-associated group A streptococci have been reported.[180–196] A review of the literature revealed more than 50 nosocomial outbreaks of GAS reported worldwide between 1966 and 1995.[180] A Canadian study group identified 20 outbreaks that occurred from 1992 through 2000 in hospitals in Ontario, Canada.[193] Historically, healthcare-associated outbreaks of GAS have involved newborns,[188] postpartum women,[180–185] patients in burn units[180,187] and geriatric units, postoperative surgical patients, and residents of long-term care facilities.[180,191,193] Outbreaks have also been reported in medical units[189] and in critical care units.[190,193] In addition to person-to-person spread, GAS may be transmitted by contaminated food. An outbreak of streptococcal pharyngitis in a hospital pediatric clinic was traced to food that had been contaminated by a healthcare worker who was a GAS carrier.[192]

Nosocomial outbreaks are often associated with colonized or infected healthcare personnel. Although nasopharyngeal carriers are thought to be particularly likely to transmit GAS, personnel implicated in group A streptococcal surgical wound infection outbreaks have been found to carry the organism in their scalp,[181] vagina,[182,183] or anus.[184,185] In one report, an outbreak of group A streptococcal surgical site infections was associated with an asymptomatic anesthesiologist who was a pharyngeal carrier.[186] The outbreak resulted from the exposure of the anesthesiologist to his infected daughter. In several reported outbreaks, the source of infection or colonization in hospital personnel was a household contact.[180,181,183,186]

It should be noted that healthcare workers either may serve as the index case or may become infected through contact with infected patients or other healthcare workers during the course of their work. In several reports, an outbreak of GAS infections occurred in healthcare workers following exposure to an infected patient.[195,196] In one report, three healthcare workers developed GAS pharyngitis after exposure in the operating room to a patient with GAS pharyngitis and necrotizing fasciitis.[195] The three healthcare workers reported their infections shortly after becoming symptomatic. An important measure for preventing and interrupting GAS outbreaks is the recognition by personnel of signs and symptoms, such as pharyngitis, that are consistent with GAS infection so that treatment may promptly be provided.

Because nosocomial infections caused by group A beta-hemolytic streptococcus are relatively uncommon and can cause significant morbidity and mortality, the occurrence of one healthcare-associated GAS infection at any site should prompt a search for other cases to detect a potential outbreak. This search can be done by reviewing laboratory reports and by asking hospital surgeons and other healthcare providers if they are aware of any GAS infections, especially surgical site infections. In its guidelines for preventing GAS infections in postpartum and postsurgical patients, the CDC recommends that "One nosocomial postpartum or postsurgical invasive GAS infection should prompt enhanced surveillance and isolate storage, whereas two cases caused by the same strain should prompt an epidemiological investigation that includes the culture of specimens from epidemiologically linked healthcare workers."[197(p950)]

The reader is referred to Chapter 4 for a discussion of the epidemiology and mode of transmission of GAS and measures that can be used to recognize, prevent, and control an outbreak of GAS. Recommendations for preventing and controlling GAS outbreaks can also be found in the CDC guideline for infection control in healthcare personnel,[25] and the reviews by Weber et al[180] and Daneman et al.[193]

Candida and *Nocardia* Species

Several outbreaks of postoperative surgical site infections caused by *Candida* species have been associated with personnel carriers. One outbreak of *Candida albicans* sternal wound infections following cardiac surgery was associated with a scrub nurse who had recurrent vaginal infections,[198] and an outbreak of *Candida tropicalis* sternal wound infections was also associated with a scrub nurse.[199] An outbreak of Candida osteomyelitis and diskitis after spinal surgery was associated with a nurse who had artificial fingernails.[200]

A few clusters of surgical site infections caused by *Nocardia farcinica* have been reported.[201,202] In one, the source was not determined,[202] and in the other the source was determined to be a colonized anesthesiologist.[201]

Gram-Negative Organisms

Outbreaks caused by gram-negative organisms such as *Pseudomonas* and *Serratia* are frequently associated with contaminated environmental reservoirs such as equipment, lotions, and solutions[89]; however, they can also be associated with onychomycosis, artificial nails, transient carriage on the hands of personnel, or by personnel who become colonized carriers.[203–205] An outbreak of *Serratia marcescens* infection and colonization in a neurosurgical ICU was associated with a healthcare worker who had psoriasis and whose hands were repeatedly colonized with *Serratia marcescens* over a prolonged period.[204] An outbreak of *P. aeruginosa* pneumonia and bloodstream infections in a neonatal intensive care unit (NICU) was associated with a healthcare worker who had otitis externa and ear cultures that grew the epidemic strain of *P. aeruginosa*.[206]

Some studies have shown that overcrowding and staff shortages can contribute to transient carriage on the hands of personnel and epidemic spread of organisms.[207] However, in many outbreaks, it is not possible to identify the source or reservoir or mode of transmission of the causative agent.[203,206,207]

Hepatitis B Virus

Transmission of HBV in the healthcare setting has long been recognized and has been associated with unsafe injection practices, contaminated equipment and medications (especially in hemodialysis settings), and direct transmission from an infected healthcare worker to a patient. Clusters of HBV infection have been traced to transmission from infected obstetricians, gynecologists, dentists, and surgeons to their patients during surgery.[208–214] Of the three most commonly recognized blood-borne pathogens—HBV, hepatitis C virus (HCV), and human immunodeficiency virus (HIV)—HBV is the most easily transmitted from person to person because an infected person can carry more than a billion HBV particles per milliliter of blood.[139] Risk factors associated with transmission of HBV from healthcare worker to patient include the presence of hepatitis B e antigen in the healthcare worker's blood, the type of surgical procedure (such as vaginal hysterectomy and cardiac, orthopedic, and major pelvic surgery), and the potential for injury of the healthcare worker (such as a needlestick during suturing) during the invasive procedure.[208,214] Twelve HBV-infected healthcare workers infected 38 patients from 1991 to 2005 in the United Kingdom and the Netherlands alone.[214] It is likely that many cases of HBV infection transmitted in healthcare settings are not recognized owing to the long incubation period, the occurrence of asymptomatic infection, and the lack of healthcare-associated HBV infection surveillance systems.[214,215]

Recommendations for preventing transmission of hepatitis B from infected healthcare providers to patients have been published by the CDC (currently being revised),[211] the SHEA,[208] United States and European consensus panels,[216,217] public health agencies, hospital associations, and others.[218,219] Each of these published guidelines provides slightly different recommendations regarding the management of HBV-infected healthcare workers who directly perform invasive procedures. In the United States there is "no uniform national policy for definitive guidance concerning whether and under what conditions infected physicians can practice."[217(1165)] However, ICPs and hospital leaders must ensure that their facility has adequate protocols in place to prevent healthcare worker-to-patient transmission of HBV, HCV, and HIV.

Because HBV in human plasma can survive for at least 1 week in the environment,[220] inanimate objects contaminated with blood can serve as vehicles for the transmission of the virus. When a cluster of healthcare-associated HBV infections is detected, and appears to be unrelated to surgery, the mode of transmission is most likely via exposure to a contaminated inanimate object rather than contact with an infected healthcare worker. When investigating an outbreak of HBV, investigators must review and observe infection control practices involving the use of needles, syringes, and multidose vials because the improper use of these items can result in the transmission of blood-borne pathogens from patient to patient.[221,222]

Outbreaks of HBV and other bloodborne pathogens related to unsafe injection practices and lack of adherence to infection prevention protocols are discussed in Chapter 5. Recommendations for safe injection practices and medication handling are also discussed in that chapter.

Hepatitis C Virus

There are several reports of clusters of HCV transmitted directly from a healthcare worker to patients.[214,223,224] In all of these cases, transmission was associated with a surgical procedure. In a review of healthcare-associated HCV infections, Perry et al. discussed 11 reports in which healthcare workers transmitted their HCV infection to 38 patients.[214]

Guidelines for preventing transmission of HCV from infected healthcare workers to patients have been published by the CDC,[225] SHEA, [208] and others.[218,219] All of these guidelines emphasize the need for infected healthcare workers to strictly follow routine infection prevention and control measures, such as standard precautions, to prevent the transmission of blood-borne pathogens. However, in the United States there is no uniform policy for the management or restriction of HCV-infected workers who perform invasive procedures.

HCV can also be transmitted from patient to patient via contaminated equipment and medications, unsafe injection practices, and medical procedures. Outbreaks of healthcare-associated HCV infection via unsafe injection practices and hemodialysis are discussed in Chapter 5 along with measures to prevent the transmission of HCV in the healthcare setting.

Human Immunodeficiency Virus

As of early 2008, worldwide, HIV transmission from an infected healthcare worker to a patient has been reported in four instances:

1. From a dentist in the United States to a patient who had an invasive dental procedure[226,227]
2. From an orthopedic surgeon in France to a patient who had a hip replacement [228]
3. From a nurse to a patient in France, with no evidence of blood exposure [229,230]
4. From an obstetrician/gynecologist in Spain to a patient who had a cesarean section[231,232]

Guidelines for preventing transmission of HIV from surgeon to patient have been published by the CDC,[211] SHEA,[208] the UK Department of Health,[233] and others.[217] Although there is no uniform national standard in the United States, all published guidelines to date have promoted the use of standard precautions, including hand hygiene and protective barriers, to minimize the exposure of patients to blood and blood-borne pathogens. They differ on the restrictions recommended for HIV-infected healthcare workers who perform invasive procedures.

Salmonella Species

Most reported hospital *Salmonella* outbreaks have been caused by improper handling of contaminated foods[234]; however, several epidemics have been traced to symptomatic dietary[235] and nursing personnel[236] and to infected patients.[237] In one outbreak, *Salmonella poona* was most likely introduced into an NICU by an asymptomatic infant whose mother was infected with *S. poona*.[237] The organism was then transmitted to two other infants via cross-infection by personnel. To prevent transmission of *Salmonella* in the healthcare setting, dietary and patient care personnel with acute gastrointestinal illness should be restricted from caring for patients and handling patient care items or food until symptoms subside.[25] Some health departments have regulations governing the restriction and culturing of healthcare workers and food handlers who have *Salmonella* infection.

Food-borne outbreaks and control measures for preventing the spread of agents such as *Salmonella* that cause gastrointestinal infections are discussed in Chapter 7.

Hepatitis A Virus

Hepatitis A virus (HAV) is most commonly transmitted in the hospital setting via the fecal-oral route by contact with feces or fecally contaminated items.[25] Transmission by ingestion of contaminated food or beverages is known to occur in hospitals but is rarely reported in the literature.[238,239] Transmission has also occurred by blood transfusion[25,240–243] and by cross-infection from a patient with asymptomatic or unrecognized HAV infection.[244,245] There is no chronic carrier state for HAV as there is for HBV and HCV. HAV is excreted in the stool, and transient viremia can occur.[24] Persons with HAV infection are most infectious during the prodromal stage, before the onset of jaundice.[24]

Several outbreaks in nurseries were traced to neonates who received blood transfusions from a donor with HAV infection.[240–242] Once introduced into the unit, HAV was transmitted by cross-infection to other infants and personnel and to parents and relatives of the infected infants. Activities that have been associated with nosocomial spread of HAV include eating and drinking in patient care areas[240,241,246,247] and failure to wash hands after caring for an infected infant.[246,247] In another outbreak, the source for nosocomial HAV was an adult patient with symptomatic HAV infection who was hospitalized for an unrelated reason, and HAV was transmitted to six healthcare workers and one patient.[244] For more information on nosocomial HAV outbreaks the reader is referred to the article by Chodick et al., who reviewed reports of outbreaks in healthcare settings that were published between 1975 and 2003.[243]

Recommendations for preventing transmission of HAV include good hand hygiene and use of standard precautions.[26] Contact precautions should be used for infants and children less than 3 years of age for the duration of hospitalization; for children 3–14 years of age for 2 weeks after onset of symptoms; and for persons over 14 years of age for 1 week after onset of symptoms.[26]

The CDC Advisory Committee on Immunization Practices (ACIP) recommends that hepatitis A vaccine, in preference to immune globulin, be administered for postexposure prophylaxis to close contacts of index patients only if an epidemiologic investigation indicates that nosocomial spread between patients or between patients and staff in a hospital has occurred.[248]

OUTBREAKS SPREAD FROM PERSON TO PERSON BY AIRBORNE AND DROPLET TRANSMISSION

Diseases Spread by Airborne Transmission

Outbreaks of nosocomial infections spread by the airborne route have long been recognized in hospitals,[249,250] although they are relatively uncommon compared to outbreaks spread by contact. Only a few diseases have been documented to be spread from person to person via a true airborne route (i.e., by airborne droplet nuclei, which are small particle residues of evaporated respiratory secretions that can remain suspended in the air and can be dispersed widely by air currents).[26,249] Three diseases caused by pathogens that can be truly airborne and have caused numerous epidemics in the healthcare setting are tuberculosis, measles, and varicella (chickenpox). Because tuberculosis outbreaks have been reported in a variety of healthcare settings, this disease is discussed in detail in Chapter 7.

Measles

Measles is one of the most contagious diseases in humans. Transmission of measles has occurred in hospitals, physicians' offices, and emergency rooms.[250–254] Measles may be introduced into the healthcare setting by infected patients or healthcare workers and is easily transmitted either via contact with respiratory secretions of infected persons or via the airborne route.[26] Infected healthcare workers can transmit the disease to patients, to other healthcare workers, and to family members. Measles is readily spread because the virus may remain airborne for prolonged periods and because infected persons with measles may shed the virus in respiratory secretions during the prodromal period before the disease is recognized.[26] Transmission from patient to patient has occurred in physicians' offices even when direct contact did not occur.[255] Fifteen of the 75 measles outbreaks reported in the United States during 1993–1996 involved transmission in a healthcare setting.[254] During 1989–1991, a major resurgence of measles occurred in the United States; however, in 1996 only 508 cases were reported, of which 65 were classified as international importations.[254]

Measles is rarely now seen in the United States owing to a highly immunized population; however, measles is still endemic in many other countries. Many physicians and healthcare providers have not seen a case of measles, and therefore it sometimes may be difficult to obtain a prompt diagnosis when a patient presents with a rash and a fever. Measles transmission in the United States is usually associated with an imported case. In 2005, 66 confirmed cases of measles were reported to the CDC, and 34 of these were from a single outbreak in Indiana associated with an unvaccinated 17 year old who returned home to the United States from Romania.[256,257] In May 2008, the CDC announced that a total of 64 confirmed measles cases had been preliminarily reported to the CDC by April 25, the most reported by this date for any year since 2001.[258] This increased incidence of measles in the United States was related to importation of measles by travelers, many of whom were returning from Europe where several outbreaks were occurring.[258] Of the 64 cases, 63 were unvaccinated or had unknown or undocumented vaccine status, one was an unvaccinated healthcare worker who was infected in a hospital, 17 (39%) were infected while visiting a healthcare facility, and one was born before 1957.

Recommendations for preventing transmission of measles have been published by the CDC[25,26,254,259] and the American Academy of Pediatrics[260] and include the following:

- Prompt recognition of persons with measles; measles should be suspected in persons with a fever and rash, regardless of age
- Prompt isolation of persons with suspected or known measles; airborne precautions should be implemented in a private room with negative airflow and nonrecirculating air[26]
- Protocols to ensure measles immunity in all healthcare workers; measles vaccine should be provided to all healthcare workers who cannot show proof of immunity, as follows:[25,254,259]
  1. Healthcare workers born before 1957 are generally considered to be immune to measles.
  2. Healthcare workers born during or after 1957 are considered immune if they have one of the following:
     - Documentation of physician-diagnosed measles
     - Documentation of two doses of live measles vaccine on or after their first birthday
     - Serologic evidence of measles immunity

Because some outbreaks have involved persons born before 1957, some experts advocate requiring proof of immunity by vaccination or serology even for those adults born before 1957.[261]

Transmission of measles can be prevented if recommendations for immunization of children, adolescents, and adults are followed. The ACIP recommendations regarding immunization of healthcare workers[259] and immunization for measles, mumps, and rubella[254] should be used when developing healthcare facility policies. In addition, some state and local health departments require measles immunity for healthcare workers, and these requirements must be incorporated into a facility's policies.

Because measles is highly communicable, one case (even a community-acquired case) should be considered a potential outbreak and should be accorded immediate action to prevent further transmission. The suspected case should promptly be reported by telephone to the local health department so that measures to prevent further spread can be implemented as soon as possible. Actions that should quickly be taken to interrupt measles transmission include the following:

- Identification and prompt isolation of persons with suspected or confirmed measles.[26] Suspected cases should promptly be reported to the health department; however, a diagnosis of measles should be verified before exposure follow-up is conducted. Serologic testing is recommended to confirm the diagnosis; however, if measles is clinically diagnosed, exposure follow-up should begin before laboratory confirmation is received. Information on the clinical and laboratory diagnosis of measles is provided in Appendix C.[10]

- Compilation of a list of all potentially exposed personnel, patients, and visitors as soon as possible, especially if the suspected case is seen in the emergency room.

- Identification of all exposed personnel, patients, and visitors. It is important to define *exposed person* before conducting contact tracing. Exposure may be defined as being in the same room (or area supplied by the same air-handling system) at the same time as a patient with measles or for up to 1 hour after the patient with measles left the room or area.

- Evaluation of immunity in all exposed personnel and patients: Guidelines for evaluating immunity can be found above and in Appendix C.

- Restriction of susceptible exposed personnel from duty, from 5 days after the first exposure to 21 days after the last exposure to measles, regardless of postexposure vaccination.[25,254]

- Isolation of exposed susceptible patients, if they are still hospitalized, using airborne precautions in a private room with negative airflow and nonrecirculating air, from 5 days after the first exposure to 21 days after the last exposure to measles.[26]

- Prompt provision of measles vaccine to susceptible persons to halt disease transmission. Note: During an outbreak, serologic testing to identify susceptible persons is not necessary.[25,254] The vaccine should be provided to those born during or after 1957 who have no documentation of complete measles vaccination or physician-documented diagnosis of measles and should be considered for those born before 1957 if they do not have serologic documentation of immunity or receipt of two doses of measles vaccine. Guidelines for providing the measles vaccine and immune globulin can be found in the ACIP recommendations for measles, mumps, and rubella immunization.[254]

Community outbreaks can result in transmission into a healthcare facility,[262,263] and nosocomial transmission can spread into the community. Outbreaks of measles in healthcare settings can be associated with significant morbidity and disruption of services. They are disruptive and costly to control due to (1) the time needed to conduct a contact investigation, (2) the lost work-days for restricted personnel who either acquire measles or who are exposed and are not immune, and (3) the cost of the measles vaccine for exposed personnel, patients, and visitors.

One of the most important measures to prevent measles transmission is to ensure that all persons who work in a healthcare setting have acceptable evidence of measles immunity.[254,263]

Varicella (Chickenpox)

Varicella-zoster virus (VZV) causes varicella (chickenpox) and zoster (shingles). Varicella is one of the most communicable diseases of humans and is readily spread from person to person via direct contact with infected lesions, droplet spread, or airborne transmission.[26,264,265] Healthcare-associated outbreaks of varicella in hospitals and physicians' offices have been well documented.[264–270] True airborne transmission has been documented in the hospital setting when susceptible patients have developed varicella even though they did not have face-to-face contact with the infected source patient.[266,268] Community outbreaks can result in healthcare-associated exposures and transmission.[267] VZV can easily be introduced into the healthcare setting by infected patients, personnel, and visitors (including the children of personnel) since infected persons may be contagious up to 2 days prior to the development of symptoms.[24,26]

Guidelines for prevention and control of VZV infections in healthcare settings have been published by the CDC,[25,26,271] the American Academy of Pediatrics,[272] and others.[264,273,274] These guidelines should be reviewed when developing hospital policies.

Measures that should be implemented in healthcare settings to prevent varicella transmission include the following:

- Implementation of protocols to ensure varicella immunity in personnel[271]
- Prompt recognition of infected patients, personnel, and visitors. Note: The diagnosis of chickenpox should be verified by infection control and/or employee health personnel before exposure follow-up and contact tracing is conducted.
- Prompt and appropriate isolation of infected patients (airborne precautions in a private room with negative airflow and nonrecirculating air)[26]
- Compilation of a list of all potentially exposed personnel, patients, and visitors as soon as possible, especially if the suspected case is seen in the emergency room
- Prompt identification of exposed persons. It is important to define *exposed person* before conducting contact tracing. Weber et al. define exposure as "being in an enclosed airspace with the source case (i.e., same room) or in intimate contact with the source in an open area during a potentially contagious stage of illness. Varicella is considered contagious beginning 48 hours prior to the onset of rash and until all lesions are dried and crusted."[264(p699)]
- Evaluation of immunity in all exposed personnel, patients, and visitors[271]

- Restriction of susceptible exposed personnel from duty beginning on the 8th day after the first exposure through the 21st day after the last exposure to chickenpox, or until all lesions are dried and crusted if varicella occurs[25,271]

- Isolation of exposed susceptible patients, if they are still hospitalized, during the period of potential infectiousness (airborne precautions in a private room with negative airflow from 8 days after the first exposure through 21 days after the last exposure)[26]

- Provision of the varicella vaccine to exposed personnel who are not immune; however, the vaccine's efficacy in preventing postexposure development of varicella is unknown, and the vaccinated personnel should be managed as if they were not immunized.[271]

Varicella exposure management, follow-up, and contact tracing can result in considerable time expenditure by infection control and employee health staff, and the exclusion of exposed susceptible personnel from duty can lead to significant cost and disruption of services for a healthcare facility.[267] Much of this disruption can be prevented if persons with varicella are promptly identified and appropriately isolated and if healthcare facilities ensure that all of their personnel are immune to varicella.[271]

Diseases Spread by Droplet Transmission

Diseases that are spread from person to person via droplet transmission are caused by pathogens that are expelled in large particle droplets of respiratory secretions by a person who is coughing, talking, or sneezing or by droplets that are produced during a procedure such as tracheal suctioning or bronchoscopy.[26] These droplets are not widely dispersed into the air and are generally said to travel several feet before settling to the ground. Diseases that have caused outbreaks in healthcare settings and that can be spread via droplet transmission include adenovirus infections,[250,275–277] mumps,[278,279] influenza,[280] parvovirus B19 infection,[281–283] rubella,[284–286] *Mycoplasma pneumoniae* infection,[287] respiratory syncytial virus (RSV) infections,[288–300] and pertussis.[301–303] Although the influenza virus has been transmitted in the acute care setting, the majority of healthcare-associated outbreaks are reported in long-term care settings, and influenza is therefore discussed in Chapter 4.

Respiratory Syncytial Virus Infection

RSV infection is most common in infants and children and, although it can cause a severe pneumonia or bronchiolitis, it usually causes a mild disease. Community outbreaks of RSV disease are seasonal, generally occurring between December and March in North America. RSV can be introduced into the hospital by infected patients, personnel, or visitors and can be easily transmitted directly from person to person via large particle aerosols during close contact with an infected person or indirectly via RSV-contaminated hands or articles.[27,288,289] The portal of entry for RSV is the conjunctiva or nasal mucosa, and transmission frequently occurs when contaminated hands touch the eyes or nose.[27] Hand hygiene is the most important measure for preventing the transmission of RSV. Outbreaks of RSV infection have most commonly been reported in pediatric units,[290] nurseries,[291,292,300] and long-term care facilities,[293,294] and in immunocompromised adults in hematology/oncology and bone marrow transplant units[295,299] and ICUs.[296] RSV infection may occur concurrently with other respiratory tract infections, making outbreaks difficult to recognize.[297,299]

Measures used to control RSV outbreaks have been published by the CDC[26,27] and include the following:

- Appropriate hand hygiene
- Adherence to contact isolation precautions, especially gloves and gowns
- Use of private rooms for infected patients; when a private room is not available, an RSV-infected patient may be cohorted in a room with another patient who has an active RSV infection but who has no other infection
- Work restrictions for personnel who have symptoms of acute upper respiratory tract infection
- Restriction of visitors who have symptoms of upper respiratory tract infection from visiting patients, especially pediatric, cardiac, and immunosuppressed patients

Pertussis

Pertussis, or whooping cough, is generally considered to be a childhood disease; however, approximately 29% of cases reported in 2004 occurred in adults 19 years of age or older and 34% in individuals between 11 and 18 years of age.[301] Disease in adults may be subclinical,[302] mild, or atypical,[303] and although pertussis has been shown to be a common cause of prolonged cough in adults, it is frequently not recognized as the etiology.[304-307] Pertussis is easily spread from person to person by direct contact with the respiratory droplets of infected persons. Multiple outbreaks of pertussis have been reported in acute care facilities,[304,308-317] and many have involved both patients and staff.[306-308,311,312,316] Outbreaks in the community may involve hospital personnel who then introduce pertussis into the hospital.[306,307,318] *Bordetella pertussis* may also be introduced into the hospital by an infected patient, parent, or visitor.[310] There has been a resurgence of pertussis in many countries, including the United States, since the 1990s,[319-321] and outbreaks in hospitals can readily occur when *B. pertussis* is circulating in the community.[307,321] Unfortunately, pertussis can be difficult to diagnose, which makes early recognition and implementation of preventive measures problematic.[322]

Guidelines for preventing the transmission of *Bordetella pertussis* and for managing pertussis exposures have been published by the CDC[25,26,323,324] and others[325,326] and include the following:

- Droplet precautions for infected patients: private room and use of masks until 5 days after patient is started on effective therapy
- Droplet precautions for suspected cases until pertussis is ruled out
- Evaluation and appropriate therapy for exposed individuals who are symptomatic, including personnel and household contacts
- Work restrictions for symptomatic personnel until 5 days of therapy are completed

- Postexposure prophylaxis for exposed individuals who are asymptomatic, including personnel and household contacts
- Implementation of a program for routine provision of pertussis vaccine to personnel to prevent infection and avoid outbreaks.[26,324]

The article by Haiduven et al. contains a pertussis workup checklist and pertussis exposure forms that can be used for managing exposures in patients and personnel.[326]

Outbreaks of pertussis occur regularly in healthcare facilities worldwide. In addition to causing significant morbidity and disruption of services, they are labor intensive and costly to control.[315–317] The number and size of pertussis outbreaks in hospitals can be reduced through routine immunization of healthcare workers, timely recognition of cases, and implementation of appropriate infection prevention and control measures.

More on Diseases Spread by the Airborne and Droplet Routes

Appendix G contains *Guidelines for the Prevention and Control of Upper and Lower Acute Respiratory Illnesses (including Influenza and Pneumonia) in Long-Term Care Facilities* developed by the Maryland Department of Health Mental Hygiene.

Exhibit 3–1 provides examples of diseases that have been responsible for outbreaks in hospitals and are caused by organisms transmitted via the airborne and droplet routes.[26] Because a detailed description of each of these diseases is beyond the scope of this chapter, for information on signs and symptoms, diagnosis, epidemiology, and infection prevention and control measures the reader is referred to the *Control of Communicable Diseases Manual* by Heymann[24] and the CDC guidelines for isolation precautions,[26] prevention of healthcare-associated pneumonia,[27] and infection control in healthcare personnel.[25]

Exhibit 3–1   Airborne and Droplet-Spread Diseases Responsible for Outbreaks in Healthcare Facilities

Airborne	Droplet
Measles	Adenovirus
Tuberculosis	Group A streptococcus
Varicella	Influenza
	Mumps
	Mycoplasma pneumoniae infection
	Erythema infectiosum (parvovirus B-19)
	Pertussis
	Rubella
	Respiratory syncytial virus infection
	Severe acute respiratory syndrome

OUTBREAKS OF GASTROENTERITIS

Outbreaks of gastroenteritis are caused by infectious and noninfectious agents and occur frequently in hospitals and long-term care settings. These agents may be spread directly from person to person or indirectly via contaminated food, water, and environmental surfaces. Gastroenteritis outbreaks are discussed in Chapter 7.

OUTBREAKS OF DISEASES THAT HAVE ENVIRONMENTAL RESERVOIRS

Legionnaires' disease (LD) and aspergillosis are two major nosocomial diseases that have airborne and droplet modes of transmission but have environmental, rather than human, reservoirs.

Legionnaires' Disease

Epidemiology

Legionella species are gram-negative bacilli that are ubiquitous in nature and live in aqueous habitats. They can be isolated from hot and cold tap water, ponds, streams, and the surrounding soil. Nosocomial cases of LD were reported shortly after the etiologic agent of LD was identified in 1977,[327,328] and multiple healthcare-associated outbreaks and clusters have since been reported.[327,329–336] Healthcare-associated LD has generally been associated with contamination of the water in cooling systems[27,334,335] or the potable hot water systems in hospitals,[27,329–333,336] and these systems may remain colonized for prolonged periods.[333] In one hospital, persistent colonization of the water supply was associated with contaminated shock absorbers installed within the pipes to decrease noise.[331]

In 2005 and 2006, 11,980 cases of LD were reported by 35 countries in Europe, and 629 of these were reported as nosocomial.[336] Sixty-six of the nosocomial cases were involved in 19 outbreaks in hospitals or healthcare facilities. Fifteen of these outbreaks were "attributed to contaminated hot or cold water systems, two to wet cooling systems, and two to an unknown source."[336]

A 1994 community outbreak of *Legionella pneumophila* pneumonia in Wilmington, Delaware, was associated with the cooling towers of a hospital.[337] Although no hospitalized patients were affected, hospital staff and persons living in the area surrounding the hospital developed LD.

Hospitals play an important role in the detection of outbreaks. Recognition of a cluster of community-acquired cases of LD by the staff of a community hospital led to the detection of an outbreak of LD among passengers of a cruise ship.[338] Because tests for *Legionella* species are not routinely performed, it is likely that many cases, both community and healthcare associated, are not recognized.

Mode of Transmission

The mode of transmission for *Legionella pneumophila* is via inhalation of the organism in aerosolized water droplets that can be produced by cooling towers, showers, room air humidifiers, and respiratory therapy nebulization devices.[27,335]

Control Measures

To avoid transmission of *Legionella* in the hospital, sterile water (not tap or distilled water) should be used to rinse and fill respiratory therapy equipment. Recommendations for preventing nosocomial LD have been published by the CDC[27] and World Health Organization[339] and include information on decontaminating potable water and cooling systems. Control measures used to interrupt outbreaks in hospitals have included hyperchlorination and superheating of the hot water system, use of sterile water in nebulizers, and use of biocides in cooling towers.[327–329,331]

Criteria for defining healthcare-associated cases have been published by a variety of organizations and public health agencies and differ slightly.[27,336,339] The incubation period for LD is generally 2–10 days, and the CDC defines healthcare-associated LD as follows:[27(pg.27)]

> Definite: Laboratory-confirmed legionellosis that occurs in a patient who has spent greater than or equal to 10 days continuously in a healthcare facility prior to onset of illness

> Possible: Laboratory-confirmed infection that occurs in a patient who has spent 2–9 days in a healthcare facility before onset of illness

The CDC recommends initiating an investigation for the source of *Legionella* spp. when healthcare-associated legionellosis is detected, as outlined in Exhibit 3–2.

An epidemiologic investigation of the source of *Legionella* spp. includes "(1) retrospective review of microbiologic and medical records,(2) active surveillance to identify all recent or ongoing cases of legionellosis, (3) identification of potential risk factors for infection (including environmental exposures, such as showering or use of respiratory-therapy equipment) by line listing of cases; analysis by time, place, and person; and comparison with appropriate controls, (4) collection of water samples from environmental sources implicated by the epidemiologic investigation and from other potential sources of aerosolized water, and (5) subtype matching between *Legionella* spp. isolated from patients and environmental samples."[27(p30)]

Much information on *Legionella* and LD can be found at www.Legionella.org.

Aspergillosis

Epidemiology and Mode of Transmission

Aspergillus species are ubiquitous in nature and can easily be cultured from the hospital environment.[340] This fungus produces spores that are approximately 3 μm in size and that can remain suspended in air for prolonged peri-

Exhibit 3–2   Response to Identification of Laboratory-Confirmed
Healthcare-Associated Legionellosis

A. In facilities with hemopoietic stem-cell transplant (HSCT) or solid-organ transplant recipients:

When one inpatient of an inpatient HSCT or solid-organ transplant unit develops a case of laboratory-confirmed definite (i.e., after >10 days of continuous inpatient stay) or possible (i.e., within 2–9 days of inpatient stay) healthcare-associated Legionnaires' disease, or when two or more patients develop laboratory-confirmed Legionnaires' disease within 6 months of each other and after having visited an outpatient transplant unit during part of the 2–10 day period before illness onset:

In consultation with the facility's infection control team, conduct a combined epidemiologic and environmental investigation to determine the source(s) of *Legionella* spp. Include but not limit the investigation to such potential sources as showers, water faucets, cooling towers, hot-water tanks, and carpet-cleaner water tanks.

B. In facilities that do not house severely immunocompromised patients (e.g., HSCT or solid-organ transplant recipients):

When a single case of laboratory-confirmed definite healthcare-associated Legionnaires' disease is identified, or when two or more cases of laboratory confirmed possible healthcare-associated Legionnaires' disease occur within 6 months of each other: Conduct an epidemiologic investigation through a retrospective review of microbiologic, serologic, and postmortem data to identify previous cases, and begin an intensive prospective surveillance for additional cases of healthcare-associated Legionnaires' disease.

Source: Adapted from Centers for Disease Control and Prevention. *Guidelines for Preventing Health-Care-Associated Pneumonia, 2003. Recommendations of CDC and the Healthcare Infection Control Practices Advisory Committee.* p. 71. http://www.cdc.gov/ncidod/dhqp/gl_hcpneumonia.html. Accessed April 19, 2008.

ods.[341] The usual portal of entry is via inhalation of aerosolized spores.[27] However, primary cutaneous aspergillosis resulting from inoculation of spores onto nonintact skin has been reported.[37,55] Immunocompromised patients are at greatest risk of developing invasive pulmonary infection, which can result in significant morbidity and mortality.[342]

Multiple outbreaks of nosocomial aspergillosis have been reported in hospitals.[37,55,340,343–350] Most outbreaks have been associated with construction or renovation in, or adjacent to, the hospital.[37,340,344–346,348] In one outbreak, exposure to a radiology suite that was undergoing extensive renovation was the only common environmental factor found among six patients who developed nosocomial aspergillosis during a 1-month period.[348] Although most outbreaks involve pulmonary aspergillosis in immunosuppressed patients,[37,343–346] there are several reports of outbreaks of primary cutaneous aspergillosis caused by contact with contaminated medical supplies, such as dressings[37,55] and intravenous arm boards.[347] In one report, an outbreak of cutaneous aspergillosis was recognized when three cases of extensive wound aspergillosis occurred in surgical and burn patients in a 3-week period. The source was traced to the outer packaging of dressing supplies (dressing trays, gauze, bandages, and tapes) that had become contaminated during renovation in the central inventory control area of the hospital.[37] An investigation of a cluster of cases of pulmonary infections with *Aspergillus fumigatus* in a transplant unit found that patient-to-patient transmission of *A. fumigatus* likely occurred from aerosolization of conidiophores during surgical dressing changes and wound debridement of a patient who had an extensive abdominal wound infected with *A. fumigatus*.[350] In addition to outbreaks of infection, pseudo-outbreaks involving aspergillosis have been reported as a result of contamination of microbiology cultures in the laboratory.[351]

Control Measures

Measures used to prevent transmission of fungal spores to patients include implementation of protocols to prevent dispersal of construction-related dust and bioaerosols,[27,89,340,352] placement of high-risk patients (e.g., those with severe and prolonged granulocytopenia) in a protected environment,[26] routine inspection and maintenance of air-handling systems in high-risk patient care areas (such as operating rooms, nurseries, ICUs, bone marrow or solid organ transplant units, and oncology units),[27] and protection of sterile supplies from contamination.

Guidelines and recommendations for controlling the airborne transmission of *Aspergillus* in the hospital have been published by the CDC,[27,89] Walsh and Dixon,[340] Carter and Barr,[352] public health agencies, and others.[353–355] Measures used to control transmission of *Aspergillus* spores during construction and renovation projects include the following:

- Construction of impermeable barriers of plastic or drywall that extend from the floor to the ceiling to control the dissemination of dust and dirt and to separate the construction site from patient care areas, the pharmacy, and areas where sterile supplies are stored
- Frequent cleaning and vacuuming of the work site and the areas adjacent to the work site
- Restriction of pedestrian traffic through the work area to prevent the tracking of dust and dirt through the facility
- Careful attention to traffic patterns of the construction crew, personnel, patients, and visitors to avoid the spread of dirt and dust through the hospital and to reduce the risk of patient exposure to infectious agents
- Evaluation of air patterns and air-handling systems in the work site and the surrounding areas to ensure that dust and spores are not disseminated through the facility via air currents
- Ventilation of construction areas so they are at negative pressure to surrounding critical areas such as patient care units and clean and sterile supply rooms.

OUTBREAKS AND PSEUDO-OUTBREAKS ASSOCIATED WITH A WATER RESERVOIR

Many outbreaks and pseudo-outbreaks in inpatient and outpatient health-care settings have been traced to a water reservoir,[356–367] including potable or drinking water, ice and ice machines, toilet water, and warm-water and sonicator baths. Table 3–6 lists several examples. Whenever outbreaks or pseudo-outbreaks are caused by nontuberculous mycobacteria or *Legionella, Pseudomonas, Flavobacterium*, or *Acinetobacter* species, an aqueous reservoir should be suspected.

For additional information on waterborne infection risks for hospitalized patients, the reader is referred to the review article by Emmerson.[368]

Potable Water

Nontuberculous mycobacteria are commonly found in municipal water supplies and are frequent causes of pseudo-outbreaks. Sniadeck et al. described an outbreak of *Mycobacterium xenopi* pseudo-infections that occurred in 13 patients over a 1-year period.[363] Acid-fast bacilli smears were negative, and only a few colonies of the organism were isolated from each of the specimens (six sputa, two bronchial washings, four urines, and one stool). None of the patients had disease that was compatible with *M. xenopi* infection. The source of the organism was believed to be the hospital's potable water system, which contaminated the specimens at the time of collection. A review of specimen collection and instrument disinfection procedures revealed the following:

1. Tap water was used to rinse a patient's mouth just prior to collecting a sputum specimen.
2. Tap water was used as a final rinse after cold sterilization of bronchoscopes.
3. Urine for mycobacterial culture was occasionally collected in previously used bedpans that had been rinsed with tap water.
4. Tap water was used for colonic irrigation.

This report highlights the need to instruct personnel to collect specimens for culture carefully in order to minimize microbial contamination, and to avoid using tap water as a final rinse when cleaning and disinfecting bronchoscopes.

Copepods and nonpathogenic freshwater microorganisms present in hospital drinking water have caused pseudo-outbreaks.[364,365] Copepods are small animals, such as *Cyclops*, that are the intermediate hosts of animal parasites of humans (e.g., the guinea worm, *Dracunculus medinensis*, and the fish tapeworm, *Diphyllobothrium latum*).

Ice

Contaminated ice machines and ice baths used to cool medical devices such as syringes have been responsible for nosocomial outbreaks.[356] An outbreak of bacteremia caused by *Flavobacterium* species was traced to syringes that were cooled in ice from the ice machine in an ICU before being used to collect arterial specimens for blood gas determination.[357] Guidelines for minimizing the

Table 3–6   Outbreaks and Pseudo-Outbreaks Associated with a Water Reservoir

Outbreak	Reservoir	Source	Year Reported/ Reference No.
Flavobacterium septicemia	Hospital potable water	Syringes cooled in ice from ice machine in intensive care unit	1975 (357)
Pseudomonas septicemia	Hospital potable water	Contaminated water bath in the operating room used to thaw fresh-frozen plasma	1981 (358)
Pseudomonas aeruginosa wound infections	Water in physical therapy department	Contaminated Hubbard tank; associated with discontinuation of using bleach to disinfect tank	1981 (359)
Mycobacterium chelonae infections	Water supply in outpatient hemo-dialysis center	Hemodialyzers that were manually reprocessed using Renalin germicide	1990 (360)
Pseudomonas pickettii bacteremia	Distilled water	Distilled water used by employee to replace Fen-tanyl during narcotic theft	1991 (48)
Gram-negative bacteremia	Hospital potable water	Pressure monitoring equip-ment left open and uncovered overnight in the operating room contaminated by house-keeping personnel who sprayed a water-disinfectant mixture when cleaning	1996 (115)
Legionellosis (one case prompted an investigation)	Hospital potable water	Contaminated ice machine	1997 (361)
Pseudo-outbreak of Pseudomonas aeruginosa	Water in hospital toilet	Fecal specimens for surveillance cultures were collected from the toilet	1997 (362)
Mycobacterium simiae colonization and one possible infection	Hospital potable water	M. simiae was recovered from hospital tap water, patients' home showers, and well supplying the hospital water	2004 (367)

risk of transmission of infectious agents by ice and ice machines have been published by the CDC[89,369] and by Burnett et al.[370]

Water Baths

Warm-water baths have frequently served as the source of outbreaks.[356] Organisms present in water baths used to thaw blood components and peritoneal dialysis solutions can easily contaminate the outer surfaces of these items and can enter the container when it is opened or punctured. Items being thawed in water baths should be placed in an impermeable plastic wrapper to avoid contamination. Alternatively, peritoneal dialysis fluid can be warmed by using a dry-heat source or a microwave oven.

OUTBREAKS OF NOSOCOMIAL PNEUMONIA IN INTENSIVE CARE UNITS

Although most nosocomial pneumonias (NPs) arise from aspiration of endogenous oropharyngeal or gastric flora, outbreaks of NP in ICUs have been caused by exogenously acquired organisms.[27,371] Outbreaks of NP can be caused by a variety of bacteria, viruses, and fungi. Organisms causing NP can be transmitted by person-to-person contact or by healthcare workers or other patients through contact with contaminated respiratory therapy devices and equipment.[27,371-378] Examples of NP outbreaks in ICUs that were spread by contact are shown in Table 3–7. Control measures used to interrupt transmission of the pathogens are also shown.

Most outbreaks of NP that are spread by cross-infection can be controlled by implementation of routine infection prevention and control practices, such as contact isolation precautions, appropriate use of gloves and hand hygiene, and intensive surveillance.[371] It is often difficult to recognize clusters and outbreaks that are caused by common pathogens, such as *S. aureus*, because these organisms may be causing endemic infections. However, outbreaks caused by unusual gram-negative organisms, such as *Burkholderia* (formerly *Pseudomonas*) *cepacia* and *Stenotrophomonas* (formerly *Xanthomonas*) *maltophilia*, are more likely to be detected because these isolates are more likely to be noticed.

Outbreaks associated with bronchoscopy and respiratory therapy solutions and equipment, such as albuterol, mechanical ventilator circuits, and nebulizers, have been discussed previously in this chapter. Most of these outbreaks can be prevented by routine use of aseptic technique when handling fluids and by adherence to proper cleaning, disinfection, and sterilization protocols for devices and equipment.

Outbreaks of *Legionella* and *Aspergillus* pneumonia associated with environmental reservoirs have occurred in ICU patients.[345,371,377-382] Control measures for these outbreaks depend on the specific reservoir and source of the organism, as outlined in Table 3–8. Information on outbreaks caused by these two pathogens was given in a previous section of this chapter.

For a comprehensive review of outbreaks of nosocomial pneumonia reported in ICU patients, including a discussion of the steps used to investigate an outbreak of NP, the reader is referred to the article by Maloney and Jarvis.[371] The CDC *Guidelines for Preventing Health Care-Associated Pneumonia* provide information on the etiology, epidemiology, pathogenesis, diagnosis, risk factors, and control measures for preventing NP.[27] They include guidelines for conducting outbreak investigations for specific pathogens. Control measures recommended by the CDC include staff education on basic infection prevention and control practices, infection surveillance, sterilization or disinfection and

Table 3–7 Reported Epidemics of Nosocomial Pneumonia (NP) in Intensive Care Unit Patients Spread by Contact Transmission, 1982–1993

Pathogen	Author (Reference No.)	Year	Study Population	Number of Patients with NP/ Colonization	Risk Factors	Patients/ Personnel	Respiratory Equipment	Control Measures*
Branhamella catarrhalis	Patterson et al[372]	1988	Intermediate care unit	8/2	Respiratory therapy Steroid use Ward location	X		1, 2, 5, 7
Influenza A virus	Centers for Disease Control[373]	1988	Med/Surg ICU**	3/NA*	NA			5
Methicillin-resistant Staphylococcus aureus	Locksley et al.[374]	1982	Hospital-wide	15/1	Mechanical ventilation ICU/ burn ward	X		1, 3, 5, 7, 8
Parainfluenza virus	Singh-Naz et al.[375]	1990	Intermediate ICN**	6/1	NA	X		1, 2, 3, 5
Pseudomonas cepacia	Weems[113]	1993	General ICU	NA/120	Mechanical ventilation Respiratory therapy		X	6
	Conly et al.[116]	1986	Medical ICU, surgical ICU	4/21	Mechanical ventilation Antimicrobial therapy	X	X	3, 4, 6
Respiratory syncytial virus and rhinovirus	Valenti et al.[297]	1982	NICU/SCN**	7/1	Endotracheal or nasogastric intubation Mechanical ventilation	X		1, 3
Xanthomonas maltophilia	Villarino et al.[376]	1992	CCU**, Trauma ICU, Med/Surg ICU	42/0	Trauma ICU Mechanical ventilation Antimicrobial therapy	X	X	1, 3, 4, 5, 6

NOTE: *Control measures: 1 = isolation precautions; 2 = cohorting of infected patients; 3 = appropriate hand washing and glove use; 4 = staff education; 5 = prospective surveillance; 6 = high-level disinfection and sterile water for respiratory equipment; 7 = appropriate antimicrobial therapy; 8 = treatment of carrier state.
**Med/Surg = medical and surgical; ICU = intensive care unit; NA = not available; ICN = intensive care nursery; NICU/SCN = neonatal intensive care and special care nursery; CCU = critical care unit.
Source: Reprinted from Maloney SA, Jarvis WR. Epidemic nosocomial pneumonia in the intensive care unit. *Chest.* 1995; 16:213.

proper handling of medical equipment and devices, installation and maintenance of special ventilation systems for patients at high risk for aspergillosis, and isolation precautions for patients with known or suspected infection.[27]

For a discussion of outbreaks of pneumonia and other infections that have been reported in neonatal intensive care units, the reader is referred to the review by Gastmeier et al.[385]

OUTBREAKS OF SICK BUILDING SYNDROME AND BUILDING-RELATED ILLNESS

Much has been published on "sick building syndrome" and indoor air pollution;[386–392] however, little has been published regarding noninfectious episodes of building-associated illnesses in healthcare facilities.[388,389,393,394] In one review of indoor air pollution, building-associated illnesses were linked to inadequate ventilation in approximately half of the cases studied, and in many cases no causal factor was found.[387] Brandt-Rauf et al. described an outbreak of eye and respiratory tract irritation in operating room personnel.[388] The outbreak was attributed to emergency generator diesel exhaust emissions that entered the ventilation system for the operating room suite; however, personnel continued to complain of symptoms after this problem was rectified and a definitive etiology for the ongoing symptoms was not identified.[388] There are also several reports of outbreaks of illness, including headache, nausea, and vomiting, in hospital personnel that were traced to vapors of xylene that had been disposed of down a drain.[393,394]

Hospital personnel in infection control, employee health, and safety management are frequently called upon to investigate clusters of complaints of symptoms and illnesses by healthcare personnel, who often attribute the problems to exposure to some factor in the workplace. Infection prevention and control personnel who are asked to investigate such incidents should follow the epidemiologic principles used to investigate outbreaks of infection and other conditions as outlined in Chapter 8. In many cases of building-related complaints, it is difficult to determine if symptoms are truly a result of building-related exposures. A review article on indoor air pollution by Gold provides helpful information that can be used when evaluating building-related complaints, and Gold suggests that the following questions be asked:[389]

1. Is the building tight?
2. Are there any significant levels of indoor air pollutants?
3. What is the overall prevalence of symptoms?
4. Are the symptoms clustered in any one work area?

When investigating building-related complaints, it is helpful to evaluate the following:

1. The work exposure histories of the personnel involved, such as exposure to chemicals, paint fumes, exhaust fumes from nearby vehicles, photocopying machines, volatile organic substances from new carpets, or mold spores from wet carpets
2. The time of day that the symptoms occur(red)

Table 3-8 Outbreaks of NP Associated with Specific Environmental Reservoirs, 1978–1994

Pathogen	Author (Reference)	Year	Study Population	Number of Patients with NP	Risk Factors	Reservoir	Source	Control Measures*
Legionella species	Fisher-Hoch et al. (377)	1981	General hospital	11	Immunosuppression; Admission to new building	Water supply and cooling system	Tap water; cooling tower	1,3
	Arnow et al. (378)	1982	General hospital	5	Immunosuppressive therapy; Jet nebulizer use	Water supply	Respiratory equipment	2,3
	Brady (379)	1988	Pediatric hospital	7	Immunosuppressive therapy; chronic lung/kidney disease	Water supply	Showers Respiratory equipment	2,4, and appropriate antimicrobial therapy
	Mastro et al. (380)	1991	General hospital	13	Chronic lung disease; Jet nebulizer use; >3 days in ICU	Water supply	Respiratory equipment	1,2
	Blatt et al. (381)	1993	Military hospital	14	Immunosuppressive therapy; nasogastric tube use; antimicrobial therapy; bed bathing	Water supply	Tap water	2.3
Aspergillus species	Arnow et al. (345)	1978	Renal unit transplantation	2	Immunosuppressive therapy; proximity to construction	Construction	Surface dust	7,,8
	Weems et al. (382)	1987	Pediatric hospital	5	Hematologic malignancy; construction activity	Construction	NA	7,8
	Arnow et al. (383)	1991	General hospital	29	Malignancy; hematology/oncology ward	Ventilation system	Ventilator filters Surface dust	5,6
	Buffington et al. (384)	1994	Pediatric hospital	7	Hematologic malignancy; construction activity	Construction	NA	5,7,8

NOTE: *Control measures: 1 = hyperchlorination and superheating of hospital water supply; 2 = sterile water for rinsing and use in respiratory equipment; 3 = prospective surveillance; 4 = staff education and shower prohibition; 5 = aggressive hospital cleaning and inspection; 6 = retrofitting of ventilation system; 7 = impermeable barriers around construction site; 8 = relocation of immunocompromised patients.
NA = not available

Source: Reprinted from Maloney SA, Jarvis WR. Epidemic nosocomial pneumonia in the intensive care unit. *Chest.* 1995;16:216.

3. The time of day that exposure(s) to possible pollutants occur(red)

4. The temporal relationship between time of exposure and onset of symptoms

5. The relationship of symptoms at and away from work; for instance, do symptoms subside on weekends or when employees are away from the workplace?

6. Physical factors, such as poor lighting

7. Psychological factors, such as job dissatisfaction, especially if no other causative factors can be found.

It is important that employers listen to, and address, the concerns of personnel and demonstrate a genuine effort to identify the cause and implement corrective measures. Such support will encourage employee productivity and workplace satisfaction and will reduce the risk of legal or regulatory actions taken by personnel against the employer.

The American College of Occupational and Environmental Medicine published an evidenced-based statement on the adverse human health effects associated with molds in the indoor environment; this is available from the *Journal of Occupational and Environmental Medicine*.[393]

NEWLY RECOGNIZED AGENTS AND SOURCES FOR HEALTHCARE-ASSOCIATED OUTBREAKS

Candida Species

Epidemiology

The *Candida* species emerged in the 1980s as an important cause of nosocomial infection in severely ill and immunocompromised patients.[396–400] The most commonly reported *Candida* species causing infection in humans are *C. albicans, C. tropicalis, C. (Torulopsis) glabrata, C. parapsilosis, C. krusei*, and *C. lusitaniae*.[396,397] Risk factors for nosocomial candidiasis include intravenous therapy (especially TPN), exposure to antibiotics, and neutropenia.[396,398,399] Although most *Candida* infections arise from a patient's endogenous flora, nosocomial transmission via contaminated intravenous fluids and medical devices and the hands of personnel has been documented.[198–200,396,398–404]

Although many reported clusters and outbreaks of *Candida* species have no identified source,[402] outbreaks have been associated with TPN,[405,406] intravenous blood pressure-monitoring devices,[407] and personnel carriers.[198–200,402,404] *Candida* species are important pathogens in NICUs. Studies demonstrate that *Candida* can be acquired by the neonate either vertically from the mother or horizontally (nosocomial) in an NICU[401–403,405] and that a mother can carry different strains of *Candida albicans* at different body sites.[403] Studies show that TPN fluids can promote growth of *Candida* species and may serve as a reservoir for infection.[405] In one NICU, an outbreak of *Candida* bloodstream infections caused by *C. albicans, C. parapsilosis*, and *C. tropicalis* was associated with a contaminated retrograde medication administration system used for TPN.[405]

Control Measures

Further epidemiologic studies are needed to identify and investigate common source outbreaks, nosocomial clusters, and instances of person-to-person transmission of *Candida* species so that the reservoirs and the modes of transmission for exogenously acquired candidiasis can be clarified.[403–408] Since little is known about the epidemiology of nosocomial *Candida* infections acquired from exogenous sources, it is difficult to identify control measures that can be used to interrupt transmission. Based on a review of the reports noted in this section, the following measures can be recommended to prevent the nosocomial spread of *Candida* species, to interrupt an outbreak, and to identify a possible cause of an outbreak:

- Since several investigators have associated outbreaks with transmission by personnel,[198–200] and since hand carriage of *Candida* species by health-care workers has been documented,[404,409] careful hand hygiene should be practiced before and after patient care, especially when caring for neonates, severely ill patients, and immunocompromised patients, and before handling intravenous solutions and related equipment. If an outbreak is suspected, personnel should be reminded of the importance of proper hand hygiene.

- Since *Candida* outbreaks have been associated with TPN[405,406] and intravenous blood pressure-monitoring devices,[407] personnel preparing and administering intravenous solutions, especially TPN, should be taught proper aseptic technique. If an outbreak is suspected, personnel practices should be observed to ensure that aseptic technique is being used.

- If a cluster or suspected increase in *Candida* infections occurs, an epidemiologic investigation should be conducted to verify the existence of an outbreak and to identify potential sources and modes of transmission as discussed in Chapter 8. If an outbreak is suspected, the laboratory should be requested to save isolates from patients for possible typing.

- If an epidemiologic investigation suggests an outbreak, control measures should be implemented based on the potential sources and possible modes of transmission identified.

- If initial control measures do not prevent transmission, culture surveys of patients, personnel, or an implicated source may be considered, based on the findings of the epidemiologic investigation; however, cultures should not be done unless the laboratory is involved in planning the specimen collection process and unless molecular typing will be done to determine the relatedness of any strains of *Candida* that are isolated.

- Because of the risk of contamination of retrograde medication administration systems, facilities using these systems need to evaluate carefully the practices used to maintain them.[405]

- Because clusters of *Candida* infections may be caused by more than one strain of *Candida*, laboratory typing methods must be chosen and interpreted carefully in conjunction with observational epidemiologic data.[410]

Identifying New Risk Factors and Sources for Infection

Emerging infectious diseases are considered to be those in which the incidence in humans increased since the 1970s or threatens to increase in the near future.[411,412] It is sobering to note that many of the diseases discussed in this text are considered emerging, or reemerging, infectious diseases, such as LD, candidiasis, cryptosporidiosis, acquired immune deficiency syndrome, HBV and HCV, and infections caused by MRSA, VRE, MDR-TB, *Clostridium difficile*, human parvovirus B19, norovirus, rotavirus, and *Pneumocystis carinii*. Two additional organisms that recently have been identified as causative agents in nosocomial outbreaks are *Escherichia coli O157:H7* and *Helicobacter pylori*.[413] Weber and Rutala noted that "The reasons for the emergence of new nosocomial pathogens include enhanced survival of immunocompromised hosts, acquisition and spread of adaptive genes (i.e., antibiotic resistance and virulence genes), enhanced ability to survive in new ecologic niches, increasing use of invasive procedures, unrecognized virulence, prior underidentification due to difficulties inculturing, and increased recognition due to taxonomic clarification."[413(p306)]

In 1998 the CDC published *Preventing Emerging Infectious Diseases: A Strategy for the 21st Century*, a plan to combat infectious diseases.[412] One of the objectives of this plan is to "identify the behaviors, environments, and host factors that put people at increased risk for infectious diseases and their sequelae."[412(p29)] Table 3–9 shows examples of new risk factors and sources for infections that were identified by CDC investigators from 1994 to 1998.[414–417] Four of the five examples given involve outbreaks of infections acquired as a result of healthcare activities in acute and home care settings. Exhibit 3–3 demonstrates an area for risk factor research that was identified by the CDC investigators: the relationship between healthcare practices and bloodstream infection rates in the acute and home care settings.[415,418–421]

Additional new and reemerging risks and organisms responsible for healthcare-associated outbreaks and pseudo-outbreaks in the early 2000s include the following:

- Biofilm formation on medical devices such as gastrointestinal endoscopes, bronchoscopes, and respiratory therapy devices that can inhibit the ability of disinfectants to destroy microorganisms, make these devices difficult to clean and disinfect, and result in the growth of organisms that can be transferred to patients[73,422,423]

- The use of probiotics (biotherapeutic agents) and the demonstration that organisms such as *Saccharomyces cerevisiae* that are used in probiotics can be transmitted to untreated patients in the same unit as a patient that is treated with a biotherapeutic preparation[424]

- *Pantoea agglomerans* (formerly *Erwniia herbicola* then *Enterobacter agglomerans*)[425–428]

- A large multistate outbreak of mumps in the United States in 2006 that resulted in infections in healthcare workers[429]

- The role of the environment and environmental surfaces in the transmission of pathogens in outbreaks[89,430,431]

Table 3–9   Examples of New Risk Factors and Sources for Infection Identified by CDC Investigations, 1994–1998

Outbreak investigations provide some of the most important opportunities for identifying risk factors for disease. The investigations described below were conducted in collaboration with many partners in state and local health departments, other federal agencies, and other organizations.

Year	Location	Problem	Finding	Implications
1994	United States	Hepatitis C[414]	Strong association with particular lots of intravenous (IV) immunoglobulin from one company	Led to requirements for viral inactivation steps and new testing procedures to ensure safety of IV and intramuscular immunoglobulin products
1994	Rhode Island	Bloodstream infections (BSIs)[415]	BSIs associated with use of inoculation devices. Findings led to CDC recommendations on the use and management of needleless devices.	First outbreak to link these devices with adverse outcomes in patients
1995	Democratic Republic of Congo	Ebola infection[416]	Transmission linked to direct contact with ill patients	No evidence of airborne transmission. Led to updating of policies for managing patients with viral hemorrhagic fever in the United States.
1996	Indiana	Vancomycin-resistant Enterococci[417]	Illness linked to prior use of antibiotics. Implementation of control measures reduced transmission	Highlighted rapid spread of this strain in the United States. Also showed feasibility and effectiveness of control measures to reduce the spread of antibiotic-resistant organisms in hospitals.
1997 –1998	New York	HIV	Cluster of cases of HIV infection in women who had sex with one HIV-positive man	HIV detection and prevention programs need to be strengthened in rural communities.

Source: Reprinted from Centers for Disease Control and Prevention. *Preventing Emerging Infectious Diseases: A Strategy for the 21st Century.* U.S. Department of Health and Human Services; 1998:30. http://www.cdc.gov/mmwr/preview/mmwrhtml/00031393.htm.

Exhibit 3–3   Bloodstream Infections in ICU and Home Healthcare Patients

Since 1993, CDC has investigated three outbreaks of bloodstream infection (BSI)[417,418] among patients in intensive care units (ICUs) that were associated with decreases in nurse-to-patient ratios. In each of these outbreaks, rates of BSI increased when the number of healthcare workers per patient decreased or when the level of training of those workers decreased. The epidemiologic relationship between nursing staff numbers and training levels and the rates of BSIs remained significant even after controlling for other factors.

Since that time, CDC has also investigated three outbreaks of BSIs among patients receiving home infusion therapy.[415,420,421] Risk factors for these outbreaks include practices related to care of the intravenous line, the use of particular types of intravenous devices, and socioeconomic factors. Interventions that involve teaching and training home healthcare providers and families of home care patients are being evaluated.

Source: Reprinted from Centers for Disease Control and Prevention. *Preventing Emerging Infectious Diseases: A Strategy for the 21st Century.* U.S. Department of Health and Human Services; 1988:31. http://www.cdc.gov/mmwr/preview/mmwrhtml/00031393.htm.

THE IMPORTANCE OF PERSONNEL AND EMPLOYEE HEALTH

Because healthcare workers (including employees, physicians, volunteers, and students) play an important role in initiating and propagating outbreaks in healthcare settings, each facility should have policies and procedures that address personnel health and include hand hygiene and personal hygiene, standard precautions, immunization, and work restrictions for certain infectious diseases. Because many outbreaks involve vaccine-preventable diseases, ICPs should ensure that the latest recommendations for healthcare worker immunization are implemented in their facility and that efforts are made to increase immunization rates in healthcare personnel.[254,259,271,315,316,324,432–434] Because immunization recommendations are frequently revised, those who are developing personnel policies should identify the latest public health recommendations on preventing diseases such as pertussis, influenza, varicella, hepatitis B, measles, mumps and rubella, and refer to the Healthcare Infection Control Practice Advisory Committee (HICPAC) guideline for infection control in healthcare personnel.[25] Appendix D contains a list of the immunizations recommended for healthcare personnel and provides the *MMWR* issue and an Internet address for the ACIP guidelines for each of the vaccines. The HICPAC summary of recommended work restrictions for personnel can be found in Appendix E.

SUMMARY

Outbreaks in acute care and other healthcare settings are caused by a variety of infectious and noninfectious agents. New, emerging and well-known pathogens will continue to evolve and present a challenge to ICPs, clinicians, and healthcare providers. Infection surveillance, prevention, and control programs in hospitals play an integral role in identifying the occurrence of infectious diseases and their risk factors, modes of transmission, and sources so that effective prevention and control measures can be identified and implemented.

REFERENCES

1. LaForce FM. The control of infections in hospitals: 1750 to 1950. In: Wenzel RP, ed. *Prevention and Control of Nosocomial Infections.* Baltimore, MD: Williams & Wilkins; 1987:1–12.

2. Stamm WE, Weinstein RA, Dixon RE. Comparison of endemic and epidemic nosocomial infections. *Am J Med.* 1981;70:393–397.

3. Haley RW, Tenney JH, Lindsey JO, Garner JS, Bennett J. How frequent are outbreaks of nosocomial infection in community hospitals? *Infect Control.* 1985;6:233–236.

4. Jarvis WR, and the Epidemiology Branch, Hospital Infections Program, Centers for Disease Control. Nosocomial outbreaks: the Centers for Disease Control's hospital infections program experience; 1980–1990. *Am J Med.* 1991;91:3B–101S–3B–106S.

5. Beck-Sague C, Jarvis W, Martone WJ. Outbreak investigations. *Infect Control Hosp Epidemiol.* 1997;18:138–145.

6. Jackson M, Fierer J. Infections and infection risk in residents of long-term care facilities: a review of the literature; 1970–1984. *Am J Infect Control.* 1985;13:63–77.

7. Nicolle LE, Garibaldi RA. Infection control in long-term-care facilities. *Infect Control Hosp Epidemiol.* 1995;16:348–353.

8. Smith P, Rusnak PG. Infection prevention and control in the long-term-care facility. *Am J Infect Control.* 1997;25:488–512.

9. Herwaldt LA, Smith SD, Carter CD. Infection control in the outpatient setting. *Infect Control Hosp Epidemiol.* 1998;19:41–74.

10. Wenzel RP, Thompson RL, Landry SM, et al. Hospital-acquired infections in intensive care unit patients: an overview with emphasis on epidemics. *Infect Control.* 1983;4:371–375.

11. Beck-Sague C, Dooley SW, Hutton MD, et al. Outbreak of multidrug-resistant *Mycobacterium tuberculosis* infections in a hospital: transmission to patients with HIV infection and staff. *JAMA.* 1992;268:1280–1286.

12. Boyle JF, Soumakis SA, Rendo A, et al. Epidemiologic analysis and genotypic characterization of a nosocomial outbreak of vancomycin-resistant enterococci. *J Clin Microbiol.* 1993;31:1280–1285.

13. Edmond MB, Wenzel RP, Pasculle W. Vancomycin-resistant *Staphylococcus aureus*: perspectives on measures needed for control. *Ann Intern Med.* 1996;124:329–334.

14. McFarland LV, Beneda HW, Clarridge JE, Raugi GJ. Implications of the changing face of *Clostridium difficile* disease for health care practitioners. *Am J Infect Control.* 2007;35:237–253.

15. Luna CM, Aruj PK. Nosocomial *Acinetobacter* pneumonia. *Respirology.* 2007;12(6):787–791.

16. Paauw A, Verhoef J, Fluit AC, et al. Failure to control an outbreak of qnrA1-positive multidrug-resistant *Enterobacter cloacae* infection despite adequate implementation of recommended infection control measures. *J Clin Microbiol.* 2007;45(5):1420–1425.

17. Wenger P, Tokars J, Brennan P, et al. An outbreak of *Enterobacter hormaechi* infection and colonization in an intensive care nursery. *Clin Infect Dis.* 1997;24:1243–1244.

18. Lederberg J, Shope R, Oaks S, eds. *Emerging Infections: Microbial Threats to Health in the United States.* Washington, DC: National Academy Press; 1992:36-41. http://www.nap.edu/catalog.php?record_id=2008. Accessed April 21, 2008.

19. Centers for Disease Control and Prevention. *Addressing Emerging Infectious Disease Threats: A Prevention Strategy for the United States.* US Dept of Health and Human Services; 1994. http://www.cdc.gov/mmwr/preview/mmwrhtml/00031393.htm. Accessed April 21, 2008.

20. Ostroff SM. Emerging infectious diseases in the institutional setting: another hot zone. *Infect Control Hosp Epidemiol.* 1996;17:484–489.

21. Merrell DS, Falkow S. Frontal and stealth attack strategies in microbial pathogenesis. *Nature*. 2004;430:250–256.

22. Smolinski MS, Hamburg MA, Lederberg J., eds. *Microbial Threats to Health: Emergence, Detection, and Response*. Executive Summary. Washington, DC: National Academies Press; 2003;1. http://www.nap.edu/catalog.php?record_id=10636. Accessed April 21, 2008.

23. Peiris JSM, Guan Y. Confronting SARS: a view from Hong Kong. *Philos Trans R Soc Lond B Biol Sci*. 2004;29;359:1075–1079. http://www.pubmedcentral.nih.gov/articlerender.fcgi?artid=1693390. Accessed April 21, 2008.

24. Heymann DL. *Control of Communicable Diseases Manual*. 18th ed. Washington, DC: APHA Press; 2005.

25. Bolyard EA, Tablan OC, Williams WW, et al. Guideline for infection control in health care personnel; 1998. *Am J Infect Control*. 1998;26:289–354. http://www.cdc.gov/ncidod/dhqp/gl_hcpersonnel.html. Accessed April 19, 2008.

26. Siegel JD, Rhinehart E, Jackson M, Chiarello L, and the Healthcare Infection Control Practices Advisory Committee. *Guideline for Isolation Precautions: Preventing Transmission of Infectious Agents in Healthcare Settings*. Atlanta, GA: CDC; June 2007. http://www.cdc.gov/ncidod/dhqp/gl_isolation.html. Accessed November 25, 2007.

27. Centers for Disease Control and Prevention. *Guidelines for Preventing Health-Care-Associated Pneumonia. Recommendations of CDC and the Healthcare Infection Control Practices Advisory Committee*. http://www.cdc.gov/ncidod/dhqp/gl_hcpneumonia.html. Accessed April 19, 2008.

28. Maki DG, Rhame FS, Mackel DC, Bennett JV. Nationwide epidemic of septicemia caused by contaminated intravenous products, I: epidemiologic and clinical features. *Am J Med*. 1976;60:471–485.

29. Centers for Disease Control and Prevention. Epidemiologic notes and reports: nosocomial bacteremias associated with intravenous fluid therapy—USA. *MMWR*. 1996;46:1227–1233.

30. Goldmann DA, Dixon RE, Fulkerson CC, et al. The role of nationwide infection surveillance in detecting epidemic bacteremia due to contaminated intravenous fluids. *Am J Epidemiol*. 1978;108:207–213.

31. Kaslow RA, Mackel DC, Mallison GF. Nosocomial pseudo-bacteremia: positive blood cultures due to contaminated benzalkonium chloride antiseptic. *JAMA*. 1976;236:2407–2409.

32. Wysowski DK, Flynt JW Jr, Goldfield M, Altman R, Davis AT. Epidemic neonatal hyperbilirubinemia and use of a phenolic disinfectant detergent. *Pediatr*. 1978;61:165–167.

33. Berkelman RL, Lewin S, Allen JR, et al. Pseudobacteremia attributed to contamination of povidone-iodine with *Pseudomonas cepacia*. *Ann Intern Med*. 1981;95:32–36.

34. Panlilio AL, Beck-Sague CM, Siegel JD, et al. Infections and pseudoinfections due to povidone-iodine solution contaminated with *Pseudomonas cepacia*. *Clin Infect Dis*. 1992;14:1078–1083.

35. Sharbaugh RJ. Suspected outbreak of endotoxemia associated with computerized axial tomography. *Am J Infect Control*. 1980;8:26–28.

36. Cleary TJ, MacIntyre DS, Castro M. *Serratia marcescens* bacteremias in an intensive care unit. *Am J Infect Control*. 1981;9:107–111.

37. Bryce EA, Walker M, Scharf S, et al. An outbreak of cutaneous aspergillosis in a tertiary-care hospital. *Infect Control Hosp Epidemiol*. 1996;17:170–172.

38. Parrott PL, Terry PM, Whitworth EN, et al. *Pseudomonas aeruginosa* peritonitis associated with contaminated poloxamer-iodine solution. *Lancet*. 1982;2:683–685.

39. Martone WJ, Williams WW, Mortensen ML, et al. Illness with fatalities in premature infants: association with intravenous vitamin E preparation, E-Ferol. *Pediatr*. 1986;78:591–600.

40. Safranek TJ, Jarvis WR, Carson LA, et al. *Mycobacterium chelonae* wound infections after plastic surgery employing contaminated gentian violet skin-marking solution. *N Engl J Med*. 1987;317:197–201.

41. Nakashima AK, McCarthy MA, Martone WJ, Anderson RL. Epidemic septic arthritis caused by *Serratia marcescens* and associated with a benzalkonium chloride antiseptic. *J Clin Microbiol*. 1987;25:1014–1018.

42. Centers for Disease Control and Prevention. *Yersinia enterocolitica* bacteremia and endotoxin shock associated with red blood cell transfusion-United States; 1987–1988. *MMWR.* 1988;37:577–578.

43. Centers for Disease Control and Prevention. Red blood cell transfusions contaminated with *Yersinia enterocolitica*—United States; 1991–1996, and initiation of a national study to detect bacteria-associated transfusion reactions. *MMWR.* 1997;46:553–556.

44. Chodick G, Ashkenazi S, Lerman Y. The risk of hepatitis A infection among healthcare workers: a review of reported outbreaks and sero-epidemiologic studies. *J Hosp Infect.* 2006;62:414–420.

45. Centers for Disease Control and Prevention Postsurgical infections associated with an extrinsically contaminated intravenous anesthetic agent—California, Illinois, Maine, and Michigan; 1990. *MMWR.* 1990;39:426–427, 433.

46. Bennett SN, McNeil MM, Bland LA, et al. Postoperative infections traced to contamination of an intravenous anesthetic, propofol. *N Engl J Med.* 1995;333:147–154.

47. Kuehnert MJ, Webb RM, Jochimsen EM, et al. *Staphylococcus aureus* bloodstream infections among patients undergoing electroconvulsive therapy traced to breaks in infection control and possible extrinsic contamination by propofol. *Anesth Analg.* 1997;85:420–425.

48. Maki DG, Klein BS, McCormick R, et al. Nosocomial *Pseudomonas pickettii* bacteremias traced to narcotic tampering. *JAMA.* 1991;265:981–986.

49. Centers for Disease Control and Prevention. Outbreak of hepatitis C associated with intravenous immunoglobulin administration—United States; October 1993–June 1994. *MMWR.* 1994;43:505–509.

50. Hamill RJ, Houston ED, Georghiou PR, et al. An outbreak of *Burkholderia cepacia* respiratory tract colonization and infection associated with nebulized albuterol therapy. *Ann Intern Med.* 1995;122:762–766.

51. Reboli AC, Koshinski R, Arias K, et al. An outbreak of *Burkholderia cepacia* lower respiratory tract infection associated with contaminated albuterol nebulization solution. *Infect Control Hosp Epidemiol.* 1996;17:741–743.

52. Trilla A, Codina C, Salles M, et al. A cluster of fever and hypotension on a surgical intensive care unit related to the contamination of plasma expanders by cell wall products of *Bacillus stearothermophilus*. *Infect Control Hosp Epidemiol.* 1995;16:335–339.

53. File TM, Tan JS, Thomson RB, et al. An outbreak of *Pseudomonas aeruginosa* ventilator-associated respiratory infections due to contaminated food coloring dye—further evidence of the significance of gastric colonization proceeding nosocomial pneumonia. *Infect Control Hosp Epidemiol.* 1995;16:417–418.

54. Anglim AM, Collmer JE, Loving J, et al. An outbreak of needlestick injuries in hospital employees due to needles piercing infectious waste containers. *Infect Control Hosp Epidemiol.* 1995;16:570–576.

55. Larkin JA, Greene JN, Sandin RL, Houston SH. Primary cutaneous aspergillosis: case report and review of the literature. *Infect Control Hosp Epidemiol.* 1996;17:365–366.

56. Orth B, Frei R, Itin PH, et al. Outbreak of invasive mycoses caused by *Paecilomyces lilacinus* from a contaminated skin lotion. *Ann Intern Med.* 1996;125:799–806.

57. Shay DK, Fann LM, Jarvis WR. Respiratory distress and sudden death associated with receipt of a peripheral parenteral nutrition admixture. *Infect Control Hosp Epidemiol.* 1997;18:814–817.

58. Archibald LK, Shah B, Schulte M, et al. *Serratia marcescens* outbreak associated with extrinsic contamination of 1% chloroxylenol soap. *Infect Control Hosp Epidemiol.* 1997;18:704–709.

59. Chetoui H, Melin P, Struelens MJ, et al. Comparison of biotyping, ribotyping, and pulsed-field gel electrophoresis for investigation of a common-source outbreak of *Burkholderia pickettii* bacteremia. *J Clin Microbiol.* 1997;35:1398–1403.

60. Mangram AJ, Archibald LK, Hupert M, et al. Outbreak of sterile peritonitis among continuous cycling peritoneal dialysis patients. *Kidney Int.* 1998;54:1367–1371. http://www.nature.com/ki/journal/v54/n4/full/4490374a.html. Accessed April 14, 2008.

61. Van Laer F, Raes D, Vandamme P, et al. An outbreak of *Burkholderia cepacia* with septicemia on a cardiology ward. *Infect Control Hosp Epidemiol.* 1998;19:112–113.

62. Centers for Disease Control and Prevention. Nosocomial *Ralstonia pickettii* colonization associated with intrinsically contaminated saline solution—Los Angeles, California, 1998. *MMWR.* 1998;47:285–286.

63. Centers for Disease Control and Prevention. Endotoxin-like reactions associated with intravenous gentamicin—California, 1998. *MMWR.* 1998;47:877–880.

64. Centers for Disease Control and Prevention. *Enterobacter cloacae* bloodstream infections associated with contaminated prefilled saline syringes—California, November 1998. *MMWR.* 1998;47:959–960.

65. Centers for Disease Control and Prevention. Nosocomial *Burkholderia cepacia* infection and colonization associated with intrinsically contaminated mouthwash—Arizona, 1996–1998. *MMWR.* 1998;47:926–928.

66. Sautter RL, Mattman LH, Legaspi, RC. *Serratia marcescens* meningitis associated with a contaminated benzalkonium chloride solution. *Infect Control.* 1984;5:223–225.

67. Matrician L, Ange G, Burns S, et al. Outbreak of nosocomial *Burkholderia cepacia* infection and colonization associated with intrinsically contaminated mouthwash. *Infect Control Hosp Epidemiol.* 2000;21:739–741.

68. Centers for Disease Control and Prevention. *Salmonella Oranienburg* Infections Associated with Fruit Salad Served in Health-Care Facilities—Northeastern United States and Canada, 2006. *MMWR.* 2007;56(39);1025–1028. http://www.cdc.gov/mmwR/preview/mmwrhtml/mm5639a3.htm. Accessed April 22, 2008.

69. Sunenshine RH, Tan ET, Terashita DM, et al. A multistate outbreak of *Serratia marcescens* bloodstream infection associated with contaminated intravenous magnesium sulfate from a compounding pharmacy. *Clin Infect Dis.* 2007;45(5):527–533.

70. Buchholz U, Richards C, Murthy R, et al. Pyrogenic reactions associated with single daily dosing of intravenous gentamicin. *Infect Control Hosp Epidemiol.* 2000;21:771–774.

71. Centers for Disease Control and Prevention. *Pseudomonas* bloodstream infections associated with a heparin/saline flush—Missouri, New York, Texas, and Michigan; 2004–2005. *MMWR.* 2005;54:269–72. http://www.cdc.gov/mmwR/preview/mmwrhtml/mm5411a1.htm. Accessed April 22, 2008.

72. Bowen AB, Braden CR. Invasive *Enterobacter sakazakii* disease in infants. *Emerg Infect Dis.* 2006 Aug;12(8):1185–1189. http://www.cdc.gov/ncidod/eid/vol12no08/05–1509.htm. Accessed April 21, 2008.

73. Jhung MA, Sunenshine RH, Noble-Wang J, et al. A national outbreak of *Ralstonia mannitolilytica* associated with use of a contaminated oxygen-delivery device among pediatric patients. *Pediatr.* 2007;119(6):1207–1209.

74. Souza Dias MB, Bernardes Habert A, Borrasca V, et al. Salvage of long-term central venous catheters during an outbreak of *Pseudomonas putida* and *Stenotrophomonas maltophilia* infections associated with contaminated heparin catheter-lock solution. *Infect Control Hosp Epidemiol.* 2008;29:125–130.

75. Centers for Disease Control and Prevention. *Exophiala* infection from contaminated injectable steroids prepared by a compounding pharmacy. *MMWR.* 2002; 51:1109–12. http://www.cdc.gov/mmwR/preview/mmwrhtml/mm5149a1.htm. Accessed April 22, 2008.

76. Civens R, Vugia DJ, Alexander R, et al. Outbreak of *Serratia marcescens* infection following injections of betamethasone compounded at a community pharmacy. *Clin Infect Dis.* 2005; 43:831–837.

77. Centers for Disease Control and Prevention. Acute allergic-type reactions among patients undergoing hemodialysis-multiple states; 2007–2008. *MMWR.* 2008;57(05);124–125. http://www.cdc.gov/mmwR/preview/mmwrhtml/mm5705a4.htm. Accessed April 22, 2008.

78. Molina-Cabrillana J, Bolanos-Rivero M, Alvarez-Leon EE, et al. Intrinsically contaminated alcohol-free mouthwash implicated in a nosocomial outbreak of *Burkholderia cepacia* colonization and infection. *Infect Control Hosp Epidemiol.* 2006;27:1181–1182.

79. Ghazal SS, Al-Mudaimeehg K, Al Fakihi EM, Asery AT. Outbreak of *Burkholderia cepacia* bacteremia in immunocompetent children caused by contaminated nebulized sulbutamol in Saudi Arabia. *Am J Infect Control*. 2006;34:394–398.

80. Hutchinson J, Runge W, Mulvet M, et al. *Burkholderia cepacia* infections associated with intrinsically contaminated ultrasound gel: the role of microbial degradation of parabens. *Infect Control Hosp Epidemiol*. 2004;25(4):291–296.

81. Matsouka DM, Costa SF, Mangini C, et al. A nosocomial outbreak of *Salmonella enteritidis* associated with lyophilized enteral nutrition. *J Hosp Infect*. 2004;58:122–127.

82. Adverse ocular reactions following transfusions—United States; 1997–1998. *MMWR*. 1998;47(03):49–50. http://www.cdc.gov/mmwR/preview/mmwrhtml/00051231.htm. Accessed April 22, 2008.

83. Pegues DA. Improving and enforcing compounding pharmacy practices to protect patients. *Clin Infect Dis*. 2006;43:838–840.

84. Weist K, Wendt C, Petersen LR, Versmold H, Ruden H. An outbreak of pyoderma among neonates caused by ultrasound gel contaminated with methicillin-susceptible *Staphylococcus aureus*. *Infect Control Hosp Epidemiol*. 2000;21:761–764.

85. Pan A, Dolcetti L, Barosi C, et al. An outbreak of *Serratia marcescens* bloodstream infections associated with misuse of drug vials in a surgical ward. *Infect Control Hosp Epidemiol*. 2006;27:79–82.

86. Gaillot O, Maruejouls C, Abachin E, et al. Nosocomial outbreak of *Klebsiella pneumoniae* producing SHV-5 extended-spectrum beta-lactamase, originating from a contaminated ultrasonography coupling gel. *J Clin Microbiol*. 1998;36:1357–1360.

87. Kimura AC, Calvet H, Higa JI, et al. Outbreak of *Ralstonia pickettii* bacteremia in a neonatal intensive care unit. *Pediatr Infect Dis J*. 2005;24(12):1099–1103.

88. Mateos I, Valencia R, Torres MJ, Cantos A, Conde M, Aznar J. Nosocomial outbreak of *Pseudomonas aeruginosa* endophthalmitis. *Infect Control Hosp Epidemiol*. 2006;27:1249–1251.

89. Sehulster L, Chinn RY, Arduino MJ, et al. Guidelines for environmental infection control in health-care facilities; 2003. Recommendations of CDC and the Healthcare Infection Control Practices Advisory Committee (HICPAC). *MMWR*. 2003;52(RR-10):1–42. http://www.cdc.gov/ncidod/dhqp/gl_environinfection.html. Accessed April 5, 2008.

90. Dixon RE, Kaslow RA, Mackel DC, Fulkerson CC, Mallinson GF. Aqueous quaternary ammonium antiseptics and disinfectants: use and misuse. *JAMA*. 1976;236:2415–2417.

91. Donowitz LG. Benzalkonium chloride is still in use. *Infect Control Hosp Epidemiol*. 1991;12:186–187.

92. France DR. Survival of *Candida albicans* in hand creams. *N Z J Med*. 1968;67:552–554.

93. Morse LJ, Williams HL, Grann FP, et al. Septicemia due to *Klebsiella pneumoniae* originating from a hand cream dispenser. *N Engl J Med*. 1967;277:472–473.

94. Morse LJ, Schonbeck LE. Hand lotions—a potential nosocomial hazard. *N Engl J Med*. 1968;278:376–378.

95. Anderson K. The contamination of hexachlorophene soap with *Pseudomonas pyocyanea*. *Med J Aust*. 1962;2:463.

96. Alonso-Echanove J, Cairns L, Richards M, et al. Nationwide outbreak of red eye syndrome associated with transfusion of leukoreduced red blood cell units. *Infect Control Hosp Epidemiol*. 2006;27:1146–1152.

97. Vonberg RP, Gastmeier P. Hospital-acquired infections related to contaminated substances. *J Hosp Infect*. 2007;65:15–23.

98. Sprach DH, Silverstein FE, Stamm WE. Transmission of infection by gastrointestinal endoscopy and bronchoscopy. *Ann Intern Med*. 1993;118:117–128.

99. Struelens MJ, Rost F, Deplano A, et al. *Pseudomonas aeruginosa* and Enterobacteriaceae bacteremia after biliary endoscopy: an outbreak investigation using DNA macrorestriction analysis. *Am J Med*. 1993;95:489–498.

100. Alvarado CJ, Stolz SM, Maki DG. Nosocomial infections from contaminated endoscopes: a flawed automated endoscope washer: an investigation using molecular epidemiology. *Am J Med.* 1991;91:272S–280S.

101. Fraser TG, Reiner S, Malczynski M, Yarnold PR, Warren J, Noskin G. Multidrug-resistant *Pseudomonas aeruginosa* cholangitis after endoscopic retrograde cholangiopancreatography: failure of routine endoscope cultures to prevent an outbreak. *Infect Control Hosp Epidemiol* 2004;25:856–859.

102. Schliessler KH, Rozendaal B, Taal C, Meawissen SGM. Outbreak of *Salmonella agona* after upper intestinal fiberoptic endoscopy. *Lancet.* 1980;2:1246.

103. Birnie GG, Quigley EM, Clements GB, Follet EAC, Watkinson G. Endoscopic transmission of hepatitis B virus. *Gut.* 1983;24:171–174.

104. Bronowicki JP, Venard V, Botte C, et al. Patient-to-patient transmission of hepatitis C virus during colonoscopy. *N Engl J Med.* 1997;337:237–240.

105. Allen JI, O'Connor AM, Olson MM, et al. Pseudomonas infection of the biliary system resulting from use of a contaminated endoscope. *Gastroenterol.* 1987;92:759–763.

106. Nelson KE, Larson PA, Schraufnagel DE, Jackson J. Transmission of tuberculosis by flexible fiberbronchoscopes. *Am Rev Respir Dis.* 1983;127:97–100.

107. Wheeler PW, Lancaster D, Kaiser AB. Bronchopulmonary cross-contamination and infection related to mycobacterial contamination of suction valves of bronchoscopes. *J Infect Dis.* 1989;159:954–958.

108. Blanc DS, Parret T, Janin B, et al. Nosocomial infections and pseudoinfections from contaminated bronchoscopes: two-year follow-up using molecular markers. *Infect Control Hosp Epidemiol.* 1997;18:134–136.

109. Gubler JG, Salfinger M, von Graevenitz A. Pseudoepidemic of nontuberculous mycobacteria due to a contaminated bronchoscope cleaning machine: report of an outbreak and review of the literature. *Chest.* 1992;101:1245–1249.

110. Agerton T, Valway S, Gore B, et al. Transmission of a highly drug-resistant strain (Strain W1) of *Mycobacterium tuberculosis*: community outbreak and nosocomial transmission via a contaminated bronchoscope. *JAMA.* 1997;278:1073–1077.

111. Cetre JC, Nicolle MC, Salord H. Outbreaks of contaminated broncho-alveolar lavage related to intrinsically defective bronchoscopes. *J Hosp Infect.* 2005;61(1):39–45.

112. Srinivasin A, Wolfenden LL, Song X, et al. An outbreak of *Pseudomonas aeruginosa* infections associated with flexible bronchoscopes. *N Engl J Med.* 2003;348:221–227.

113. Weems JJ. Nosocomial outbreak of *Pseudomonas cepacia* associated with contamination of reusable electronic ventilator temperature probes. *Infect Control Hosp Epidemiol.* 1993;14:583–586.

114. Loukil C, Saizou C, Doit C, et al. Epidemiologic investigation of *Burkholderia cepacia* acquisition in two pediatric intensive care units. *Infect Control Hosp Epidemiol.* 2003;24: 707–710.

115. Rudnick JR, Beck-Sague CM, Anderson RL, Schable B, Miller JM, Jarvis WR. Gram-negative bacteremia in open-heart-surgery patients traced to probable tap-water contamination of pressure-monitoring equipment. *Infect Control Hosp Epidemiol.* 1996;17:281–285.

116. Conly JM, Klass L, Larson L, et al. *Pseudomonas cepacia* colonization and infection in intensive care units. *Can Med Assoc J.* 1986;134:363–366.

117. Beck-Sague CM, Jarvis WR. Epidemic bloodstream infections associated with pressure transducers: a persistent problem. *Infect Control Hosp Epidemiol.* 1989;10:54–59.

118. Centers for Disease Control and Prevention. Guidelines for the prevention of intravascular catheter-related infections. *MMWR.* 2002;51(No. RR-10):1-36. http://www.cdc.gov/mmwr/PDF/rr/rr5110.pdf.Accessed April 28, 2008.

119. Centers for Disease Control. Hepatitis B associated with jet gun injection—California. *MMWR.* 1986;35:373–376.

120. Centers for Disease Control. Nosocomial transmission of hepatitis B virus associated with a spring-loaded finger stick device—California. *MMWR.* 1990;39:610–613.

121. Centers for Disease Control and Prevention. Nosocomial hepatitis B virus infection associated with reusable fingerstick blood sampling devices—Ohio and New York City; 1996. *MMWR*. 1997;46:217–221.

122. Hamill RJ, Wright CE, Andres N, Koza MA. Urinary tract infection following instrumentation for urodynamic testing. *Infect Control Hosp Epidemiol*. 1989;10:26–32.

123. Climo MW, Pastor A, Wong ES. An outbreak of *Pseudomonas aeruginosa* related to contaminated urodynamic equipment. *Infect Control Hosp Epidemiol*. 1997;18:509–510.

124. Gillespie K, Arnold J, Noble-Wang B, et al. Outbreak of *Pseudomonas aeruginosa* infections after transrectal ultrasound-guided prostate biopsy. *Urology*. 2007;69:912–914.

125. Yardy GW, Cox RA. An outbreak of *Pseudomonas aeruginosa* infection associated with contaminated urodynamic equipment. *J Hosp Infect*. 2001;47:60–63.

126. Livornese L, Dias S, Samel C, et al. Hospital-acquired infection with vancomycin-resistant *Enterococcus faecium* transmitted by electronic thermometers. *Ann Intern Med*. 1992; 117:112–116.

127. Karanfil LV, Murphy M, Josephson A, et al. A cluster of vancomycin-resistant *Enterococcus faecium* in an intensive care unit. *Infect Control Hosp Epidemiol*. 1992;13:195–200.

128. Arnow PM, Garcia-Houchins S, Neagle MB, Bova JL, Dillon JJ, Chou T. An outbreak of bloodstream infections arising from hemodialysis equipment. *J Infect Dis*. 1998;178:783–791.

129. Maragakis LL, Bradley KL, Song X, et al. Increased catheter-related bloodstream infection rates after the introduction of a new mechanical valve intravenous access port. *Infect Control Hosp Epidemiol*. 2006;27:67–70.

130. Rupp ME, Sholtz LA, Jourdan DR, et al. Outbreak of bloodstream infection temporally associated with the use of an intravascular needleless valve. *Clin Infect Dis*. 2007;44(11): 1408–1414.

131. Corne P, Godreuil S, Jean-Pierre H, et al. Unusual implication of biopsy forceps in outbreaks of *Pseudomonas aeruginosa* infections and pseudo-infections related to bronchoscopy. *J Hosp Infect*. 2005;61(1):20–26.

132. Van der Zweit WC, Parlevliet GA, Savelkoul PH, et al. Outbreak of *Bacillus cereus* infections in a neonatal intensive care unit traced to balloons used in manual ventilation. *J Clin Microbiol*. 2000;38:4131–4136. http://www.pubmedcentral.nih.gov/picrender.fcgi?artid=87553& blobtype=pdf. Accessed April 25, 2008.

133. Trick WE, Kioski CM, Howard KM, et al. Outbreak of *Pseudomonas aeruginosa* ventriculitis among patients in a neurosurgical intensive care unit. *Infect Control Hosp Epidemiol*. 2000;21:204–208.

134. Durante L, Zulty JC, Israel E, et al. Investigation of an outbreak of bloody diarrhea: association with endoscopic cleaning solution and demonstration of lesions in an animal model. *Am J Med*. 1992;92:476–480.

135. Burtin P, Ruget O, Petit R, Boyer J. Gluteraldehyde-induced proctitis after anorectal ultrasound examination: a higher risk of incidence than expected? *Gastrointest Endosc*. 1993;39:859–860.

136. Beck-Sague CM, Jarvis WR, Bland LA, Arduino MJ, Aguero SM, Verosic G. Outbreak of gram-negative bacteremia and pyrogenic reactions in a hemodialysis center. *Am J Nephrol*. 1990;10:397–403.

137. Welbel SF, Schoendorf K, Bland LA, et al. An outbreak of gram-negative bloodstream infections in chronic hemodialysis patients. *Am J Nephrol*. 1995;15:1–4.

138. Flaherty JP, Garcia-Houchins S, Chudy R, Arnow PM. An outbreak of gram-negative bacteremia traced to contaminated O-rings and reprocessed dialyzers. *Ann Intern Med*. 1993;119:1072–1078.

139. Centers for Disease Control and Prevention. Outbreaks of hepatitis B virus infection among hemodialysis patients—California, Nebraska, and Texas; 1994. *MMWR*. 1996;45:285–289.

140. Band JD, Ward JI, Fraser DW. Peritonitis due to a *Mycobacterium chelonei*-like organism with intermittent chronic peritoneal dialysis. *J Infect Dis*. 1982;145:9–17.

141. Berkelman RL, Godley J, Weber JA, et al. *Pseudomonas cepacia* peritonitis associated with contamination of automatic peritoneal dialysis machines. *Ann Intern Med*. 1982;96:456–458.

142. Kayabas U, Bayraktar M, Otlu B, et al. An outbreak of *Pseudomonas aeruginosa* because of inadequate disinfection procedures in a urology unit: A pulsed-field gel electrophoresis-based epidemiologic study. *Am J Infect Control.* 2008;36:33–38.

143. Pena C, Dominguez MA, Pujol M, Verdaguer R, Gudiol F, Ariza J. An outbreak of carbapenem-resistant *Pseudomonas aeruginosa* in a urology ward. *Clin Microbiol Infect.* 2003;9:938–943.

144. Centers for Disease Control and Prevention. Transplantation-transmitted tuberculosis—Oklahoma and Texas; 2007. *MMWR.* 2008;57:333–336.

145. Singh N, Paterson DL. *Mycobacterium tuberculosis* infection in solid-organ transplant recipients: impact and implications for management. *Clin Infect Dis.* 1998;27:1266–1277.

146. Young L, Sable A, Price CS. Epidemiologic, clinical, and economic evaluation of an outbreak of clonal multidrug-resistant *Acinetobacter baumannii* infection in a surgical intensive care unit. *Infect Control Hosp Epidemiol.* 2007;28:1247–1254.

147. Schabrun S, Chipchase L, Rickard H. Are therapeutic ultrasound units a potential vector for nosocomial infection? *Physiother Res Int.* 2006;11(2):61–71.

148. Kronman MP, Baden HP, Jeffries HE, Heath J, Cohen GA, Zerr DM. An investigation of *Aspergillus* cardiac surgical site infections in 3 pediatric patients. *Am J Infect Control.* 2007;35:332–327.

149. Berthelot P, Carricajo A, Aubert G, Akhavan H, Gazielly D, Lucht F. Outbreak of postoperative shoulder arthritis due to propionibacterium acnes infection in nondebilitated patients. *Infect Control Hosp Epidemiol.* 2006;27:987–990.

150. Weber DJ, Rutala WA. Lessons from outbreaks associated with bronchoscopy. *Infect Control Hosp Epidemiol.* 2001;22:403–408.

151. Kaczmarek RG, Moore RM, McCrohan J, et al. Multi-state investigation of the actual disinfection/sterilization of endoscopes in health care facilities. *Am J Med.* 1992;92:257–261.

152. Gorse GJ, Messner RL. Infection control practices in gastrointestinal endoscopy in the United States: a national survey. *Infect Control Hosp Epidemiol.* 1991;12:289–296.

153. Multidisciplinary guideline for reprocessing flexible gastrointestinal gastroscopes. *Endoscopy.* 2003;58:1–8. http://www.asge.org/WorkArea/showcontent.aspx?id=3376. Accessed April 28, 2008.

154. Honeybourne D, Newmann CS. An audit of bronchoscopy practice in the United Kingdom: a survey of adherence to national guidelines. *Thorax.* 1997;52:709–713.

155. American Society for Gastroenterology. Infection control during gastrointestinal endoscopy. *Gastrointest Endosc.* 1999;49:836–841.

156. Culver DA, Gordon SM, Mehta AC. Infection control in the bronchoscopy suite: a review of outbreaks and guidelines for prevention. *Am J Respir Crit Care Med.* 2003;167:1050–1056. http://ajrccm.atsjournals.org/cgi/reprint/167/8/1050. Accessed April 28, 2008.

157. Bassett DCJ, Stokes KJ, Thomas WRG. Wound infection with *Pseudomonas multivorans.* A waterborne contaminant of disinfectant solutions. *Lancet.* 1970;1:1188–1191.

158. Everett ED, Pearson S, Rogers W. Rhizopus surgical wound infection associated with elasticized adhesive tape dressing. *Arch Surg.* 1979;114:738–739.

159. Keys TF, Haldorson AM, Rhodes KH, Roberts GD, Fifer EZ. Nosocomial outbreak of Rhizopus infections associated with Elastoplast wound dressings—Minnesota. *MMWR.* 1978;27:33–34.

160. Pearson RD, Valenti WM, Steigbigel RT. Clostridium perfringens wound infections associated with elastic bandages. *JAMA.* 1980;244:1128–1130.

161. Mitchell RG, Hayward AC. Postoperative urinary tract infections caused by contaminated irrigating fluid. *Lancet.* 1966;1:793–795.

162. Geiss HK, Schmitt J, Frank SC. Bleeding after cardiovascular surgery caused by detergent residues in laparotomy sponges. *Infect Control Hosp Epidemiol.* 1997;18:579–581.

163. Courtright P, Lewallen S, Holland SP, Wendt TM. Corneal decompensation after cataract surgery: an outbreak investigation in Asia. *Ophthalmol.* 1995;102:1461–1465.

164. Pegues CF. Outbreak investigations: red-eyed rabbits and community service. *Infect Control Hosp Epidemiol.* 2006;27:1143–1145

165. Hugonnet S, Dosso A, Dharan S, et al. Outbreak of endophthalmitis after cataract surgery: the importance of the quality of the surgical wound. *Infect Control Hosp Epidemiol.* 2006; 27:1246–1248.

166. Mateos I, Valencia R, Torres MJ, Cantos A, Conde M, Aznar J. Nosocomial outbreak of *Pseudomonas aeruginosa* endophthalmitis. *Infect Control Hosp Epidemiol.* 2006; 27:1249–1251.

167. Labarca JA, Trick WE, Peterson CL, et al. A multistate nosocomial outbreak of *Ralstonia pickettii* colonization associated with an intrinsically contaminated respiratory care solution. *Clin Infect Dis.* 1999;29:1281–1286.

168. Maroye P, Doermann HP, Rogues AM, Gachie JP, Megraud F. Investigation of an outbreak of *Ralstonia pickettii* in a paediatric hospital by RAPD. *J Hosp Infect.* 2000;44:276–272.

169. Moreira BM, Leobons MBGP, Pellegrino FLPC, et al. *Ralstonia pickettii* and *Burkholderia cepacia* complex bloodstream infections related to infusion of contaminated water for injection. *J Hosp Infect.* 2005;60:51–55.

170. Sheretz RJ, Bassetti S, Bassetti-Wyss B. "Cloud" Health-Care Workers. *Emerg Infect Dis.* 2001;7:241–244.

171. Vonberg R-P, Stamm-Balderjahn S, Hansen S, et al. How often do asymptomatic healthcare workers cause methicillin-resistant *Staphylococcus aureus* outbreaks? A systematic evaluation. *Infect Control Hosp Epidemiol.* 2006;27:1123–1127.

172. Wenzel RP. Healthcare workers and the incidence of nosocomial infection: can treatment of one influence the other? a brief review. *J Chemother.* 1994;4:33–40.

173. Dineen P, Drudin L. Epidemics of postoperative wound infection associated with hair carriers. *Lancet.* 1973;2:1157–1159.

174. Kreiswirth BN, Kravitz GR, Schlievert PM, Novick RP. Nosocomial transmission of a strain of *Staphylococcus aureus* causing toxic shock syndrome. *Ann Intern Med.* 1986;105:704–707.

175. Faibis F, Laporte C, Fiacre A, et al. An outbreak of methicillin-resistant *Staphylococcus aureus* surgical-site infections initiated by a healthcare worker with chronic sinusitis. *Infect Control Hosp Epidemiol.* 2005;26:213–215.

176. Belani A, Sheretz RJ, Sullivan ML, Russell BA, Reumen PD. Outbreak of staphylococcal infection in two nurseries traced to a single carrier. *Infect Control.* 1986;7:487–490.

177. Mean M, Mallaret MR, Andrini P, et al. A neonatal specialist with recurrent methicillin-resistant *Staphylococcus aureus* (MRSA) carriage implicated in the transmission of MRSA to newborns. *Infect Control Hosp Epidemiol.* 2007;28:625–628.

178. Sheretz RJ, Reagan DR, Hampton KD, et al. A cloud adult: the *Staphylococcus aureus-virus* interaction revisited. *Ann Intern Med.* 1996;124:539–547.

179. Centers for Disease Control and Prevention. Surveillance for food-borne disease outbreaks—United States,; 1998–2002. Surveillance Summaries; 2006. *MMWR.* 2006;55(SS-10):9.

180. Weber DJ, Rutala WA, Denny FW. Management of healthcare workers with pharyngitis or suspected streptococcal infections. *Infect Control Hosp Epidemiol.* 1996;17:753–761.

181. Mastro TD, Farley TA, Elliot JA, et al. An outbreak of surgical wound infections due to group A streptococcus carried on the scalp. *N Engl J Med.* 1990;32:968–972.

182. Stamm WE, Feeley JC, Facklam RR. Wound infections due to group A streptococcus traced to a vaginal carrier. *J Infect Dis.* 1978;138:287–292.

183. Berkelman RL, Martin D, Graham DR, et al. Streptococcal wound infections caused by a vaginal carrier. *JAMA.* 1982;247:2680–2682.

184. Schaffner W, Lefkowitz LB Jr, Goodman JS, Koenig MG. Hospital outbreak of infections with group A streptococci traced to an asymptomatic anal carrier. *N Engl J Med.* 1969;280:1224–1225.

185. Viglionese A, Nottebart VF, Bodman HA, Platt R. Recurrent group A streptococcal carriage in a health care worker associated with widely separated nosocomial outbreaks. *Am J Med.* 1991;91(suppl 3B):329S–333S.

186. Paul SM, Genese C, Spitalny K. Postoperative group A beta-hemolytic streptococcus outbreak with the pathogen traced to a member of a healthcare worker's household. *Infect Control Hosp Epidemiol.* 1990;11:643–646.

187. Ridgway EJ, Allen KD. Clustering of group A streptococcal infections on a burns unit: important lessons in outbreak management. *J Hosp Infect.* 1993;25:173–182.

188. Isenberg HD, Tucci V, Lipsitz P, Facklam RR. Clinical laboratory and epidemiological investigations of a *Streptococcus pyogenes* cluster epidemic in a newborn nursery. *J Clin Microbiol.* 1984;19:366–370.

189. Ramage L, Green K, Pyskir D, Simor AE. An outbreak of fatal infections due to group A streptococcus on a medical ward. *Infect Control Hosp Epidemiol*. 1996;17:429–431.

190. Lannigan R, Hussain Z, Austin TW. *Streptococcus pyogenes* as a cause of nosocomial infection in a critical care unit. *Diagn Microbiol Infect Dis*. 1985;3:337–341.

191. Schwartz B, Elliott JA, Butler JC, et al. Clusters of invasive group A streptococcal infections in family, hospital, and nursing home settings. *Clin Infect Dis*. 1992;15:277–284.

192. Decker MD, Lavely GB, Hutcheson RH, Schaffner W. Foodborne streptococcal pharyngitis in a hospital pediatrics clinic. *JAMA*. 1985;253:679–681.

193. Daneman N, Green KA, Low DE, et al., and the Ontario Group A Streptococcal Study Group. Surveillance for hospital outbreaks of invasive group A streptococcal infections in Ontario, Canada; 1992 to 2000. *Ann Intern Med*. 2007;147(4):234–241. http://www.annals.org/cgi/reprint/147/4/234.pdf. Accessed April 22, 2008.

194. Felkenr M, Pascoe N, Shupe-Rickecker K, Goodman E. The wound care team: a new source of group a streptococcal nosocomial transmission. *Infect Control Hosp Epidemiol*. 2005; 26(5):462–465.

196. Chandler RE, Lee LL, Townes JM, Taplitz RA. Transmission of Group A *Streptococcus* limited to healthcare workers with exposure in the operating room. *Infect Control Hosp Epidemiol*. 2006; 27:1159–1163.

196. Kakis A, Gibbs L, Eguia J, et al. An outbreak of group A streptococcal infection among health care workers. *Clin Infect Dis*. 2002;35(11):1353–1359.

197. Prevention of Invasive Group A Streptococcal Infections Workshop Participants. Prevention of invasive group A streptococcal disease among household contacts of case patients and among postpartum and postsurgical patients: recommendations from the Centers for Disease Control and Prevention. *Clin Infect Dis*. 2002;35:950–959.

198. Pertowski CA, Baron RC, Lasker BA, Werner SB, Jarvis WR. Nosocomial outbreak of *Candida albicans* sternal wound infections following cardiac surgery traced to a scrub nurse. *J Infect Dis*. 1995;172:817–822.

199. Isenberg HD, Tucci V, Cintron F, et al. Single source outbreak of *Candida tropicalis* complicating coronary bypass surgery. *J Clin Microbiol*. 1989;27:2426–2428.

200. Parry MF, Grant B, Yukena M, et al. *Candida* osteomyelitis and diskitis after spinal surgery: an outbreak that implicates artificial nail use. *Clin Infect Dis*. 2001; 32:352–357. http://www.journals.uchicago.edu/doi/pdf/10.1086/318487. Accessed April 25, 2008.

201. Wegener PN, Brown JM, McNeil MM, Jarvis WR. *Nocardia farcinica* sternotomy site infections in patients following open heart surgery. *J Infect Dis*. 1998;178:1539–1543.

202. Exmelin L, Malbruny B, Vergnaud M, Provost F, Boiron P, Morel C. Molecular study of nosocomial nocardiosis outbreak involving heart transplant recipients. *J Clin Microbiol*. 1996;34:1014–1016.

203. Maragakis LL, Winkler A, Tucker MG, et al. Outbreak of multidrug-resistant *Serratia marcescens* infection in a neonatal intensive care unit. *Infect Control Hosp Epidemiol*. 2008;29:418–423.

204. de Vries JJC, Baas WH, vander Ploeg K, Heesink A, Degener JE, Arends JP. Outbreak of *Serratia marcescens* colonization and infection traced to a healthcare worker with long-term carriage on the hands. *Infect Control Hosp Epidemiol*. 2006; 27:1153–1158.

205. Zawacki A, O'Rourke E, Potter-Boyne G, et al. An outbreak of *Pseudomonas aeruginosa* pneumonia and bloodstream infection associated with intermittent otitis externa in a healthcare worker. *Infect Control Hosp Epidemiol*. 2004;25:1083–1089.

206. Friedman ND, Kotsanas D, Brett J, Billah B, Korman TM. Investigation of an outbreak of *Serratia marcescens* in a neonatal unit via a case control study and molecular typing. *Am J Infect Control*. 2008;36:22–28.

207. Liu S-C, Leu H-S, Yen M-Y, Lee P-I, Chou M-C. Study of an outbreak of *Enterobacter cloacae* sepsis in a neonatal intensive care unit: the application of epidemiologic chromosome profiling by pulsed-field gel electrophoresis. *Am J Infect Control*. 2002;30:381–385.

208. AIDS/TB Committee of the Society for Healthcare Epidemiology of America. Management of healthcare workers infected with hepatitis B virus, hepatitis C virus, human immunodefi-

ciency virus, or other bloodborne pathogens. *Infect Control Hosp Epidemiol*. 1997;18:349–363.

209. Bell D, Shapiro CN, Chamberland ME, Ciesielski CA. Preventing bloodborne pathogen transmission from healthcare workers to patients: the CDC perspective. *Surg Clin North Am*. 1995;75:1189–1203.

210. Prentice MB, Flower AJE, Morgan GM, et al. Infection with hepatitis B virus after open heart surgery. *BMJ*. 1992;304:761–764.

211. Centers for Disease Control. Recommendations for preventing transmission of human immunodeficiency virus and hepatitis B virus to patients during exposure-prone invasive procedures. *MMWR*. 1991;40(RR-8):1–9. http://www.cdc.gov/mmwR/preview/mmwrhtml/00014845.htm. Accessed April 30, 2008.

212. Spijkerman IJB, van Doorn L-J, Janssen MHW, et al. Transmission of hepatitis B virus from a surgeon to his patients during high-risk and low risk surgical procedures during 4 years. *Infect Control Hosp Epidemiol*. 2002;23:306–312.

213. Redd JT, Baumbach J, Kohn W, Nainan O, Khristova M, Williams I. Patient-to-patient transmission of hepatitis B virus associated with oral surgery. *J Infect Dis*. 2007;195:1311–1314.

214. Perry JL, Pearson RD, Jagger J. Infected health care workers and patient safety: a double standard. *Am J Infect Control*. 2006;34:313–319.

215. Allos BM, Schaffner W. Transmission of hepatitis B in the health care setting: the elephant in the room...or the mouse? *J Infect Dis*. 2007;195:1245–1247.

216. Mele A, Ippolito G, Craxì A, et al. Risk management of HBsAG or anti-HCV positive healthcare workers in hospital. *Dig Liver Dis*. 2001;33:795–802.

217. Reitsma AM, Closen ML, Cunningham M, et al. Infected physicians and invasive procedures: safe practice management. *Clin Infect Dis*. 2005;40:1665–1672. http://www.journals.uchicago.edu/doi/pdf/10.1086/429821. Accessed April 30, 2008.

218. United Kingdom Department of Health. Guidance for health care workers: protection against infection with blood-borne viruses. Recommendations of the Expert Advisory Group on AIDS and the Advisory Group on Hepatitis. London, UK: Her Majesty's Stationery Office, 1993. http://www.dh.gov.uk/assetRoot/04/01/44/74/04014474.pdf. Accessed April 30, 2008.

219. Gunson RN, Shouval D, Roggendorf M, et al. Hepatitis B virus (HBV) and hepatitis C virus (HCV) infections in health care workers (HCW): guidelines for prevention of transmission of HBV and HCV from HCW to patients. *J Clin Virol*. 2003;27:213–230.

220. Bond WW, Favero MS, Petersen NJ, Gravelle CR, Ebert JW, Maynard JE. Survival of hepatitis B virus after drying and storage for one week. *Lancet*. 1981;27:550–551.

221. Oren I, Hershow RC, Ben-Porath E, et al. A common-source outbreak of fulminant hepatitis B in a hospital. *Ann Intern Med*. 1989;110:691–698.

222. Centers for Disease Control and Prevention. Improper infection-control practices during employee vaccination programs—District of Columbia and Pennsylvania, 1993. *MMWR*. 1993;42:969–971.

223. Esteban JI, Gomez J, Martell M, et al. Transmission of hepatitis C virus by a cardiac surgeon. *N Engl J Med*. 1996;334:555–560.

224. Lot F, Delarocque-Astagneau E, Thiers V, et al. Hepatitis C virus transmission from a healthcare worker to a patient. *Infect Control Hosp Epidemiol*. 2007;28:227–229.

225. Centers for Disease Control and Prevention. Recommendations for prevention and control of hepatitis C virus (HCV) infection and HCV-related chronic disease. *MMWR*. 1998;47(RR-19):1–39.

226. Centers for Disease Control. Update: transmission of human immunodeficiency virus infection during an invasive dental procedure—Florida. *MMWR*. 1991;40:21–33.

227. Scully C, Greenspan JS. Human immunodeficiency virus (HIV) transmission in dentistry. *J Dent Res*. 2006;85:794–800.

228. Lot F, Seguier JC, Fegueux S, et al. Probable transmission of HIV from an orthopedic surgeon to a patient in France. *Ann Intern Med*. 1999;130:1–6.

229. Goujon CP, Schneider VM, Grofti J, et al. Phylogenetic analyses indicate an atypical nurse-to-patient transmission of human immunodeficiency virus type 1. *J Virol*. 2000;74:2525–2532.

230. Astagneau P, Lot F, Fegueux S, et al. Lookback investigation of patients potentially exposed to HIV type I after a nurse-to-patient transmission. *Am J Infect Control.* 2002;30:242–245.

231. Bosch X. Second case of doctor-to-patient HIV transmission. *Lancet Infect Dis.* 2003;3:261.

232. Mallolas J, Arnedo M, Pumarola T. Transmission of HIV-1 from an obstetrician to a patient during a caesarean section. *AIDS.* 2006;20:285–287.

233. UK Department of Health. *HIV Infected Health Care Workers: A Consultation Paper on Management and Patient Notification.* London, UK: Department of Health; 2002. http://www .dh.gov.uk/assetRoot/04/01/85/96/04018596.pdf. Accessed April 30, 2008..

234. Centers for Disease Control. Foodborne nosocomial outbreak of *Salmonella* reading—Connecticut. *MMWR.* 1991;40:804–806.

235. Opal SM, Mayer KH, Roland F, Brondum J, Heelan J, Lyhte L. Investigation of a food-borne outbreak of salmonellosis among hospital employees. *Am J Infect Control.* 1989;17:141–147.

236. Perlino CA, Parrish CM, Terry PM. *Salmonella infantis* outbreak in neonates in an intermediate intensive care nursery. Presented at: Third Decennial International Conference on Nosocomial Infections; July 31–August 3, 1990; Atlanta, GA. Abstract 62.

237. Stone A, Shaffner M, Sautter R. *Salmonella poona* infection and surveillance in a neonatal nursery. *Am J Infect Control.* 1993;21:270–273.

238. Meyers JD, Romm FJ, Tihen WS, Bryan JA. Food-borne hepatitis A in a general hospital: epidemiologic study of an outbreak attributed to sandwiches. *JAMA.* 1975;231:1049–1053.

239. Eisenstein AB, Aach RD, Jacobsohn W, Goldman A. An epidemic of infectious hepatitis in a general hospital: probable transmission by contaminated orange juice. *JAMA.* 1963;185:171–174.

240. Rosenblum LS, Villarino ME, Naina OV, et al. Hepatitis A outbreak in a neonatal intensive care unit: risk factors for transmission and evidence of prolonged viral excretion among preterm infants. *J Infect Dis.* 1991;164:476–482.

241. Azimi PH, Roberto RR, Guralnik J, et al. Transfusion-acquired hepatitis A in a premature infant with secondary nosocomial spread in an intensive care nursery. *Am J Dis Child.* 1986;140:23–27.

242. Noble RC, Kane MA, Reeves SA, Roeckel I. Posttransfusion hepatitis A in a neonatal intensive care unit. *JAMA.* 1984;252:2711–2715.

243. Chodick G, Ashkenazi S, Lerman Y. The risk of hepatitis A infection among healthcare workers: a review of reported outbreaks and sero-epidemiologic studies. *J Hosp Infect.* 2006;62:414–420.

244. Goodman RA, Carder CC, Allen JR, Orenstein WA, Finton RJ. Nosocomial hepatitis A transmission by an adult patient with diarrhea. *Am J Med.* 1982;73:220–226.

245. Petrosillo N, Raffaele B, Martini L, et al. A nosocomial and occupational cluster of hepatitis A virus infection in a pediatric ward. *Infect Control Hosp Epidemiol.* 2002;23:343–345.

246. Doebbeling BN, Li N, Wenzel RP. An outbreak of hepatitis A among health care workers: risk factors for transmission. *Am J Public Health.* 1993;83:1679–1684.

247. Drusin LM, Sohmer M, Groshen SL, Spiritos MD, Senterfit LB, Christenson WN. Nosocomial hepatitis A infection in a pediatric intensive care unit. *Arch Dis Child.* 1987;62:690–695.

248. Centers for Disease Control and Prevention. Update: prevention of hepatitis A after exposure to hepatitis A virus and in international travelers. Updated recommendations of the Advisory Committee on Immunization Practices (ACIP). *MMWR.* 2007;56(41);1080–1084. http://www.cdc.gov/mmwR/preview/mmwrhtml/mm5641a3.htm. Accessed May 2, 2008.

249. Eickhoff TC. Airborne nosocomial infection: a contemporary perspective. *Infect Control Hosp Epidemiol.* 1994;15:663–672.

250. Sepkowicz KA. Occupationally acquired infections in health care workers, pt I. *Ann Intern Med.* 1996;125:826–834.

251. Atkinson WL. Measles and healthcare workers. *Infect Control Hosp Epidemiol.* 1994;15:5–7.

252. Gurevich I, Barzarga RA, Cuhna BA. Measles: lessons from an outbreak. *Am J Infect Control.* 1992;20:319–325.

253. Rank EL, Brettman L, Katz-Pollack H, DeHertogh D, Neville D. Chronology of a hospital-wide measles outbreak: lessons learned and shared from an extraordinary week in late March 1989. *Am J Infect Control.* 1992;20:315–318.

254. Centers for Disease Control and Prevention. Measles, mumps, and rubella—vaccine use and strategies for elimination of measles, rubella, and congenital rubella syndrome and control of mumps: recommendations of the Advisory Committee on Immunization Practices (ACIP). *MMWR*. 1998;47(RR-8):1–57. http://www.cdc.gov/MMWR/preview/MMWRhtml/00053391.htm. Acessed April 6, 2008.

255. Bloch AB, Orenstein WA, Ewing WM, et al. Measles outbreak in a pediatric practice: airborne transmission in an office setting. *Pediatr*. 1985;75:676–683.

256. Centers for Disease Control and Prevention. Import-associated measles outbreak—Indiana, May–June 2005. *MMWR*. 2005;54(42):1073–1075. http://www.cdc.gov/mmwr/preview/mmwrhtml/mm5442a1.htm. Accessed April 5, 2008.

257. Parker AA, Staggs W, Dayan GH, et al. Implications of a 2005 measles outbreak in Indiana for sustained elimination of measles in the United States. *N Engl J Med*. 2006;355(5):447–455. http://content.nejm.org/cgi/content/abstract/355/5/447. Accessed April 5, 2008.

258. Centers for Disease Control and Prevention. Measles—United States, January 1–April 25, 2008. *MMWR*. 2008;57(Early Release):1–4. http://www.cdc.gov/mmwr/preview/mmwrhtml/mm57e501a1.htm?s_cid=mm57e501a1_e. Accessed May 1, 2008.

259. Centers for Disease Control and Prevention. Immunization of health-care workers: recommendations of the Advisory Committee on Immunization Practices (ACIP) and the Hospital Infection Control Practices Advisory Committee (HICPAC). *MMWR*.1997;6(RR-18):1–42. http://www.cdc.gov/mmwr/preview/mmwrhtml/00050577.htm. Accessed April 6, 2008.

260. American Academy of Pediatrics. Measles. In: Peter G, ed. *2006 Red Book: Report of the Committee on Infectious Diseases*. 24th ed. Elk Grove Village, IL: American Academy of Pediatrics; 2006.

261. Uckay I, Hugonnet S, Kaiser L, Sax H, Pittet D. Age limit does not replace serologic testing for determination of immune status for measles. *Infect Control Hosp Epidemiol*. 2007;28:1117–1120.

262. Rivera ME, Mason WH, Ross LA, Wright HT Jr. Nosocomial measles infection in a pediatric hospital during a community-wide epidemic. *J Pediatr*. 1991;119:183–186.

263. Houck P, Scott-Johnson G, Krebs L. Measles immunity among community hospital employees. *Infect Control Hosp Epidemiol*. 1991;12:663–668.

264. Weber DJ, Rutala WA, Hamilton H. Prevention and control of varicella-zoster infections in healthcare facilities. *Infect Control Hosp Epidemiol*. 1996;17:694–705.

265. Sawyer MH, Chamberlain CJ, Wu YN, Aintablian N, Wallace MR. Detection of varicella-zoster virus DNA in air samples from hospital rooms. *J Infect Dis*. 1994;169:91–94.

266. Leclair JM, Zaia JA, Levin MJ, Congdon RG, Goldmann DA. Airborne transmission of chickenpox in a hospital. *N Engl J Med*. 1980;302:450–453.

267. Faoagali JL, Darcy D. Chickenpox outbreak among the staff of a large, urban adult hospital: costs of monitoring and control. *Am J Infect Control*. 1995;23:247–250.

268. Gustafson TL, Lavely GB, Brawner ER, Hutcheson RH, Wright PF, Schaffner W. An outbreak of airborne nosocomial varicella. *Pediatr*. 1982;70:550–556.

269. Apisarnthanarak A, Kitphati R, Tawatsupha P, et al. Outbreak of varicella-zoster virus infection among Thai healthcare workers. *Infect Control Hosp Epidemiol*. 2007;28:430–434.

270. Yehia A, Aly N, Al Obaid I, Al-Qulooshi N, Zahed Z. Occupationally related outbreak of chickenpox in an intensive care unit. *Med Princ Pract*. 2007;16:399–401.

271. Centers for Disease Control and Prevention. Prevention of varicella: recommendations of the Advisory Committee on Immunization Practices (ACIP). *MMWR*. 2007;56(RR-04):1–40.

272. American Academy of Pediatrics. Varicella-zoster. In: Peter G, ed. *2006 Red Book: Report of the Committee on Infectious Diseases*. 24th ed. Elk Grove Village, IL: American Academy of Pediatrics; 2006.

273. Brawley RL, Wenzel RP. An algorithm for chickenpox exposure. *Pediatr Infect Dis J*. 1984;3:502–504.

274. Stover BH, Bratcher DF. Varicella-zoster virus: infection, control and prevention. *Am J Infect Control*. 1998;26:369–381.

275. Levandowski RA, Rubenis M. Nosocomial conjunctivitis caused by adenovirus Type 4. *J Infect Dis*. 1981;143:28–31.

276. Brummit CF, Cherrington JM, Katzenstein DA. Nosocomial adenovirus infections: molecular epidemiology of an outbreak due to adenovirus 3a. *J Infect Dis.* 1988;158:423–432.

277. Birenbaum E, Linder N, Varsano N, et al. Adenovirus type 8 conjunctivitis outbreak in a neonatal intensive care unit. *Arch Dis Child.* 1993;68:610–611.

278. Wharton M, Cochi SL, Hutcheson RH, Schaffner W. Mumps transmission in hospitals. *Arch Intern Med.* 1990;150:47–49.

279. Fischer PR, Brunetti C, Welch V, Christenson JC. Nosocomial mumps: report of an outbreak and its control. *Am J Infect Control.* 1996;24:13–18.

280. Buxton Bridges C, Kuehnert MJ, Hall CB. Transmission of influenza: implications for control in health care setting. *Clin Infect Dis.* 2003;37:1094–1101.

281. Shishiba T, Matsunaga Y. An outbreak of erythema infectiosum among hospital staff members including a patient with pleural fluid and pericardial effusion. *J Am Acad Dermatol.* 1993;29:265–267.

282. Seng C, Watkins P, Morse D, et al. Parvovirus B19 outbreak on an adult ward. *Epidemiol Infect.* 1994;113:345–353.

283. Pillay D, Patou G, Hurt S, Kibbler CC, Griffiths PD. Parvovirus B19 outbreak in a children's ward. *Lancet.* 1992;339:107–109.

284. Poland GA, Nichol KL. Medical students as sources of rubella and measles outbreaks. *Arch Intern Med.* 1990;150:44–46.

285. Fliegel PE, Weinstein WM. Rubella outbreak in a prenatal clinic: management and prevention. *Am J Infect Control.* 1982;10:29–33.

286. Polk FB, White JA, DeGirolami PC, Modlin JF. An outbreak of rubella among hospital personnel. *N Engl J Med.* 1980;303:541–545.

287. Klausner JD, Passaro D, Rosenberg J, et al. Enhanced control of *Mycoplasma pneumoniae* pneumonia with azithromycin prophylaxis. *J Infect Dis.* 1998;177:161–166.

288. Hall CB. Nosocomial viral respiratory infections: perennial weeds on pediatric wards. *Am J Med.* 1981;70:670–676.

289. Hall CB, Douglas RG Jr. Possible transmission by fomites of respiratory syncytial virus. *J Infect Dis.* 1980;141:98–102.

290. Hall CB. Respiratory syncytial virus: its transmission in the hospital environment. *Yale J Biol Med.* 1982;55:219–223.

291. Hall CB. The nosocomial spread of respiratory syncytial viral infections. *Annu Rev Med.* 1983;34:311–319.

292. Snydman DR, Greer C, Meissner HC, McIntosh K. Prevention of nosocomial transmission of respiratory syncytial virus in a newborn nursery. *Infect Control Hosp Epidemiol.* 1988;9:105–108.

293. Falsey AR. Noninfluenza respiratory virus infection in long-term care facilities. *Infect Control Hosp Epidemiol.* 1991;12:602–608.

294. Sorvillo FJ, Huie SF, Strassburg MA, Butsumyo A, Shandera WAX, Fannin SL. An outbreak of respiratory syncytial virus pneumonia in a nursing home for the elderly. *J Infect.* 1984;9:252–256.

295. Harrington RD, Hooton TM, Hackman RC, et al. An outbreak of respiratory syncytial virus in a bone marrow transplant center. *J Infect Dis.* 1992;165:987–993.

296. Guidry GG, Black-Payne CA, Payne DK, Jamison RM, George RB, Bocchini JA Jr. Respiratory syncytial virus infection among intubated adults in a university intensive care unit. *Chest.* 1991;100:1377–1384.

297. Valenti WM, Clarke TA, Hall CB, et al. Concurrent outbreaks of rhinovirus and respiratory syncytial virus in an intensive care nursery: epidemiology and associated risk factors. *J Pediatr.* 1982;100:722–726.

298. Goldmann DA. Epidemiology and prevention of pediatric viral respiratory infections in health-care institutions. *Emerg Infect Dis.* 2001;7:249–253.

299. Jalal H, Bibby DF, Bennett J, et al. Molecular investigations of an outbreak of parainfluenza virus type 3 and respiratory syncytial virus infections in a hematology unit. *J Clin Microbiol.* 2007;45:1690–1696.

300. Halasa NB, Williams JV, Wilson GJ, Walsh WF, Schaffner W, Wright PF. Medical and economic impact of a respiratory syncytial virus outbreak in a neonatal intensive care unit. *Pediatr Infect Dis J*. 2005;24(12):1040–1044.

301. Broder KR, Cortese MM, Iskander JK, et al. Preventing tetanus, diphtheria, and pertussis among adolescents: use of tetanus toxoid, reduced diphtheria toxoid and acellular pertussis vaccines recommendations of the Advisory Committee on Immunization Practices (ACIP). *MMWR Recomm Rep*. 2006; 55:1–34.

302. Long SS, Welkon CJ, Clark JL. Widespread silent transmission of pertussis in families: antibody correlates of infection and symptomatology. *J Infect Dis*. 1990;161:480–486.

303. Black S. Epidemiology of pertussis. *Pediatr Infect Dis J*. 1997;16:S85–S89.

304. Weber DJ, Rutala WA. Pertussis: an underappreciated risk for nosocomial outbreaks. *Infect Control Hosp Epidemiol*. 1998;19:825–828.

305. Cherry JD. Nosocomial pertussis in the nineties. *Infect Control Hosp Epidemiol*. 1995;16:553–555.

306. Bryant K, Humbaugh K, Brothers K, et al. Measures to control an outbreak of pertussis in a neonatal intermediate care nursery after exposure to a healthcare worker. *Infect Control Hosp Epidemiol*. 2006;27:541–545.

307. Boulay BR, Murray CJ, Ptak J, Kirkland KB, Montero J, Talbot EA. An outbreak of pertussis in a hematology-oncology care unit: implications for adult vaccination policy. *Infect Control Hosp Epidemiol*. 2006; 27:92–95.

308. Linneman CC Jr, Ramundo N, Perlstein PH, Minton SD, Englender GS. Use of pertussis vaccine in an epidemic involving hospital staff. *Lancet*. 1975;2:540–543.

309. Valenti WM, Pincus PH, Messner MK. Nosocomial pertussis: possible spread by a hospital visitor. *Am J Dis Child*. 1980;134:520–521.

310. Kurt TL, Yeager AS, Guenette S, Dunlop S. Spread of pertussis by hospital staff. *JAMA*. 1972;221:264–267.

311. Bassinet L, Matrat M, Njamkepo E, et al. Nosocomial pertussis outbreak among adult patients and healthcare workers. *Infect Control Hosp Epidemiol*. 2004;25:995–997.

312. Pascual FB, McCall CL, McMurtray A, et al. Outbreak of pertussis among healthcare workers in a hospital surgical unit. *Infect Control Hosp Epidemiol*. 2006;27(6):546–552.

313. Bonmarin I, Poujol I, Lévy-Bruhl D. Nosocomial infections and community clusters of pertussis in France, 2000–2005. *Eur Surveill*. 2007;12(11). http://www.eurosurveillance.org/em/v12n11/1211–226.asp. Accessed May 1, 2008.

314. Vranken P, Pogue M, Romalewski C, Ratard R. Outbreak of pertussis in a neonatal intensive care unit—Louisiana, 2004. *Am J Infect Control*. 2006;34:550–554.

315. Calugar A, Ortega-Sanchez IR, Tiwari T, et al. Nosocomial pertussis: costs of an outbreak and benefits of vaccinating health care workers. *Clin Infect Dis*. 2006;42(7):981–988.

316. Daskalaki I, Hennessey P, Hubler R, Long SS. Resource consumption in the infection control management of pertussis exposure among healthcare workers in pediatrics. *Infect Control Hosp Epidemiol*. 2007;28:412–417.

317. Baggett HC, Duchin JS, Shelton W. Two nosocomial pertussis outbreaks and their associated costs—King County, Washington, 2004. *Infect Control Hosp Epidemiol*. 2007;28:537–543.

318. Christie CD, Glover AM, Wilke MJ, Marx ML, Reising SF, Hutchinson NM. Containment of pertussis in the regional pediatric hospital during the greater Cincinnati epidemic of 1993. *Infect Control Hosp Epidemiol*. 1995;16:556–563.

319. Tam TWS, Bentsi-Enchill A. The return of the 100-day cough: resurgence of pertussis in the 1990s. *CMAJ*. 1998;159(6):695–596.

320. de Melker HE, Schellekens JFP, Neppelenbroek SE, et al. Reemergence of pertussis in the highly vaccinated population of the Netherlands: observations on surveillance data. *Emerg Infect Dis*. 2000;6:348–335.

321. Wirsing von König C, Riffelman M,. Pertussis: An old disease in new clothes [Epub ahead of print]. *Eur Surveill*. 2007;12(9). http://www.eurosurveillance.org/em/v12n09/1209–221.asp. Accessed May 2, 2008.

322. Centers for Disease Control and Prevention. Outbreaks of respiratory illness mistakenly attributed to pertussis—New Hampshire, Massachusetts, and Tennessee, 2004–2006. *MMWR*. 2007;56(33);837–842.

323. Centers for Disease Control and Prevention. *Guidelines for the Control of Pertussis Outbreaks*. Centers for Disease Control and Prevention: Atlanta, GA, 2000. (Amendments made in 2005 and 2006). http://www.cdc.gov/vaccines/pubs/pertussis-guide/guide.htm. Accessed May 1, 2008.

324. Centers for Disease Control and Prevention. CDC. Preventing tetanus, diphtheria, and pertussis among adults: use of tetanus toxoid, reduced diphtheria toxoid and acellular pertussis vaccine. Recommendations of the Advisory Committee on Immunization Practices (ACIP), supported by the Healthcare Infection Control Practices Advisory Committee (HICPAC), for use of Tdap among health-care personnel. *MMWR*. 2006;55(No. RR-17).

325. Rutala WA, Weber DJ. Management of healthcare workers exposed to pertussis. *Infect Control Hosp Epidemiol*. 1994;15:411–415.

326. Haiduven DJ, Hench CP, Simpkins SM, Stevens DA. Standardized management of patients and employees exposed to pertussis. *Infect Control Hosp Epidemiol*. 1998;19:861–864.

327. Haley CE, Cohen ML, Halter J, Meyer RD. Nosocomial Legionnaires' disease: a continuing common-source epidemic at Wadsworth Medical Center. *Ann Intern Med*. 1979;90:583–586.

328. Thacker SB, Bennett JV, Tsai TF, et al. An outbreak in 1965 of severe respiratory illness caused by the Legionnaires' disease bacterium. *J Infect Dis*. 1978;138:512–519.

329. Mermel LA, Josephson SL, Giorgio CH, Dempsey J, Parentau S. Association of Legionnaires' disease with construction: contamination of potable water? *Infect Control Hosp Epidemiol*. 1995;16:76–81.

330. Doebbeling BN, Ishak MA, Wade BH, et al. Nosocomial *Legionella micdadei* pneumonia: 10 years experience and a case-control study. *J Hosp Infect*. 1989;13:289–298.

331. Memish ZA, Oxley C, Contant J, Garber GE. Plumbing system shock absorbers as a source of *Legionella pneumophila*. *Am J Infect Control*. 1992;20:305–309.

332. Venezia RA, Agresta MD, Hanley EM, Urquhart K, Schoonmaker D. Nosocomial legionellosis associated with aspiration of nasogastric feedings diluted in tap water. *Infect Control Hosp Epidemiol*. 1994;15:529–533.

333. Centers for Disease Control and Prevention. Sustained transmission of nosocomial Legionnaires' disease—Arizona and Ohio. *MMWR*. 1997;46:416–421.

334. Dondero TJ, Rendtorff RC, Mallison GF, et al. An outbreak of Legionnaires' disease associated with a contaminated cooling tower. *N Engl J Med*. 1980;302:365.

335. Arnow PM, Chou T, Weil D, et al. Nosocomial Legionnaires' disease caused by aerosolized tap water from respiratory devices. *J Infect Dis*. 1982;146:460–467.

336. Ricketts K, Joseph C, Legionnaires' disease in Europe: 2005–2006 [Epub ahead of print]. *Eur Surveill* 2007;12(12). http://www.eurosurveillance.org/em/v12n12/1212–224.asp. Accessed July 29, 2008.

337. Brown CM, Nuorti P, Breiman RF, et al. A community outbreak of Legionnaires' disease linked to hospital cooling towers: an epidemiological method to calculate dose of exposure. *Int J Epidemiol*. 1999;28:353–359.

338. Guerrero IC, Filippone C. A cluster of Legionnaires' disease in a community hospital—a clue to a larger epidemic. *Infect Control Hosp Epidemiol*. 1996;17:177–178.

339. Bartram J, Chartier Y, Lee JV, Pond K, Surman-Lee S, eds. *Legionella and the Prevention of Legionellosis*. Geneva, Switzerland: World Health Organization; 2007. http://www.who.int/water_sanitation_health/emerging/legionella/en/index.html. Accessed May 2, 2008.

340. Walsh TJ, Dixon DM. Nosocomial aspergillosis: environmental microbiology, hospital epidemiology, diagnosis, and treatment. *Eur J Epidemiol*. 1989;5:131–142.

341. Cole EC, Cook CE. Characterization of infectious aerosols in health care facilities: an aid to effective engineering controls and preventive strategies. *Am J Infect Control*. 1998;26:453–464.

342. Pannuti CS, Gingrich RD, Pfaller MA, Wenzel RP. Nosocomial pneumonia in adult patients undergoing bone marrow transplantation: a 9-year study. *J Clin Oncol*. 1991;9:77–84.

343. Rotstein C, Cummings KM, Tidings J, et al. An outbreak of invasive aspergillosis among allogeneic bone marrow transplants: a case-control study. *Infect Control.* 1985;6:347–355.

344. Opal SM, Asp AA, Cannady PB Jr, Morse PL, Burton LJ, Hammer PG II. Efficacy of infection control measures during a nosocomial outbreak of disseminated aspergillosis associated with hospital construction. *J Infect Dis.* 1986;153:634–637.

345. Arnow PM, Anderson RL, Mainous D, et al. Pulmonary aspergillosis during hospital renovation. *Am Rev Respir Dis.* 1978;118:49–53.

346. Flynn PM, Williams BG, Hetherington SV, Williams BF, Giannini MA, Pearson TA. *Aspergillus terreus* during hospital renovation. *Infect Control Hosp Epidemiol.* 1993;14:363–365.

347. McCarty JM, Flam MJ, Pulen G, et al. Outbreak of primary cutaneous aspergillosis related to intravenous arm boards. *J Pediatr.* 1986;108:721–724.

348. Hopkins CC, Weber DJ, Rubin RH. Invasive *Aspergillus* infection: possible non-ward common source within the hospital environment. *J Hosp Infect.* 1989;13:19–25.

349. Thio CL, Smith D, Merz WG, et al. Refinements of environmental assessment during an outbreak investigation of invasive aspergillosis in a leukemia and bone marrow transplant unit. *Infect Control Hosp Epidemiol.* 2000;21(1):18–23.

350. Pegues DSA, Lasker BA, McNeil MM, et al. Cluster of cases of invasive aspergillosis in a transplant intensive care unit: evidence of person-to-person airborne transmission. *Clin Infect Dis.* 2002;34:412–416. http://www.journals.uchicago.edu/doi/pdf/10.1086/338025. Accessed May 2, 2008.

351. Hruszkewycz V, Ruben B, Hypes CM, Bostic GD, Staszkiewicz J, Band JD. A cluster of pseudofungemia associated with hospital renovation adjacent to the microbiology laboratory. *Infect Control Hosp Epidemiol.* 1992;13:147–150.

352. Carter CD, Barr BA. Infection control issues in construction and renovation. *Infect Control Hosp Epidemiol.* 1997;18:587–596.

353. Maryland Department of Health and Mental Hygiene, Community Health Administration. *Guidelines for Prevention and Control of Nosocomial Pulmonary Aspergillosis, 1999.* http://www.cha.state.md.us/edcp/guidelines/aspers2.html. Accessed May 2, 2008.

354. Carreras E. Preventing exposure to molds. *Clin Microbiol Infect.* 2006;12(suppl 7):77–83. http://www.blackwell-synergy.com/doi/abs/10.1111/j.1469–0691.2006.01608.x. Accessed May 2, 2008.

355. Gangneux J-P, Bretagne S, Cordonnier C, et al. Prevention of nosocomial fungal infection: the French approach. *Clin Infect Dis.* 2002;35:343–345. http://www.journals.uchicago.edu/doi/pdf/10.1086/341318. Accessed May 2, 2008.

356. Rutala WA, Weber DJ. Water as a reservoir of nosocomial pathogens. *Infect Control Hosp Epidemiol.* 1997;18:609–616.

357. Stamm WE, Colella JJ, Anderson RL, Dixon RE. Indwelling arterial catheters as a source of nosocomial bacteremia: an outbreak caused by *Flavobacterium* species. *N Engl J Med.* 1975;292:1099–1102.

358. Casewell MW, Slater NGP, Cooper JE. Operating theatre water baths as a cause of *Pseudomonas* septicaemia. *J Hosp Infect.* 1981;2:237–240.

359. McGuckin MB, Thorpe RJ, Abrutyn E. Hydrotherapy: an outbreak of *Pseudomonas aeruginosa* wound infections related to Hubbard tank treatments. *Arch Phys Med Rehabil.* 1981;62:283–285.

360. Lowry PW, Beck-Sague CM, Bland LA, et al. *Mycobacterium chelonae* infection among patients receiving high-flux dialysis in a hemodialysis clinic in California. *J Infect Dis.* 1990;161:85–90.

361. Graman PS, Quinlan GA, Rank JA. Nosocomial legionellosis traced to a contaminated ice machine. *Infect Control Hosp Epidemiol.* 1997;18:637–640.

362. Verweij PE, Bilj D, Melchers W, et al. Pseudo-outbreak of multiresistant *Pseudomonas aeruginosa* in a hematology unit. *Infect Control Hosp Epidemiol.* 1997;18:128–131.

363. Sniadack DH, Ostroff SM, Karlix MA, et al. A nosocomial pseudo-outbreak of *Mycobacterium xenopi* due to a contaminated potable water supply: lessons in prevention. *Infect Control Hosp Epidemiol.* 1993;14:636–641.

364. Van Horn KG, Tatz JS, Li KI, Newman L, Wormser GP. Copepods associated with a perirectal abscess and copepod pseudo-outbreak in stools for ova and parasite examinations. *Diagn Microbiol Infect Dis*. 1992;15:561–565.

365. Klotz SA, Normand RE, Kalinsky RG. "Through a drinking glass and what was found there": pseudocontamination of a hospital's drinking water. *Infect Control Hosp Epidemiol*. 1992;13:477–481.

366. Muyldermans G, de Smet F, Pierard D, et al. Neonatal infections with *Pseudomonas aeruginosa* associated with a water-bath used to thaw fresh frozen plasma. *J Hosp Infect*. 1998; 9(4):309–314.

367. Conger NG, O'Connell RJ, Laurel VL, et al. *Mycobacterium simiae* outbreak associated with a hospital water supply. *Infect Control Hosp Epidemiol*. 2004;25:1050–1055.

368. Emmerson AM. Emerging waterborne infections in health-care settings. *Emerg Infect Dis*. 2007;7:272–276. http://www.cdc.gov/ncidod/eid/vol7no2/emmerson.htm. Accessed May 2, 2008.

369. Manangan LP, Anderson RL, Arduino MJ, Bond WW. Sanitary care and maintenance of ice-storage chests and ice-making machines in health care facilities. *Am J Infect Control*. 1998;26(2):111–112.

370. Burnett IA, Weeks GR, Harris DM. A hospital study of ice-making machines: their bacteriology, design, usage, and upkeep. *J Hosp Infect*. 1994;28:305–313.

371. Maloney SA, Jarvis WR. Epidemic nosocomial pneumonia in the intensive care unit. *Chest*. 1995;16:209–223.

372. Patterson TF, Patterson JE, Masecar BL, et al. A nosocomial outbreak of *Branhamella catarrhalis* confirmed by restriction endonuclease analysis. *J Infect Dis*. 1988;157:996–1001.

373. Centers for Disease Control. Suspected nosocomial influenza cases in an intensive care unit. *MMWR*. 1988;37:3–4.

374. Locksley RM, Cohen ML, Quinn TC, et al. Multiply antibiotic-resistant *Staphylococcus aureus*: introduction, transmission, and evolution of nosocomial infection. *Ann Intern Med*. 1982;97:317–324.

375. Singh-Naz N, Willy M, Riggs N. Outbreak of para-influenza virus type 3 in a neonatal nursery. *Pediatr Infect Dis J*. 1990;9:31–33.

376. Villarino ME, Stevens LE, Schable BS, et al. Risk factors for epidemic *Xanthomonas* infection/colonization in intensive care unit patients. *Infect Control Hosp Epidemiol*. 1992;13:201–206.

377. Fisher-Hoch SP, Tobin JO, Nelson AM, et al. Investigation and control of Legionnaires' disease in a district general hospital. *Lancet*. 1981;1:933–936.

378. Arnow PM, Chou T, Weil D, et al. Nosocomial Legionnaires' disease caused by aerosolized tap water from respiratory devices. *J Infect Dis*. 1982;146:460–467.

379. Brady MT. Nosocomial Legionnaires' disease in a children's hospital. *J Pediatr*. 1988;115: 46–58.

380. Mastro TD, Fields BS, Breiman RF, et al. Legionnaires' disease and use of medication nebulizers. *J Infect Dis*. 1991;163:667–671.

381. Blatt SP, Parkinson MD, Pace E, et al. Nosocomial Legionnaires' disease: aspiration as a primary mode of disease acquisition. *Am J Med*. 1991;95:16–22.

382. Weems JJ, Davis BJ, Tablan OC, et al. Construction activity: an independent risk factor for invasive aspergillosis and zygomycosis in patients with hematologic malignancy. *Infect Control*. 1987;8:71–75.

383. Arnow PM, Sadigh M, Costas C, et al. Endemic and epidemic aspergillosis associated with in-hospital replication of *Aspergillus* organisms. *J Infect Dis*. 1991;164:998–1002.

384. Buffington J, Reporter R, Lasker B, et al. Investigation of an epidemic of invasive aspergillosis: utility of molecular typing with the use of random amplified polymorphic DNS probes. *Pediatr Infect Dis J*. 1994;13:386–393.

385. Gastmeier P, Loui A, Stamm-Balderjahn S, et al. Outbreaks in neonatal intensive care units—They are not like others. *Am J Infect Control*. 2007;35:172–176.

386. Samet JM, Marbury MC, Spengler JD. Health effects and sources of indoor air pollution, pt. 1. *Am Rev Respir Dis*. 1987;136:1486–1508.

387. Samet JM, Marbury MC, Spengler JD. Health effects and sources of indoor air pollution, pt. 2. *Am Rev Respir Dis*. 1988;137:221–242.

388. Brandt-Rauf PW, Andrews LR, Schwarz-Miller J. Sick-hospital syndrome. *J Occup Med*. 1991;33:737–739.

389. Gold DR. Indoor air pollution. *Clin Chest Med*. 1992;13:215–229.

390. Hodgson M. Indoor environmental exposures and symptoms. *Environ Health Perspect*. 2002;110:(Suppl 4):663–667. http://www.ehponline.org/members/2002/suppl-4/663–667hodgson/hodgson-full.html. Accessed May 3, 2008.

391. Jaakkola MS, Yang L, Ieromnimon A, Jaakkola JJK. Office work exposures and respiratory and sick building syndrome symptoms. *Occup Environ Med*. 2007;64(3):178–184. [Erratum in: *Occup Environ Med*. 2007 Jun;64(6):428.] http://oem.bmj.com/cgi/content/full/64/3/178. Accessed May 3, 2008.

392. Donnell HD Jr, Bagby JR, Harmon RG, et al. Report of an illness outbreak at the Harry S Truman State Office Building. *Am J Epidemiol*. 1989;129(3):550–558.

393. Klaucke DN, Johansen M, Vogt RL. An outbreak of xylene intoxication in a hospital. *Am J Ind Med*. 1982;3(2):173–178.

394. Klauck D, Vogt R. A case exercise: outbreak investigation at a Vermont community hospital. *J Public Health Manag Pract*. 2005;11(4):301–305.

395. Hardin BD, Kelman BJ, Saxon A. ACOEM evidence-based statement. adverse human health effects associated with molds in the indoor environment. *J Occup Environ Med*. 2003;45(5):70–478. http://www.joem.org/pt/re/joem/fulltext.00043764-200305000-00006.htm; jsessionid=LcDNJvXVnnDgJvDR7d155vzr6LtQRhMWdVdf03HSSnmK1JL6D3Wt!1379360954!181195629!8091!-1?&fullimage=true. Accessed May 3, 2008.

396. Pfaller MA. Nosocomial candidiasis: emerging species, reservoirs, and modes of transmission. *Clin Infect Dis*. 1996;22(suppl 2):S89–S94.

397. Jarvis WR. Epidemiology of nosocomial fungal infections with emphasis on *Candida* species. *Clin Infect Dis*. 1995;20:1526–1530.

398. Pfaller MA, Diekma DJ. Epidemiology of invasive candidiasis: a persistent public health problem. *Clin Microbiol Rev*. 2007;20(1):133–163. http://www.pubmedcentral.nih.gov/articlerender.fcgi?tool=pubmed&pubmedid=17223626. Accessed May 3, 2008.

399. Perlroth J, Choi B, Spellberg B. Nosocomial fungal infections: epidemiology, diagnosis, and treatment. *Med Mycol*. 2007;45(4):321–346.

400. Pappas PG. Invasive candidiasis. *Infect Dis Clin North Am*. 2006;20(3):485–506.

401. Waggoner-Fountain LA, Whit Walker M, Hollis RJ, et al. Vertical and horizontal transmission of unique *Candida* species to premature newborns. *Clin Infect Dis*. 1996:22:803–808.

402. Fowler SL, Rhoten B, Springer SC, Messer SA, Hollis RJ, Pfaller MA. Evidence for person-to-person transmission of *Candida lusitaniae* in a neonatal intensive care unit. *Infect Control Hosp Epidemiol*. 1998;19:343–345.

403. Reef SE, Lasker BA, Butcher DS. Nonperinatal nosocomial transmission of *Candida albicans* in a neonatal intensive care unit: prospective study. *J Clin Microbiol*. 1998;36:1255–1259.

404. van Asbeck EC, Huang YC, Markham AN, Clemons KV, Stevens DA. *Candida parapsilosis* fungemia in neonates: genotyping results suggest healthcare workers hands as source, and review of published studies. *Mycopathologia*. 2007;164(6):287–293.

405. Sheretz RJ, Gledhill KS, Hampton KD, et al. Outbreaks of *Candida* bloodstream infections associated with retrograde medication administration in a neonatal intensive care unit. *J Pediatr*. 1992;120:455–461.

406. Solomon SL, Khabbaz R, Parker RH, et al. An outbreak of *Candida parapsilosis* bloodstream infections in patients receiving parenteral nutrition. *J Infect Dis*. 1984;149:96–102.

407. Solomon SL, Alexander H, Eley JW, et al. Nosocomial fungemia in neonates associated with intravascular pressure monitoring devices. *Pediatr Infect Dis J*. 1986;5:680–685.

408. Faix RG, Finkel DJ, Andersen RD, Hostetter MK. Genotypic analysis of a cluster of systemic *Candida albicans* infections in a neonatal intensive care unit. *Pediatr Infect Dis J.* 1995;14:1063–1068.

409. Strausbaugh LJ, Sewell DL, Ward TT, Pfaller MA, Heitzman T, Tjoelker R. High frequency of yeast carriage on hands of hospital personnel. *J Clin Microbiol.* 1994;32:2299–2300.

410. Khatib R, Thirumoorthi MC, Riederer KM, Sturm L, Oney LA, Baran J. Clustering of *Candida* infections in the neonatal intensive care unit: concurrent emergence of multiple strains simulating intermittent outbreaks. *Pediatr Infect Dis J.* 1998;17:130–134.

411. Institute of Medicine. *Emerging Infections: Microbial Threats to Health in the United States.* Washington, DC: National Academy Press; 1994.

412. Centers for Disease Control and Prevention. *Preventing Emerging Infectious Diseases: A Strategy for the 21st Century.* Atlanta, GA: US Dept of Health and Human Services; 1998. http://www.cdc.gov/MMWR/PDF/rr/rr4715.pdf. Accessed May 3, 2008.

413. Weber DJ, Rutala WA. The emerging nosocomial pathogens *Cryptosporidium, Escherichia coli* O157:H7, *Helicobacter pylori,* and hepatitis C: epidemiology, environmental survival, efficacy of disinfection, and control measures. *Infect Control Hosp Epidemiol.* 2001;22:306–315.

414. Bresee JS, Mast EE, Coleman PJ, et al. Hepatitis C virus infection associated with administration of intravenous immune globulin: a cohort study. *JAMA.* 1996;276:1563–1567.

415. Danzig LE, Short LJ, Collins K, et al. Bloodstream infections associated with a needleless intravenous infusion system in patients receiving home infusion therapy. *JAMA.* 1995;273:1862–1864.

416. Dowell SF, Mukunu R, Ksiazek TG, Khan AS, Rollin PE, Peters CJ, and the Ebola Hemorrhagic Fever Study Group. Transmission of Ebola hemorrhagic fever: a study of risk factors in family members—Kikwit, Zaire. *J Infect Dis.* 1999;179:S87–S91.

417. Jochimsen EM, Fish L, Manning K, et al. Evaluation and control of vancomycin-resistant enterococci at an Indianapolis hospital. Presented at: Seventh Annual Meeting of the Society for Healthcare Epidemiology of America; April 27–29, 1997; St. Louis, MO. Abstract 54.

418. Fridkin SK, Pear SM, Williamson TH, Galgiani JN, Jarvis WR. The role of understaffing in central venous catheter-associated bloodstream infections. *Infect Control Hosp Epidemiol.* 1996;17:150–158.

419. Archibald LK, Manning ML, Bell LM, Banerjee S, Jarvis WR. Patient density, nurse-to-patient ratio and nosocomial infection risk in a pediatric cardiac intensive care unit. *Pediatr Infect Dis J.* 1997;16:1045–1048.

420. Kellerman S, Shay DK, Howard J, et al. Bloodstream infections in home infusion patients: the influence of race and needleless intravascular access devices. *J Pediatr.* 1996;129:711–717.

421. Do A, Ray B, Barnett B, et al. Evaluation of the role of needleless devices (ND) in bloodstream infections. Presented at: 1996 Annual Meeting of the American Society of Microbiology, 36th Interscience Conference on Antimicrobial Agents and Chemotherapy; September 1996; New Orleans, LA. Abstract J61.

422. Donlan RM. Biofilms and device-associated infections. *Emerg Infect Dis.* 2002;7:277–281. http://www.cdc.gov/ncidod/eid/vol7no2/donlan.htm. Accessed May 3, 2008.

423. Lindsay D, von Holy A. Bacterial biofilms within the clinical setting: what healthcare professionals should know. *J Hosp Infect.* 2006;64:313–325.

424. Cassone M, Serra P, Mondello F, et al. Outbreak of *Saccharomyces cerevisiae* subtype boulardii fungemia in patients neighboring those treated with a probiotic preparation of the organism. *J Clin Microbiol.* 2003;41:5340–5343.

425. Bicudo EL, Macedo VO, Carrara MA, Castro FFS, Rage RI. Nosocomial outbreak of *Pantoea agglomerans* in a pediatric urgent care center. *Braz J Infect Dis.* 207;11:281–284. http://www.scielo.br/pdf/bjid/v11n2/23.pdf. Accessed April 23, 2008.

426. Habsah H, Zeehaida M, Van Rostenberghe H. An outbreak of *Pantoea* spp. in a neonatal intensive care unit secondary to contaminated parenteral nutrition. *J Hosp Infect.* 2005;61(3):213–218.

427. Van Rostenberghe H, Noraida R, Wan Pauzi WI, et al. The clinical picture of infection with *Pantoea* species. *Jpn J Infect Dis*. 2006;59:120–121. http://www.nih.go.jp/JJID/59/120.pdf. Accessed May 4, 2008.

428. Koo H-K, Kim J-S, Eom J-S, et al. Pseudooutbreak of *Pantoea* species bacteremia associated with contaminated cotton pledgets. *Am J Infect Control*. 2006;34:443–446.

429. Centers for Disease Control and Prevention. Update: multistate outbreak of mumps—United States, January 1–May 2, 2006. *MMWR*. 2006;55(20):559–563. http://www.cdc.gov/mmwR/preview/mmwrhtml/mm5520a4.htm. Accessed May 4, 2008.

430. Boyce J. Environmental contamination makes an important contribution to hospital infection. *J Hosp Infect*. 2007;65(Suppl 2):50–54.

431. Hayden MK, Blom DW, Lyle EA, Moore CG, Weinstein RA. Risk of hand or glove contamination after contact with patients colonized with vancomycin-resistant *Enterococcus* or the colonized patient's environment. *Infect Control Hosp Epidemiol*. 2008;29:149–154.

432. Centers for Disease Control and Prevention. Influenza vaccination of health-care personnel recommendations of the Healthcare Infection Control Practices Advisory Committee (HICPAC) and the Advisory Committee on Immunization Practices (ACIP). *MMWR Recommendations and Reports*. 2006;55(RR-02);1–16. http://www.cdc.gov/MMWR/PREVIEW/MMWRHTML/rr5502a1.htm. Accessed May 4, 2008.

433. Centers for Disease Control and Prevention. Notice to readers: updated recommendations of the Advisory Committee on Immunization Practices (ACIP) for the control and elimination of mumps. *MMWR*. 2006;55(22);629–630. http://www.cdc.gov/mmwR/preview/mmwrhtml/mm5522a4.htm. Accessed May 4, 2008.

434. Centers for Disease Control and Prevention. *Epidemiology and Prevention of Vaccine-Preventable Diseases. The Pink Book*. 10th ed. Atlanta, GA: CDC; 2008. http://www.cdc.gov/vaccines/pubs/pinkbook/default.htm. Accessed May 4, 2008.

SUGGESTED READING AND RESOURCES

Readings

APIC Text of Infection Control and Epidemiology. Washington, DC: Association for Professionals in Infection Control and Epidemiology; 2005.

American Academy of Pediatrics. *2006 Red Book: Report of the Committee on Infectious Diseases*. 24th ed. Elk Grove Village, IL: American Academy of Pediatrics; 2006. http://www.aap.org.

Block SS, ed. *Disinfection, Sterilization, and Preservation*. 4th ed. Philadelphia, PA: Lea & Febiger; 1991.

Biosafety in Microbiological and Bio-Medical Laboratories. 4th ed. Atlanta, GA: US Dept of Health and Human Services, Public Health Service; 1999. http://www.cdc.gov/OD/ohs/biosfty/bmbl4/bmbl4toc.htm. Accessed May 4, 2008.

Atkinson W, Hamborsky J, McIntyre L, Wolfe S, eds. *Epidemiology and Prevention of Vaccine-Preventable Diseases. The Pink Book*. 10th ed. Washington DC: Public Health Foundation, 2008. http://www.cdc.gov/vaccines/pubs/pinkbook/default.htm. Accessed May 4, 2008.

Heymann DL. *Control of Communicable Diseases Manual*. 18th ed. Washington, DC: APHA Press; 2005.

Institute of Medicine. *Emerging Infections: Microbial Threats to Health in the United States*. Washington, DC: National Academy Press; 1994.

U.S. Department of Labor, Occupational Safety and Health Administration. Occupational Exposure to Bloodborne Pathogens (Final Rule). 1910 C.F.R. § 1030 (1991).

Preventing Emerging Infectious Diseases: A Strategy for the 21st Century. Atlanta, GA: US Dept of Health and Human Services; 1998. http://www.cdc.gov/mmwr/preview/mmwrhtml/00031393.htm. Accessed April 21, 2008.

Rutala WA, Weber DJ. Disinfection and sterilization in health care facilities: what clinicians need to know. *Clin Infect Dis*. 2004;39(5):702–709. http://www.journals.uchicago.edu/doi/abs/10.1086/423182. Accessed April 5, 2008.

United Kingdom Department of Health. Guidance for health care workers: protection against infection with blood-borne viruses. Recommendations of the Expert Advisory Group on AIDS and the Advisory Group on Hepatitis. London, UK: Her Majesty's Stationery Office; 1993. http://www.dh.gov.uk/assetRoot/04/01/44/74/04014474.pdf. Accessed April 30, 2008.

Centers for Disease Control and Prevention. Guideline for hand hygiene in health-care settings. Recommendations of the Healthcare Infection Control Practices Advisory Committee and the HICPAC/SHEA/APIC/IDSA Hand Hygiene Task Force. *MMWR.* 2002;51(No. RR-16). http://www.cdc.gov/mmwr/preview/mmwrhtml/rr5116a1.htm. Accessed April 5, 2008.

Centers for Disease Control and Prevention. Immunization of health-care workers: recommendations of the Advisory Committee on Immunization Practices (ACIP) and the Hospital Infection Control Practices Advisory Committee (HICPAC). *MMWR.* 1997;46(RR-18):1–42.

Bolyard EA, Tablan OC, Williams WW, et al. Guideline for infection control in health care personnel, 1998. *Am J Infect Control.* 1998;26:289–354. http://www.cdc.gov/ncidod/dhqp/gl_hcpersonnel .html. Accessed April 19, 2008.

Siegel JD, Rhinehart E, Jackson M, Chiarello L, and the Healthcare Infection Control Practices Advisory Committee, *2007 Guideline for Isolation Precautions: Preventing Transmission of Infectious Agents in Healthcare Settings.* Atlanta, GA: CDC; 2007. http://www.cdc.gov/ncidod/ dhqp/gl_isolation.html. Accessed November 25, 2007.

Centers for Disease Control and Prevention. *Guidelines for Preventing Health-Care-Associated Pneumonia, 2003. Recommendations of CDC and the Healthcare Infection Control Practices Advisory Committee.* Atlanta, GA: CDC; 2003. http://www.cdc.gov/ncidod/dhqp/gl_hcpneumonia .html. Accessed April 19, 2008.

Centers for Disease Control and Prevention. Recommendations for preventing transmission of human immunodeficiency virus and hepatitis B virus to patients during exposure-prone invasive procedures. *MMWR.* 1991;40(RR-8):1–9. http://www.cdc.gov/mmwR/preview/ mmwrhtml/00014845.htm. Accessed April 30, 2008.

Centers for Disease Control and Prevention. Guidelines for the prevention of intravascular catheter-related infections. *MMWR.* 2002;51(No. RR-10):1–36. http://www.cdc.gov/mmwr/ PDF/rr/rr5110.pdf. Accessed April 28, 2008.

Sehulster L, Chinn RY, Arduino MJ, et al. Guidelines for environmental infection control in health-care facilities, 2003. Recommendations of CDC and the Healthcare Infection Control Practices Advisory Committee (HICPAC). *MMWR.* 2003;52(RR-10):1–42. http://www.cdc.gov/ncidod/dhqp/gl_environinfection.html. Accessed April 5, 2008.

Appendix A of this text contains "Methods for Sterilizing and Disinfecting Patient-Care Items and Environmental Surfaces" reprinted from: CDC. Guidelines for infection control in dental health-care settings, 2003. *MMWR.* 2003:52(RR-17).

Resources

CDC recommended infection control guidelines for dentistry: Information on dental infection control issues as well as consensus evidence-based recommendations. See also the slide set and accompanying speaker notes. http://www.cdc.gov/oralhealth/ or http://www.cdc.gov/oralhealth/ infectioncontrol/guidelines/ppt.htm. Accessed April 14, 2008.

CDC Vaccines and Immunizations

- General information: http://www.cdc.gov/vaccines/default.htm
- Immunization schedules, recommendations and guidelines, and information for healthcare workers: http://www.cdc.gov/vaccines/recs/schedules/default.htm Accessed April 6, 2008.
- General recommendations on immunization: Recommendations of the Advisory Committee on Immunization Practices (ACIP). *MMWR.* 2006;55(No. RR-15).
- Prevention of varicella: Recommendations of the Advisory Committee on Immunization Practices (ACIP). *MMWR.* 2007;56(No. RR-4).

CDC Infection control in health care settings: http://www.cdc.gov/ncidod/dhqp/

CDC Dialysis-associated infections: Infection prevention and control guidelines and links to outbreak reports and surveillance data. http://www.cdc.gov/ncidod/dhqp/dpac_dialysis_pc.html. Accessed April 11, 2008.

Disinfection and Sterilization.org: Guidelines and resources on cleaning, disinfection, and sterilization in healthcare settings: http://disinfectionandsterilization.org.

Food and Drug Administration (FDA) Adverse Event Reporting System

MedWatch—The FDA Safety Information and Adverse Event Reporting System. http://www .fda.gov/medwatch.

Agencies and Organizations

The following national agencies and organizations have guidelines, position papers, and standards that can be used for developing infection prevention and control programs in the acute care setting. Information on obtaining copies of these guidelines can be obtained by telephoning the organization or accessing their Web site.

American College of Occupational and Environmental Medicine (ACOEM)
25 Northwest Point Blvd, Suite 700
Elk Grove Village, IL 60007-1030
Telephone: 847/818-1800, Fax: 847/818-9266
http://www.acoem.org

American Society for Gastrointestinal Endoscopy (ASGE)
13 Elm St
Manchester, MA 01944-1314
Telephone: 978-526-8330
http://www.asge.org

Multidisciplinary guideline for reprocessing flexible gastrointestinal gastroscopes. *Endoscopy.* 2003;58:1–8. http://www.asge.org/WorkArea/showcontent.aspx?id=3376. Accessed April 28, 2008.

Association for Professionals in Infection Control and Epidemiology (APIC)
1275 K St NW, Suite 1000
Washington, DC 20005-4006
Telephone: 202-789-1890
http://www.apic.org

Association for the Advancement of Medical Instrumentation (AAMI)
3330 Washington Blvd, Suite 400
Arlington, VA 22201-4598
Telephone: 800-332-2264, ext. 217
http://www.aami.org

Provides standards for dialysis water quality, storage, and distribution and standards for disinfection and sterilization in healthcare settings.

Association of periOperative Registered Nurses (AORN)
2170 South Parker Rd, Suite 300
Denver, CO 80231-5711
Telephone: 800-755-2676
http://www.aorn.org

Provides standards for operating rooms and for cleaning, disinfection, and sterilization of equipment.

Centers for Disease Control and Prevention (CDC)
1600 Clifton Rd
Atlanta, GA 30033
http://www.cdc.gov

The *Morbidity and Mortality Weekly Report (MMWR)* and most of the CDC guidelines noted in this chapter can be downloaded from this Web site.

Immunization Action Coalition
1573 Selby Avenue, St. Paul, MN 55104
(651) 647-9009
http://www.immunize.org and http://www.vaccineinformation.org

CHAPTER 4

Outbreaks Reported in Long-Term Care Settings

Kathleen Meehan Arias

> Outbreaks of infection are common in long-term care facilities, and a wide variety have been reported . . . Effective implementation of control programs should limit the occurrence and extent of outbreaks.[1]

INTRODUCTION

The term *long-term care facility* (LTCF) encompasses a variety of institutions: nursing homes (NHs), skilled nursing facilities (SNFs), psychiatric hospitals, rehabilitation centers, pediatric chronic care facilities, and facilities for persons with intellectual and developmental disabilities. In addition to freestanding LTCFs, many acute care hospitals have affiliated long-term subacute care units. Conversely, many LTCFs have ventilator and subacute care units. These specialty care settings are known as long-term acute care because they provide comprehensive nursing and medical care for an extended period of time to persons who cannot be managed in a nursing or home health care setting.[2] The majority of LTCFs in the United States are nursing homes. Of the estimated 2.5 million Americans who reside in an LTCF, approximately 1.6 million elderly and disabled residents receive care in nearly 17,000 NHs in the United States.[3] These numbers are expected to increase as the baby-boom generation ages. An estimated 25–43% of persons who reach the age of 65 years will likely spend some time in an NH.[4,5] Most persons admitted to an NH generally have a chronic disease or a disability or have reached an advanced age and require nursing and medical care, and 90% of those who reside in NHs are over 65 years of age.[6]

The purpose of this chapter is to review reports of outbreaks that have occurred in long-term care settings and discuss effective infection prevention and control measures. These reports were identified by conducting a Medline search of English-language publications from 1985 through 2007, by reviewing the table of contents of selected publications, and by reading the references listed in relevant articles and infection prevention and control textbooks. Almost all of the identified outbreaks occurred in NHs. Perhaps this is because the frail elderly population that resides in NHs is more likely to develop a nosocomial or healthcare-associated infection (HAI) than the mostly younger, more mobile residents of other types of LTCFs. Little has been published about epidemic infections in pediatric LTCFs, and only a few reports from pediatric settings are noted.[7] The reports of outbreaks in LTCFs highlight the importance of having a routine surveillance program that can identify the occurrence of both facility-acquired and community-acquired infections. Personnel who are responsible for infection prevention and control programs in long-term care settings should be familiar with the types of outbreaks that have been reported in LTCFs and should implement prevention and control measures to prevent similar occurrences in their facility. Although this chapter describes outbreaks that occurred in LTCFs, many of the reported etiologic agents and disease syndromes, especially gastrointestinal and respiratory illnesses, are associated with endemic and epidemic infections in both the long-term care and acute care settings. Therefore, practitioners in long-term care settings should be familiar with outbreaks reported in a variety of healthcare settings, including those reported in acute care settings.

Several agents that have been found to cause outbreaks in a variety of healthcare settings are discussed in Chapter 7. These include *Mycobacterium tuberculosis*, *Sarcoptes scabiei*, norovirus, *Clostridium difficile*, the influenza viruses, and multidrug-resistant organisms such as methicillin-resistant *Staphylococcus aureus* (MRSA) and vancomycin-resistant *Enterococcus* (VRE). There are many reports of outbreaks of VRE in hospitals, especially in patients in intensive care units. Although VRE is often found to colonize LTCF residents, and is responsible for causing sporadic infections in residents, there are few published reports of VRE outbreaks in an LTCF.[8,9]

The Suggested Reading and Resources section at the end of this chapter provides additional information on infectious diseases and infection prevention and control in LTCFs.

ENDEMIC INFECTIONS

Elderly patients in hospitals and LTCFs are particularly susceptible to infection, and HAIs have long been recognized in this population.[6,10,11,13] The overall nosocomial infection rates reported in LTCFs vary widely because of differences in definitions used to classify infections, duration of study, data collection methods, format for data presentation (incidence versus prevalence), population characteristics, and level of nursing intensity (e.g., intermediate SNFs versus nursing facilities). Reported overall prevalence rates range from 1.6 to 32.7 infections per 100 residents per month,[6,10,14] and incidence rates range from 10.7% to 20.7% or 2.6 to 7.1 infections per 1000 resident-days.[6] An estimated 1.6 million to 3.8 million HAIs per year occur in NH patients in the United States.[15] It is important to remember that "classification of an infection as nosocomial does not imply that the LTCF caused the infection, that the infecting organism was acquired in the LTCF, or that it was preventable, but simply that it occurred in the LTCF."[6(p490)]

The most common endemic infections in LTCFs are urinary tract infections (UTIs), respiratory tract infections (pharyngitis, sinusitis, pneumonia, bronchitis, and influenza), skin and soft tissue infections (cellulitis and infected pressure ulcers), gastroenteritis, and conjunctivitis.[6,12,13,16,17]

Risk Factors for Infection

Factors that place residents at risk for infection include indwelling urinary catheters (UTI); incontinence (infected pressure ulcers); decreased mental status (aspiration pneumonia and pressure ulcers); age-related decline in cell-mediated immunity (reactivation of latent infections such as tuberculosis or herpes zoster); decreased cough reflex (aspiration pneumonia); and underlying diseases such as congestive heart failure, chronic obstructive pulmonary disease, and diabetes mellitus.[6,13] Invasive devices such as intravascular catheters, tracheostomy tubes, feeding tubes, and mechanical ventilators, which are well-recognized risk factors for HAIs, are commonly used in many LTCFs.[1] Other factors that predispose LTCF residents to infection include poor nutritional status, functional impairment leading to decreased mobility, epidermal thinning, poor vascular circulation, and decreased gastric acidity. In addition, the LTCF is the resident's home and socializing, which increases direct contact with other residents and healthcare workers, is encouraged.[13]

EPIDEMIC INFECTIONS

The majority of reported infectious disease outbreaks in LTCFs involve respiratory and gastrointestinal infections.[10,11,13,18] Exhibit 4–1 lists the types of infections and etiologic agents responsible for outbreaks in long-term care facilities.

Exhibit 4–1   Etiologic Agents of Outbreaks Reported in Long-Term Care Facilities

Respiratory Infections	*Gastrointestinal Infections*
Adenovirus	*Aeromonas hydrophilia*
Bordetella pertussis	*Bacillus cereus* (food poisoning)
Chlamydia pneumoniae	*Campylobacter jejuni*
Group A streptococcus	*Clostridium botulinum* (food poisoning)
Hemophilus influenzae	*Clostridium difficile*
Human metapneumovirus	*Clostridium perfringens* (food poisoning)
Influenza A and B	*Entamoeba histolytica*
Legionella species	*Escherichia coli* O157:H7
Mycobacterium tuberculosis	*Giardia lamblia*
Neisseria meningitidis	Norovirus
Parainfluenza virus	Rotavirus
Respiratory syncytial virus	*Salmonella* species
Rhinovirus (common cold virus)	*Shigella* species
Streptococcus pneumoniae	*Staphylococcus aureus* (food poisoning)
Skin Infections	*Conjunctivitis*
Group A streptococcus	Group A streptococcus
Methicillin-resistant *Staphylococcus aureus*	Adenovirus
Sarcoptes Scabiei	

RECOGNIZING AND CONFIRMING AN OUTBREAK IN THE LONG-TERM CARE SETTING

An outbreak is defined as the occurrence of more cases of a disease or event than expected during a specified period of time in a given area or among a specific group of people. A cluster is a group of cases of a disease or health-related event that are closely related in time and place, although the number of cases in a cluster may or may not exceed the expected number. Outbreaks and clusters of disease in healthcare facilities may go undetected unless they result in considerable morbidity or mortality or are caused by an unusual organism. An active, ongoing surveillance program, as discussed in Chapter 2, is essential to detect an outbreak or a cluster in an LTCF. Methods that can be used to investigate, control, and prevent outbreaks are discussed in Chapter 8.

Many health departments and public health agencies have guidelines for identifying and controlling outbreaks in LTCFs, and these guidelines are frequently posted on the agency's Web site.[19–22] Many of these guidelines have criteria for defining the occurrence of an outbreak in an LTCF: case definitions; line-listing forms to record cases among residents and personnel; information on collecting appropriate specimens to confirm a clinical diagnosis; and control measures that can be used to interrupt an outbreak. For example, the Centers for Disease Control and Prevention (CDC) provides the following criteria for defining a cluster and an outbreak of acute febrile respiratory illness in an LTCF:[18]

- Cluster: Three or more cases of acute febrile respiratory illness (AFRI) occurring within a 48- to 72-hour period in residents who are in close proximity to each other (e.g., in the same area of the facility)
- Outbreak: A sudden increase of AFRI cases over the normal background rate or when any resident tests positive for influenza. One case of confirmed influenza by any testing method in an LTCF.

Very few LTCFs have on-site laboratories and radiology services and, owing to the nature of the population, diagnostic testing is not frequently performed. Many suspected infections are treated empirically, and a definitive diagnosis may not be made. The imprecision in clinical and laboratory diagnosis inherent in LTCFs makes recognition and confirmation of an outbreak more difficult than in the acute care setting. In addition, investigations of outbreaks in facilities with an elderly, debilitated population are complicated by the fact that many of the residents cannot give a clear history of the development of symptoms or exposures to risk factors such as food or beverages consumed or contact with other residents. These facts should be kept in mind when conducting routine surveillance and when investigating a cluster or potential outbreak in an LTCF.

OUTBREAKS OF RESPIRATORY DISEASE

Outbreaks of respiratory disease in the long-term care setting have involved a variety of viral and bacterial agents including influenza A and B viruses, rhinovirus, respiratory syncytial virus (RSV), parainfluenza virus, human metapneumovirus, adenovirus, *Mycobacterium tuberculosis, Streptococcus pneumoniae,* group A streptococcus, *Hemophilus influenzae, Bordetella pertussis, Legionella* species, *Chlamydia pneumoniae,* and *Neisseria meningitidis.*[23-65] The etiologic agent for many cases of respiratory disease in LTCFs is not definitively diagnosed because bacterial and viral cultures and serologic studies are not routinely performed. Serologic and culture surveys performed in LTCFs have demonstrated that viral agents are often responsible for sporadic cases and epidemics of acute respiratory illness such as cough, nasal congestion, pharyngitis, or wheezing.[66-68] Reported outbreaks of pertussis in LTCFs are rare; however, it is likely that many go undetected because many adult cases are mild or asymptomatic. Examples of respiratory infectious disease outbreaks in LTCFs are shown in Table 4-1.

Streptococcus Pneumoniae

Epidemiology and Mode of Transmission

Streptococcus pneumoniae (the pneumococcus) is commonly found in the upper respiratory tract of children and adults worldwide. It can cause a variety of illnesses: invasive infections such as bacteremia and meningitis, lower respiratory tract infections such as pneumonia, and upper respiratory tract infections such as otitis media and sinusitis.[69] Children 2 years and younger and adults 65 years and older are at increased risk for pneumococcal infection. Persons who have chronic cardiovascular, pulmonary, or liver diseases are also at risk for developing pneumococcal infection and frequently develop severe disease and complications.[69] *S. pneumoniae* is the most common bacterial cause of community-acquired and NH-acquired pneumonia.[32,69,70] The organism is transmitted from person to person by direct oral contact, by droplet spread, or by contact with articles that have been freshly soiled with respiratory secretions.[71]

There are several reports of outbreaks of pneumococcal disease in LTCFs.[29-35,72] The attack rates among residents in these outbreaks ranged from 7.4% to 23%,[29-35,72] and deaths resulting from pneumococcal infection were reported in a majority of the facilities. In most of the reported outbreaks, less than 10% of the residents had previously received the pneumococcal vaccine, and underutilization of the vaccine was considered to be a contributing factor to the outbreak.[31,32,72] In recent years, drug-resistant strains of *Streptococcus pneumoniae* have been responsible for both sporadic and epidemic infections in LTCFs.[29,33,35]

Control Measures

Immunization of those at greatest risk of infection is the most important measure used to prevent pneumococcal disease. Identified risk groups include all persons 65 years of age or older and residents of NHs and other chronic care facilities.[32,69] Although there are few published recommendations for controlling outbreaks of pneumococcal disease in LTCFs, several reports indicate that prompt immunization of unvaccinated residents resulted in decreased transmission and termination of the outbreak.[30,32,69] Using information

Table 4–1   Outbreaks of respiratory disease reported in long-term care facilities

Agent	Major Symptoms of Disease Reported	Comments	Year Reported/ Reference
Adenovirus type 7	Fever, increased tracheal secretions, pneumonia, wheezing, tracheitis, chest congestion	84% of residents in a specialty hospital of an LTCF were infected: 30 were confirmed cases of adenovirus infection and 12 were suspected cases; 26 residents were hospitalized and 7 died; adenoviruses can cause severe and fatal respiratory disease in immunocompromised patients.	2004[60]
Influenza A	Nasal congestion, fever, muscle aches, fatigue, sore throat, headache	53% attack rate in residents (74/139) of LTCF with 15% case fatality (11/74); 31% attack rate in staff (55/175) with one staff member hospitalized; occurred in highly immunized population (85% residents and 84% staff had been immunized prior to outbreak).	2006[25]
Influenza A	Cough, coryza, sore throat, fever	First cases occurred in five unvaccinated nurses; 11% attack rate in personnel (34/309) and 13% attack rate in residents (25/192) in one building; 2 residents died.	1999[23]
Influenza B	Fever, cough, pneumonia	Occurred in 300-bed extended care NH; 28 resident cases (10% attack rate); 9% attack rate among immunized residents (20/220) and 12% among nonimmunized residents (8/66); 3 residents died; 43% staff not immunized; many staff members had influenza-like illness.	2001[24]
Streptococcus pneumoniae	Pneumonia, bacteremia	Nine cases in 108 NH residents; all cases occurred in elderly residents who had not received pneumococcal vaccine; only 49% of residents had received pneumococcal vaccine at time of first case.	2003[31]

Table 4–1   (*Continued*)

Agent	Major Symptoms of Disease Reported	Comments	Year Reported/ Reference
Streptococcus pneumoniae—multidrug-resistant (MDR)	Pneumonia, bacteremia	Between December 27, 1995, and January 30, 1996, five cases of MDR pneumococcal disease occurred in an 80-bed AIDS care unit of LTCF; nasopharyngeal cultures collected in March from 6 of 65 residents were positive for MDR pneumococcus; none of 70 staff cultured were positive; two case patients died; MDR pneumococcus continued to circulate in the unit through December 1999.	2005[35]
Mycobacterium tuberculosis	Persistent cough	Source was highly infectious NH resident; 30% (49/161) of tuberculin-negative residents became infected and eight developed tuberculosis; 15% (21/138) of tuberculin-negative employees became infected and one developed clinical tuberculosis.	1981[27]
Mycobacterium tuberculosis		NH outbreak detected by tuberculin skin testing (TST) program when TST conversions occurred in residents and personnel; began in one NH and spread to second NH, a local hospital, and community; a nurse exposed in hospital to source case developed tuberculous cervical abscess and one employee in NH developed pulmonary TB.	2002[26]
Group A streptococcus (GAS)—invasive	Sepsis, pneumonia, cellulitis	Eight cases in LTCF residents (six died); screening found 11/112 residents (10%) and 8/95 staff (9%) culture-positive for GAS; risk factors for infection and carriage were skin treatment and having roommate that was case or carrier.	2005[37]

Continues

Table 4–1   (*Continued*)

Agent	Major Symptoms of Disease Reported	Comments	Year Reported/ Reference
Group A streptococcus—noninvasive	Pharyngitis	Occurred in LTCF for developmentally disabled; 57 of 251 residents affected (42 confirmed, 15 probable); 10 confirmed cases in staff.	2006[36]
Respiratory syncytial virus (RSV)	Rhinorrhea, cough, fever, pneumonia, malaise, anorexia	Outbreaks of RSV in NH residents can result in considerable morbidity and mortality.	1990[46] 2003[59]
Bordetella pertussis	Prolonged cough	NH outbreak occurred during a community outbreak; 38 residents were seropositive (nine ill, 29 asymptomatic) and seven employees were seropositive (five ill, two asymptomatic).	1991[49]
Rhinovirus	Upper and lower respiratory illnesses	56 residents and 26 staff of an LTCF developed respiratory illness; rhinovirus produced severe illness in some residents; 15 residents developed pneumonia, and 12 residents died.	2005[43]
Parainfluenza virus	Cough, fever, pneumonia	Respiratory illness outbreak affected 25 of 49 residents in a skilled nursing facility; resulted in considerable morbidity and mortality; three residents hospitalized and four died.	2000[55]
Neisseria meningitidis	Fever, bacteremia, meningitis	First published report of an LTCF as the setting for a meningococcal outbreak; index case was a nurse with respiratory illness and meningitis; two patients developed meningococcemia (one died) and a nursing assistant developed meningitis.	1998[58]

Table 4–1   (*Continued*)

Agent	Major Symptoms of Disease Reported	Comments	Year Reported/ Reference
Legionella pneumophila	Pneumonia	Four residents of an LTCF developed Legionnaires' disease; no *Legionella* was isolated from multiple water samples collected throughout the LTCF; three additional cases were detected in community residents; outbreak strain was isolated from cooling tower approximately 0.4 km from the LTCF; LTCF outbreak occurred as part of wider community outbreak associated with industrial cooling tower.	2007[52]
Chlamydia pneumoniae	Cough, wheezing, sore throat, hoarseness, rhinorrhea, nasal obstruction, bronchitis, pneumonia	Respiratory illness with significant morbidity occurred in 53% (31/59) residents and 22% (9/41) staff in a NH for elderly patients; one resident case died.	2006[57]
Human metapneumo-virus	Cough, pneumonia	26 residents and 13 staff of an LTCF developed acute respiratory illness; eight residents (31%) developed pneumonia and two residents (5%) were hospitalized.	2007[65]

NH = nursing home; LTCF = long-term care facility

published by the CDC on preventing pneumococcal disease, and measures reported to be effective in controlling the reported outbreaks, the following measures are recommended to prevent and control the transmission of *S. pneumoniae* in LTCFs[18,20,72–74]:

- Develop and implement a protocol for assessing vaccination status and for immunizing residents, if needed, at the time of admission.[73]
- Document administration of pneumococcal vaccine in the resident's medical record. This will aid in the rapid assessment of susceptible residents if an outbreak occurs.

- Conduct routine surveillance for acute upper and lower respiratory tract illness in residents and employees. Use standardized surveillance criteria (case definitions) for disease.

- Whenever possible, encourage ill residents to cover their mouth and nose when coughing or sneezing and to wash their hands after coughing or sneezing.

- When possible, restrict employees with acute respiratory illness from direct care of residents (at the very least, instruct these employees to wash their hands before caring for a resident and to use tissues to cover their mouth and nose when coughing or sneezing).

- If pneumonia is suspected, or a resident has a febrile respiratory illness, perform appropriate diagnostic tests, such as chest X-ray and throat or sputum cultures, to establish the diagnosis and to determine the etiologic agent.

- Keep an updated, ongoing surveillance log of residents and employees who meet the case definition for an acute respiratory disease.

- If an outbreak is suspected, develop a line listing of residents with pneumococcal disease.

- Use standard precautions when caring for a resident with pneumococcal disease.[74]

Additional information on investigating, preventing, and controlling outbreaks of pneumococcal pneumonia can be found in Appendix G.[22] Appendix G is available for download at this text's Web site: http://www.jbpub.com/catalog/9780763757793/.

Neisseria Meningitidis

Epidemiology and Mode of Transmission

Neisseria meningitidis (the meningococcus) is one of the leading causes of bacterial meningitis in the United States.[75,76] Most cases of meningococcal disease are sporadic—less than 2% of cases in the United States occur during an outbreak.[75] *N. meningitidis* colonizes the nasopharynx and is transmitted from person to person via direct contact with respiratory secretions and droplets.[74,75]

Outbreaks of meningococcal disease have long been recognized in communities and in organizations such as primary and secondary schools, colleges, military barracks, and correctional facilities[75,76]; however, outbreaks in the healthcare setting are rare. Between July 1994 and June 2002, a total of 76 outbreaks were identified in the United States and nine of those were reported to occur in NHs.[75] A search of the literature uncovered only one additional published report of an outbreak of meningococcal disease in a healthcare facility, and that occurred in an SNF in Florida in 1997.[58] The index case in that outbreak was a nurse who was hospitalized with confusion and fever and suspected meningitis after a 2-week illness. Shortly after his hospitalization, a 90-year-old patient in the wing where the nurse was assigned developed meningococcemia and died and a 56-year-old nursing assistant developed meningococcal meningitis. The nursing assistant had cared for the 90-year-old case patient. Ciprofloxacin prophylaxis was administered to all 114 of the facility's staff members and all but one of the 104 residents. Shortly thereafter, the one patient who refused prophylaxis was hospitalized with meningococcemia. At the recommendation of a community physician, the facility provided antibiotic prophylaxis to approximately 250 visitors and collected nasopharyngeal cultures from all available patients postprophylaxis—all cultures were negative for *Neisseria meningitidis*. The CDC investigators noted that mass prophylaxis was justified for the facility's staff and patients but was not needed for the 250 casual contacts and that culturing of patients or staff was an inappropriate response to the outbreak.[58]

Control Measures

Two measures that can be used to prevent meningococcal disease are chemoprophylaxis and vaccination. For information on the use of chemoprophylaxis and vaccination, the reader is referred to the CDC Advisory Committee on Immunization Practices (ACIP) recommendations on control and prevention of meningococcal disease.[75,76] The primary tool that is used to prevent the development of disease is the identification and chemoprophylaxis of close contacts of persons with meningococcal disease.

Based on the ACIP recommendations[75,76] and the findings from the report of the nursing home outbreak,[58] the following measures are recommended to identify and control an outbreak of meningococcal disease in a healthcare facility:

- Conduct routine surveillance to identify persons with meningococcal disease. Case definitions are given in the ACIP recommendations[75] and in Appendix B. Appendix B is available for download at this text's Web site: http://www.jbpub.com /catalog/9780763757793/.

- Identify close contacts of a person with meningococcal disease. Close contacts are defined as persons "directly exposed to the patient's oral secretions (e.g., through kissing, mouth-to-mouth resuscitation, endotracheal intubation, or endotracheal tube management)."[75(p4)]

- Provide chemoprophylaxis as soon as possible to close contacts. The ACIP guidelines recommend using rifampin, ciprofloxacin, or ceftriaxone for chemoprophylaxis.[75]

- Report cases of laboratory-confirmed meningococcal disease to the local or state health department. In many states meningococcal disease should be reported immediately by telephone to the health department.

- Use droplet precautions (private room and masks) for persons with known or suspected meningococcal meningitis, meningococcal pneumonia, or meningococcemia (meningococcal sepsis) until 24 hours after appropriate antimicrobial therapy is given.[74]

- In some outbreaks, postexposure vaccination of the population at risk for developing meningococcal disease should be considered, as discussed in the ACIP guidelines.[75]

- Instruct the laboratory to type (serogroup) the organism and to save the isolate(s) of *N. meningitidis* for confirmation of serogrouping and possible subtyping.[75,76]
- Do not collect oropharyngeal or nasopharyngeal cultures from residents, contacts, or personnel because cultures are not needed when investigating outbreaks or for determining who should receive antimicrobial prophylaxis.[75,76]

Outbreaks of Respiratory Disease Caused by Other Organisms

Other organisms that have been reported to cause outbreaks of respiratory disease in LTCFs include RSV,[10,47,59] rhinovirus (common cold virus),[43–45] *Bordetella pertussis*,[48,49,77,78] adenovirus,[60–64] *Chlamydia pneumoniae*,[56,57] *Mycobacterium tuberculosis*,[26–28] and parainfluenza virus.[55] Each of these agents can affect both residents and personnel and can result in significant morbidity. Both endemic and epidemic infections caused by these organisms are likely to go unrecognized because specific diagnostic testing is rarely done.[66] Control measures to prevent transmission of these agents include recognition of illness in both residents and personnel and consistent use of good hygienic practices such as hand hygiene and using tissues to cover the mouth and nose when coughing or sneezing.

Pertussis should be suspected in persons who have a prolonged cough (regardless of age), especially if pertussis is reported in the community.[77,78] Since chemoprophylactic agents are recommended to prevent development of disease in close contacts of persons with pertussis, early recognition and contact tracing are important.[79] Guidelines for preventing transmission of *Bordetella pertussis* and for managing outbreaks of pertussis are discussed in Chapter 3.

Legionella species have caused outbreaks in the community, hospitals, and NHs.[50–54] In one report, an investigation of a cluster of Legionnaires' disease in LTCF residents led to the identification of a community-wide outbreak whose source was traced to an industrial cooling tower located 0.4 kilometer from the LTCF.[52] Prevention and control measures for *Legionella* are discussed in Chapter 3, and for *Mycobacterium tuberculosis* they are discussed in Chapter 7.

OUTBREAKS OF GASTROINTESTINAL DISEASE

Sporadic and epidemic cases of diarrhea occur frequently in LTCFs, and they can be associated with significant morbidity and mortality.[9,18,80,81] Outbreaks of infectious gastroenteritis in the long-term care setting have been caused by a variety of bacteria, viruses, and parasites: *Salmonella* species, *Clostridium difficile*, *Shigella* species, *Bacillus cereus*, *Aeromonas hydrophilia*, *Staphylococcus aureus*, *Campylobacter jejuni*, *Clostridium perfringens* and *C. botulinum*, *Escherichia coli* O157:H7, norovirus, rotavirus, *Giardia lamblia*, and *Entamoeba histolytica,* as noted in Exhibit 4–1.

The organisms that cause epidemic diarrhea in LTCFs can be spread by contact with a contaminated item (such as soiled laundry), by contact with an infected or colonized person, or by consumption of contaminated food or beverages. Some organisms, such as *Salmonella* and *Giardia lamblia*, can be transmitted by both the contact and food-borne routes.

Food-borne outbreaks in NHs and other LTCFs accounted for 2% of all food-borne outbreaks and 19% of outbreak-related deaths reported to the CDC from 1975 through 1987.[81] From 1998 through 2002, *Salmonella* and norovirus were the most commonly reported pathogens responsible for food-borne outbreaks in LTCFs.[82] Outbreaks of gastrointestinal illness in LTCFs are difficult to investigate because diagnostic tests are infrequently performed to identify an infectious agent, and those tests that are done are frequently negative. In addition, many residents in LTCFs are poor historians and are unable to remember risk factors for infection such as consumption of a particular food or contact with an infectious resident.

Each LTCF should have an ongoing education program to instruct personnel how to properly handle, prepare, and store food, and when, why, and how to wash their hands and use standard precautions.[5] The identification, investigation, prevention, and control of outbreaks of food-borne and gastrointestinal disease are discussed in detail in Chapter 7. Many state health department Web sites have information on detecting, preventing, investigating, and controlling outbreaks of gastrointestinal disease.[21,22] The Maryland Department of Health and Mental Hygiene's Guidelines for the Epidemiological Investigation of Gastroenteritis Outbreaks in Long-Term Care Facilities are reprinted in Appendix H. Appendix H is available for download at this text's Web site: http://www.jbpub.com/catalog/9780763757793/.

OUTBREAKS OF CONJUNCTIVITIS

Conjunctivitis is a common nosocomial ailment in NHs, and in recent years there have been frequent reports of conjunctivitis outbreaks in various long-term care settings.[62,83–89] The reported incidence of endemic episodes of conjunctivitis varies widely from 0.08 to 3.5 per 1000 patient-days.[90] Conjunctivitis may be caused by microbial pathogens, allergies, or other irritative responses. The etiology of infective conjunctivitis in long-term care residents has not been well elucidated. Boustcha and Nicolle reported that *Staphylococcus aureus* and *Branhamella catarrhalis* were the most commonly isolated bacterial pathogens during a prospective study of episodes of conjunctivitis in residents of an LTCF.[90] They noted that no bacterial pathogen was isolated from the majority of cases, and these may possibly have been caused by viruses or *Chlamydia* (laboratory tests for these agents were not performed). Brennen and Muder studied the clinical characteristics of 20 episodes of MRSA-associated conjunctivitis that occurred in 19 patients over a 3-year period in a 432-bed LTCF.[91] These were infections that occurred in a facility in which MRSA had been endemic for at least 6 years, and nine of the patients who developed conjunctivitis from which MRSA was isolated had documented prior colonization of other body sites with MRSA.[91]

Reported outbreaks of conjunctivitis in LTCFs have been caused by group A streptococcus, adenovirus, and *Hemophilus influenzae*.[83,85–89] The etiologic agents that can cause conjunctivitis are spread via direct person-to-person contact, contact with respiratory secretions, contact with contaminated environmental surfaces, and use of contaminated eyedrops.[71,74] In several reports, both endemic and epidemic conjunctivitis appeared to occur most often in debilitated patients and those with cognitive impairment.[84,85,90] In several reports, residents in NHs developed conjunctivitis in concurrence with a widespread outbreak of group A streptococcal disease.[41,86]

In reports of outbreaks of conjunctivitis in LTCFs, the most successful measures shown to interrupt transmission were strict adherence to good hand hygiene practices by healthcare workers, use of aseptic technique when providing eye care and touching respiratory secretions, use of a disinfectant that inactivates adenovirus, recognition of an outbreak, and restricting the movement of infected residents that had cognitive impairment.[85,87]

Outbreaks of conjunctivitis in LTCFs cause considerable discomfort and pain, frequently involve both residents and staff, and can result in substantial disruption and cost.[83,88,89] Piednoir et al. reported on the direct costs associated with an outbreak of adenoviral conjunctivitis on one unit in a 340-bed LTCF affiliated with a large university hospital.[88] In this outbreak, 29 residents (attack rate 29/57 = 50.8%) and 12 staff members were infected during an 8-week period. Direct costs associated with related medical care, the outbreak investigation, prevention and control measures, and lost productivity (staff absenteeism) amounted to approximately US $30,000.[88]

OUTBREAKS CAUSED BY GROUP A STREPTOCOCCUS

Epidemiology and Mode of Transmission

Although group A beta-hemolytic streptococcus (*Streptococcus pyogenes*) most commonly causes pharyngitis, it can also cause invasive disease such as pneumonia, sepsis, cellulitis, wound infection, and toxic shock-like syndrome.[36,37,39,71,92] Some serotypes of group A streptococci are primarily associated with pharyngeal and minor skin infections such as impetigo, while others readily cause invasive diseases such as sepsis and pneumonia.[92] The elderly are particularly prone to developing invasive disease, and mortality rates from group A streptococcal bacteremia have been reported to be as high as 60% in this population.[93] Person-to-person transmission generally occurs by direct contact with an infected or colonized person, although food-borne outbreaks of streptococcal pharyngitis have also occurred.[71] Little has been published on the risk factors for acquisition, mode of transmission, and effective control measures to prevent transmission of group A streptococci in LTCFs.

Outbreaks of invasive and noninvasive group A streptococcal infections in LTCFs have been reported.[36–41,86,92,93] The reports of these outbreaks identified several risk factors for nosocomial acquisition and disease: sharing a room with an infected resident, being bedridden, requiring extensive nursing care, having contact with a culture-positive nurse or with an infected resident, and having decubitus ulcers.[92,93] Outbreaks of group A strep can involve both residents and staff.[36,40,92] In all of the reported LTCF outbreaks, the organism was thought to be spread by direct contact with an infected or colonized person or by cross-infection due to poor infection prevention and control practices, such as lack of hand hygiene or failure to change gloves between residents. In two outbreaks nursing personnel with symptomatic group A streptococcal pharyngitis had direct contact with residents who subsequently became infected, and these personnel may have been responsible for introducing the organism into their facilities.[40,92]

Control Measures

The following measures are recommended to recognize and control outbreaks of group A streptococcus in an LTCF[40,86,93]:

- Conduct routine ongoing surveillance for healthcare-associated group A streptococcal infections so that single cases, clusters, and outbreaks can be detected and control measures can be promptly implemented.
- Provide timely diagnosis and antimicrobial therapy for persons with pharyngitis or other streptococcal infections.
- Educate personnel about the importance of reporting pharyngitis in themselves and in residents.
- Restrict personnel with group A streptococcal infections from resident care activities until 24 hours after they have received appropriate therapy.[94]
- Enforce good infection prevention and control practices (hand hygiene and glove use for wound care), especially when caring for an infected resident.
- Ensure that personnel use standard precautions when caring for minor wounds; however, if a resident has a major group A streptococcal wound infection (i.e., one that cannot be covered or has drainage that cannot be contained), in addition to standard precautions use contact and droplet precautions (private room or cohort with another resident with known or suspected group A streptococcal infection, gloves and mask for direct care, proper hand hygiene, and a gown for contact with the resident). Contact and droplet precautions are needed only until 24 hours after appropriate antimicrobial therapy has been given.[74]
- Use droplet precautions for group A streptococcal pneumonia and standard precautions for mild cutaneous and other streptococcal infections.[74]
- Initiate an outbreak investigation if two nosocomial group A streptococcal infections occur in a short time period among residents of an LTCF.
- Instruct the laboratory to save group A streptococcal isolates for serotyping if an outbreak or cluster occurs (i.e., more than two healthcare-associated cases).
- Obtain assistance in conducting an outbreak investigation from the local or state health department.
- Consider prophylactic antimicrobials if an outbreak is ongoing or involves severe infections.[93]
- Use a case definition and construct a line listing of infected and colonized persons. Case definitions for streptococcal toxic-shock syndrome and invasive group A streptococcal disease can be found in Appendix B. Appendix B is available for download at this text's Web site: http://www.jbpub.com/catalog/9780763757793/.

SUMMARY

Residents and patients in LTCFs are at risk for developing HAIs (nosocomial). Preventing the transmission of infectious agents in LTCFs presents a challenge because LTCF residents are frequently ambulatory and may have profound physical and mental disabilities. Personnel responsible for managing the infection prevention and control program in an LTCF should establish a routine infection surveillance program and ensure that evidence-based infection prevention practices are implemented and used to reduce the risk of infection in both residents and personnel.[5,9,19–22,69,73–76,94,95] An effective surveillance program should be able to detect and quantify the occurrence of infections so that clusters and outbreaks can be identified and control measures can be instituted as soon as possible to prevent further transmission. The infection prevention program should include the participation of personnel, residents, and visitors of the facility. All should be instructed on proper hand hygiene, respiratory hygiene and cough etiquette, and other infection prevention measures.[95,96] Outbreaks in LTCFs can be avoided if personnel, residents, and visitors routinely follow basic infection prevention measures.

REFERENCES

1. Nicolle LE. Infection control in long-term care facilities. *Clin Infect Dis.* 2000;31(3):752–756.
2. Eskildsen MA. Long-term acute care: a review of the literature. *J Am Geriatr Soc.* 2007;55(5):775–779.
3. Health Care Financing Administration (HCFA). *Medicare Fact Sheet.* May 16, 1999.
4. American Medical Association. White paper on elderly health. *Arch Intern Med.* 1990;150:2459–2472.
5. Kemper P, Murtaugh CM. Lifetime use of nursing home care. *N Engl J Med.* 1991;324:595–600.
6. Smith PW, Rusnak PG. Infection prevention and control in the long-term-care facility. *Am J Infect Control.* 1997;25:488–512.
7. Harris J. Infection control in pediatric extended care facilities. *Infect Control Hosp Epidemiol.* 2006;27:598–603.
8. Pacio GA, Visintainer P, Maguire G, Wormser GP, Raffalli J, Montecalvo MA. Natural history of colonization with vancomycin-resistant *Enterococci*, methicillin resistant *Staphylococcus aureus*, and resistant gram-negative bacilli among long-term-care facility residents. *Infect Control Hosp Epidemiol.* 2003;24:246–250.
9. Armstrong-Evans M, Litt M, McArthur MA, et al. Control of transmission of vancomycin-resistant *Enterococcus faecium* in a long-term-care facility. *Infect Control Hosp Epidemiol.* 1999;20:312–317.
10. Nicolle LE, Garibaldi RA. Infection control in long-term-care facilities. *Infect Control Hosp Epidemiol.* 1995;16:348–353.
11. Loeb M, McGeer A, McArthur M, Peeling RW, Petric M, Simor AE. Surveillance for outbreaks of respiratory tract infections in nursing homes. *CMAJ.* 2000;162(8):1133–1137.
12. Bentley DW, Bradley S, High K, Schoenbaum S, Taler G, Yoshikawa TT. Practice guideline for evaluation of fever and infection in long-term care facilities. *J Am Geriatr Soc.* 2001;49(2):210–222.
13. Nicolle LE. Preventing infections in non-hospital settings: Long-term care. *Emerg Infect Dis.* 2001;7:205–207. http://www.cdc.gov/ncidod/eid/vol7no2/nicolle.htm. Accessed October 5, 2008.

14. Smith PW, Daly PB, Roccaforte JS. Current status of nosocomial infection control in extended care facilities. *Am J Med.* 1991;91:3B-281S–3B-285S.

15. Strausbaugh LJ. Infection control in long-term care: news from the front. *Am J Infect Control.* 1999;27:1–3.

16. Yoshikawa TT, Norman DC. Approach to fever and infection in the nursing home. *J Am Geriatr Soc.* 1996;44:74–82.

17. Muder RR. Pneumonia in residents of long-term care facilities: epidemiology, etiology, management, and prevention. *Am J Med.* 1998;105:319–330.

18. Strausbaugh LJ, Sukumar SR, Joseph CL. Infectious disease outbreaks in nursing homes: an unappreciated hazard for frail elderly persons. *Clin Infect Dis.* 2003;36(7):870–876.

19. Centers for Disease Control and Prevention. Infection control measures for preventing and controlling influenza transmission in long-term care facilities. http://www.cdc.gov/flu/professionals/ infectioncontrol/longtermcare.htm. Accessed October 27, 2007.

20. Ontario Ministry of Health and Long-Term Care, Public Health Division and Long-Term Care Homes Branch. A guide to the control of respiratory infection outbreaks in long-term care homes. Published 2004 http://www.health.gov.on.ca/english/providers/pub/pub_menus/ pub_pubhealth.html. Accessed October 27, 2007.

21. California Department of Health Services, Division of Communicable Disease Control, Resources and Publications. http://www.dhs.ca.gov/ps/dcdc/disb/disbindex.htm. Accessed April 24, 2008.

22. Maryland Department of Health & Mental Hygiene, Epidemiology & Disease Control Program, Community Health Administration. Guidelines for long term care facilities. http:// www.cha.state.md.us/edcp/html/cd_guide.html. Accessed November 20, 2007.

23. Centers for Disease Control and Prevention. Update: influenza activity—United States, 1998–99 season. *MMWR.* 1999;48:177–181.

24. Public Health Agency of Canada. Experience with oseltamivir in the control of a nursing home influenza B outbreak. *Can Commun Dis Rep.* 2001;27:37–40. http://www.phac-aspc .gc.ca/publicat/ccdr-rmtc/01pdf/cdr2705.pdf. Accessed November 20, 2007.

25. Mitchell R, Huynh V, Pak J, et al. Influenza outbreak in an Ontario long-term care home, January 2005. *Can Commun Dis Rep.* 2006;32:257–262. http://www.phac-aspc.gc.ca/publicat/ ccdr-rmtc/index.html. Accessed October 5, 2008.

26. Ijaz K, Dillaha JA, Yang Z, Cave MD, Bates JH. Unrecognized tuberculosis in a nursing home causing death with spread of tuberculosis to the community. *J Am Geriatr Soc.* 2002;50:1213–1218.

27. Stead WW. Tuberculosis among elderly persons: an outbreak in a nursing home. *Ann Intern Med.* 1981;94:606–610.

28. Brenner C, Muder RR, Muraca PW. Occult endemic tuberculosis in a chronic care facility. *Infect Control Hosp Epidemiol.* 1988;9:548–552.

29. McNeeley DF, Lyons J, Conte S. Labowitz A, Layton M. A cluster of drug-resistant *Streptococcus pneumoniae* among nursing home patients. *Infect Control Hosp Epidemiol.* 1998;19:476–477.

30. Sheppard DC, Bartlett KA, Lampiris HW. *Streptococcus pneumoniae* transmission in chronic-care facilities: description of an outbreak and review of management strategies. *Infect Control Hosp Epidemiol.* 1998;19:851–853.

31. Tan CG, Ostrawski S, Bresnitz EA. A preventable outbreak of pneumococcal pneumonia among unvaccinated nursing home residents in New Jersey during 2001. *Infect Control Hosp Epidemiol.* 2003;24:848–852.

32. Centers for Disease Control and Prevention. Outbreaks of pneumococcal pneumonia among unvaccinated residents in chronic-care facilities—Massachusetts, October 1995, Oklahoma, February 1996, and Maryland, May-June 1996. *MMWR.* 1997;46:60–62.

33. McNeeley DF, Lyons J, Conte S. Labowitz A, Layton M. A cluster of drug-resistant *Streptococcus pneumoniae* among nursing home patients. *Infect Control Hosp Epidemiol.* 1998;19:476–477.

34. Gleich S, Morad Y, Echague R, et al. *Streptococcus pneumoniae* serotype 4 outbreak in a home for the aged: report and review of recent outbreaks. *Infect Control Hosp Epidemiol.* 2000; 21(11):711–717.

35. Carter RJ, Sorenson G, Heffernan R, et al. Failure to control an outbreak of multidrug-resistant *Streptococcus pneumoniae* in a long-term-care facility: emergence and ongoing transmission of a fluoroquinolone-resistant strain. *Infect Control Hosp Epidemiol.* 2005;26:248–255.

36. Dworkin MS, Park L, Barringer J, Curtis R. An outbreak of noninvasive group A streptococcal disease in a facility for the developmentally disabled. *Am J Infect Control.* 2006;34:296–300.

37. Greene CM, Van Beneden CA, Javadi M, et al. Cluster of deaths from group A streptococcus in a long-term care facility—Georgia, 2001. *Am J Infect Control.* 2005;33(2):108–113.

38. Smith A, Li A, Tolomeo O, Tyrrell GJ, Jamieson F, Fisman D. Mass antibiotic treatment for group A streptococcus outbreaks in two long-term care facilities. *Emerg Infect Dis.* 2003; 9(10):1260–1265.

39. Arnold KE, Schweitzer JL, Wallace B, et al. Tightly clustered outbreak of group A streptococcal disease at a long-term care facility. *Infect Control Hosp Epidemiol.* 2006;27(12):1377–1384.

40. Harkness GA, Bentley DW, Mottley M, Lee J. *Streptococcus pyogenes* outbreak in a long-term care facility. *Am J Infect Control.* 1992;20:142–148.

41. McNutt LA, Casiano-Colon AE, Coles FB, et al. Two outbreaks of primarily noninvasive group A streptococcal disease in the same nursing home, New York, 1991. *Infect Control Hosp Epidemiol.* 1992;13:748–751.

42. Nazir J, Urban C, Mariano N, et al. Quinolone-resistant *Haemophilus influenzae* in a long-term care facility: clinical and molecular epidemiology. *Clin Infect Dis.* 2004;38(11):1564–1569.

43. Louie JK, Yagi S, Nelson FA, et al. Rhinovirus outbreak in a long-term care facility for elderly persons associated with unusually high mortality. *Clin Infect Dis.* 2005;41(2):262–265.

44. Wald TG, Shult P, Krause P, Miller BA, Drinka P, Gravenstein S. A rhinovirus outbreak among residents of a long-term care facility. *Ann Intern Med.* 1995;123:588–593.

45. Hicks LA, Shepard CW, Britz PH, et al. Two outbreaks of severe respiratory disease in nursing homes associated with rhinovirus. *J Am Geriatr Soc.* 2006;54(2):284–289.

46. Osterweil D, Norman D. An outbreak of influenza-like illness in a nursing home. *J Am Geriatr Soc.* 1990;38:659–662.

47. Sorvillo FJ, Huie SF, Strassburg M, Butsumyo A, Shandera WX, Fannin SL. An outbreak of respiratory syncytial virus pneumonia in a nursing home for the elderly. *J Infect.* 1984;9:252–259.

48. Ferson MJ, Morgan K, Robertson PW, Hampson AW, Carter I, Rawlinson WD. Concurrent summer influenza and pertussis outbreaks in a nursing home in Sydney, Australia. *Infect Control Hosp Epidemiol.* 2004;25:962–966.

49. Addiss DG, Davis JP, Meade BD. A pertussis outbreak in a Wisconsin nursing home. *J Infect Dis.* 1991;164:704–710.

50. Loeb M, Simor AE, Mandell L, et al. Two nursing home outbreaks of respiratory infection with *Legionella sainthelensi. J Am Geriatr Soc.* 1999;47:547–552.

51. Stout JE, Brennen C, Muder RR. Legionnaires' disease in a newly constructed long-term care facility. *J Am Geriatr Soc.* 2000;48(12):1589–1592.

52. Phares CR, Russell E, Thigpen MC, et al. Legionnaires' disease among residents of a long-term care facility: the sentinel event in a community outbreak. *Am J Infect Control.* 2007;35(5):319–323.

53. Gilmour MW, Bernard K, Tracz DM, et al. Molecular typing of a *Legionella pneumophila* outbreak in Ontario, Canada. *J Med Microbiol.* 2007;56(Pt 3):336–341.

54. Seenivasan MH, Yu VL, Muder RR. Legionnaires' disease in long-term care facilities: overview and proposed solutions. *J Am Geriatr Soc.* 2005;53(5):875–880.

55. Todd Faulks J, Drinka PJ, Shult P. A serious outbreak of parainfluenza type 3 on a nursing unit. *J Am Geriatr Soc.* 2000;48(10):1216–1218.

56. Troy CJ, Peeling RW, Ellis AG, et al. *Chlamydia pneumoniae* as a new source of infectious outbreaks in nursing homes. *JAMA.* 1997;277:1214–1218. [Published erratum appears in *JAMA* 1997;278:118].

57. Nakashima K, Tanaka T, Kramer MH, et al. Outbreak of *Chlamydia pneumoniae* infection in a Japanese nursing home, 1999–2000. *Infect Control Hosp Epidemiol.* 2006;27(11):1171–1177.

58. Centers for Disease Control and Prevention. Outbreaks of group B meningococcal disease—Florida, 1995 and 1997. *MMWR.* 1998;47:883–837.

59. Ellis SE, Coffey CS, Mitchel EF Jr, Dittus RS, Griffin MR. Influenza and respiratory syncytial virus-associated morbidity and mortality in the nursing home population. *Am Geriatr Soc.* 2003;51(6):761–767.

60. Calder JAM, Erdman DD, Ackelsberg J, et al. Adenovirus type 7 genomic-type variant, New York City, 1999. *Emerg Infect Dis.* 2004;10:149–152. http://www.cdc.gov/ncidod/EID/vol10no1/02-0605.htm. Accessed November 20, 2007.

61. Uemura T, Kawashitam T, Ostuka Y, Tanaka Y, Kusubae R, Yoshinaga M. A recent outbreak of adenovirus type 7 infection in a chronic inpatient facility for the severely handicapped. *Infect Control Hosp Epidemiol.* 2000;21:559–560.

62. James L, Vernon MO, Jones RC, et al. Outbreak of human adenovirus type 3 infection in a pediatric long-term care facility Illinois, 2005. *Clin Infect Dis.* 2007;45(4):416–420.

63. Sanchez MP, Erdman DD, Torok TJ, Freeman CJ, Matyas BT. Outbreak of adenovirus 35 pneumonia among adult residents and staff of a chronic care psychiatric facility. *J Infect Dis.* 1997;176(3):760–763.

64. Gerber S, Erdman DD, Pur PS, et al. Outbreak of adenovirus genome type 7d2 infection in a pediatric chronic-care facility and tertiary-care hospital. *Clin Infect Dis.* 2001;32:694–700.

65. Louie JK, Schnurr DP, Chao-Yang Pan, et al. A summer outbreak of human metapneumovirus infection in a long-term care facility. *J Infect Dis.* 2007;196(5):705–708.

66. Falsey AR, Treanor JJ, Betts RF, Walsh EE. Viral respiratory infections in the institutionalized elderly: clinical and epidemiologic findings. *J Am Geriatr Soc.* 1992;40:115–119.

67. Falsey AR. Noninfluenza respiratory virus infection in long-term care facilities. *Infect Control Hosp Epidemiol.* 1991;12:602–608.

68. Drinka PJ, Gravenstein S, Langer E, Krause P, Shult P. Mortality following isolation of various respiratory viruses in nursing home residents. *Infect Control Hosp Epidemiol.* 1999;20:812–815.

69. Centers for Disease Control and Prevention. Prevention of pneumococcal disease: recommendations of the Advisory Committee on Immunization Practices (ACIP). *MMWR.* 1997;46(RR-8):1–24. http://www.cdc.gov/mmwr/preview/mmwrhtml/00047135.htm. Accessed November 20, 2007.

70. Marrie TJ, Slater KL. Nursing home-acquired pneumonia. Treatment options. *Drugs Aging.* 1996;8:338–348.

71. Heymann, David L. *Control of Communicable Diseases Manual.* 18th ed. Washington, DC: American Public Health Association; 2004.

72. Quick RE, Hoge CW, Hamilton DJ, Whitney CJ, Borge M, Kobayaski JM. Underutilization of penumococcal vaccine in nursing homes in Washington state: report of a serotype-specific outbreak and a survey. *Am J Med.* 1993;94:149–152.

73. CDC and the Healthcare Infection Control Practices Advisory Committee. Guidelines for preventing health-care-associated pneumonia, 2003. *MMWR.* 2004;53(RR03):1-36. http://www.cdc.gov/ncidod/dhqp/index.html. Accessed November 20, 2007.

74. Siegel JD, Rhinehart E, Jackson M, Chiarello L, and the Healthcare Infection Control Practices Advisory Committee. 2007 guideline for isolation precautions: preventing transmission of infectious agents in healthcare settings. http://www.cdc.gov/ncidod/dhqp/index.html. Accessed November 20, 2007.

75. Centers for Disease Control and Prevention. Prevention and control of meningococcal disease: recommendations of the Advisory Committee on Immunization Practices (ACIP). *MMWR.* 2005;54(RR-7):1–21. http://www.cdc.gov/mmwr/preview/mmwrhtml/rr5407a1.htm. Accessed November 20, 2007.

76. Centers for Disease Control and Prevention. Control and prevention of meningococcal disease and control and prevention of serogroup C meningococcal disease: evaluation and management

of suspected outbreaks: recommendations of the Advisory Committee on Immunization Practices (ACIP). *MMWR*. 1997;46(No. RR-5):13–21. http://www.cdc.gov/mmwr/preview/ind97_rr .html. Accessed November 20, 2007.

77. Edwards KM, Talbot TR. The challenges of pertussis outbreaks in healthcare facilities: is there a light at the end of the tunnel? *Infect Control Hosp Epidemiol*. 2006;27:537–540.

78. Weber DJ, Rutala WA. Pertussis: an underappreciated risk for nosocomial outbreaks. *Infect Control Hosp Epidemiol*. 1998;19:825–828.

79. Centers for Disease Control and Prevention. Recommended antimicrobial agents for the treatment and postexposure prophylaxis of pertussis: 2005 CDC guidelines. *MMWR*. 2005;54(No. RR-14):1–16.

80. Bennett RG. Diarrhea among residents of long-term care facilities. *Infect Control Hosp Epidemiol*. 1993;14:397–404.

81. Levine WC, Smart JF, Archer DL, Bean NH, Tauxe RV. Foodborne disease outbreaks in nursing homes, 1975 through 1987. *JAMA*. 1991;266:2105–2109.

82. Centers for Disease Control and Prevention. Surveillance for foodborne disease outbreaks, United States, 1998–2002. Surveillance Summaries. *MMWR*. 2006;55(No. SS-10):1–42.

83. Dominguez-Berjon MF, Hernando-Briongos P, Miguel-Arroyo PJ, Echevarria JE, Casas I. Adenovirus transmission in a nursing home: analysis of an epidemic outbreak of keratoconjunctivitis. *Gerontology*. 2007;53(5):250–254.

84. Garibaldi RA, Brodine S, Matsumiya S. Infections among patients in nursing homes—policies, prevalence, and problems. *N Engl J Med*. 1981;305:731–735.

85. Buffington J, Chapman LE, Stobierski MG, et al. Epidemic keratoconjunctivitis in a chronic care facility: risk factors and measures for control. *J Am Geriatr Soc*. 1993;41(11):1177–1181.

86. Ruben FL, Norden CW, Heisler B, Korica Y. An outbreak of *Streptococcus pyogenes* infections in a nursing home. *Ann Intern Med*. 1984;101:494–496.

87. Van Dort M, Walden C, Walker ES, Reynolds SA, Levy F, Sarubbi FA. An outbreak of infections caused by non-typeable *Haemophilus influenzae* in an extended care facility. *J Hosp Infect*. 2007;66(1):59–64.

88. Piednoir E, Bureau-Chalot F, Merle C, Gotzamanis A, Wuibout J, Bajolet O. Direct costs associated with a nosocomial outbreak of adenoviral conjunctivitis infection in a long-term care institution. *Am J Infect Control*. 2002;30(7):407–410.

89. Sendra-Gutierrez JM, Martin-Rios D, Casas I, Saez P, Tovar A, Moreno C. An outbreak of adenovirus type 8 keratoconjunctivitis in a nursing home in Madrid. *Euro Surveill*. 2004;9(3):27–30. http://www.eurosurveillance.org/em/v09n03/0903-225.asp. Accessed November 20, 2007.

90. Boustcha E, Nicolle LE. Conjunctivitis in a long-term care facility. *Infect Control Hosp Epidemiol*. 1995;16:210–216.

91. Brennen C, Muder RR. Conjunctivitis associated with methicillin-resistant *Staphylococcus aureus* in a long-term care facility. *Am J Med*. 1990;88:5-14N-5-17N.

92. Schwartz B, Ussery XT. Group A streptococcal outbreaks in nursing homes. *Infect Control Hosp Epidmiol*. 1992;13:742–747.

93. Auerbach SB, Schwartz B, Williams D, et al. Outbreak of invasive group A streptococcal infections in a nursing home: lessons on prevention and control. *Arch Intern Med*. 1992;152:1017–1022.

94. Centers for Disease Control and Prevention. Guideline for infection control in health care personnel, 1998. *Am J Infect Control*. 1998;26:289-354. http://www.cdc.gov/ncidod/dhqp/ index.html. Accessed November 20, 2007.

95. Centers for Disease Control and Prevention. Guideline for hand hygiene in health-care settings: recommendations of the Healthcare Infection Control Practices Advisory Committee and the HICPAC/SHEA/APIC/IDSA Hand Hygiene Task Force. *MMWR*. 2002;51(No. RR-16):1–45. http://www.cdc.gov/ncidod/dhqp/index.html. Accessed November 20, 2007.

96. Centers for Disease Control and Prevention. Respiratory hygiene/cough etiquette in health care facilities. http://www.cdc.gov/flu/professionals/infectioncontrol/resphygiene.htm. Accessed November 20, 2007.

SUGGESTED READING AND RESOURCES

California Department of Health Services, Division of Communicable Disease Control, Resources and Publications. http://www.dhs.ca.gov/ps/dcdc/disb/disbindex.htm. Accessed April 24, 2008.

Centers for Disease Control and Prevention. *Epidemiology and Prevention of Vaccine-Preventable Diseases*. The Pink Book. Atkinson W, Hamborsky J, McIntyre L, Wolfe S, eds. 10th ed. Washington DC: Public Health Foundation; 2007. http://www.cdc.gov/ncidod/dhqp/index.html. Accessed November 20, 2007.

Centers for Disease Control and Prevention, Division of Healthcare Quality Promotion. Infection control in healthcare settings resources. http://www.cdc.gov/ncidod/dhqp/index.html. Accessed November 20, 2007.

Centers for Disease Control and Prevention. Respiratory hygiene/cough etiquette in health care facilities. http://www.cdc.gov/flu/professionals/infectioncontrol/resphygiene.htm. Accessed November 20, 2007

Colorado Department of Public Health and Environment. Protocols for prevention, treatment and management of infectious diseases for Colorado long term care and rehabilitation facilities. http://www.cdphe.state.co.us/hf/protocols.htm. Accessed November 20, 2007.

Maryland Department of Health and Mental Hygiene, Office of Epidemiology and Disease Control Programs. Guidelines for long-term care facilities. http://www.edcp.org/html/cd_guide.html. Accessed November 20, 2007.

Ontario Ministry of Health and Long-Term Care. Public Health Division and Long-Term Care Homes Branch. A guide to the control of respiratory infection outbreaks in long-term care homes, 2004. http://www.health.gov.on.ca/english/providers/pub/pub_menus/pub_pubhealth .html. Accessed November 20, 2007.

Smith PW, ed. *Infection Control in Long-Term Care Facilities*. 2nd ed. Albany, NY: Delmar Publishers; 1994.

Strausbaugh LJ. Emerging health care-associated infections in the geriatric population. *Emerg Infect Dis*. 2001;7(2):268–271. http://www.cdc.gov/ncidod/eid/vol7no2/strausbaugh.htm. Accessed November 20, 2007.

Strasbaugh LF, Joseph C. Epidemiology and prevention of infections in long-term care facilities. In: Mayhall G, ed. Hospital epidemiology. Baltimore, MD: Williams & Wilkins; 1996.

Smith PW, Rusnak PG. Infection prevention and control in the long-term care facility. *Am J Infect Control*. 1997;25:488–512.

CHAPTER 5

Outbreaks Reported in Ambulatory Care Settings

Kathleen Meehan Arias

> Infection control staff must develop programs that address the special needs of the ambulatory care setting, because this is where most medical care will be given in the 21st century.[1(p42)]

INTRODUCTION

Despite the general belief that the risk of transmission of infectious diseases and other illnesses in the ambulatory healthcare setting is low, numerous outbreaks caused by a variety of bacterial, fungal, viral, and chemical agents have been reported in outpatient settings.[1,2] Many therapeutic, diagnostic, and surgical procedures formerly performed in the inpatient hospital setting are now routinely done in freestanding or hospital-sponsored outpatient facilities such as same-day or ambulatory surgery centers. As more healthcare services move from inpatient to outpatient facilities, the potential for healthcare-associated infections (HAIs) and other adverse events in the ambulatory care setting increases.

This chapter reviews outbreaks that have been reported in ambulatory care settings. One can use the findings of these outbreak investigations to identify risk factors that may be contributing to a similar outbreak and to identify prevention and control measures. For the purposes of this chapter, the ambulatory care setting is defined as one in which a patient does not remain overnight for healthcare services. Examples include physicians' offices, ambulatory surgery centers, dental offices, hemodialysis and peritoneal dialysis centers, chemotherapy facilities, outpatient clinics, and procedure suites (e.g., gastrointestinal endoscopy and bronchoscopy).

Little is known about the incidence of HAIs in the ambulatory care setting because infection surveillance is not performed as often in outpatient settings as it is in the acute care setting, and the populations at risk (i.e., the denominator numbers needed to calculate rates) are frequently difficult to define. Unlike the routine surveillance methods used to detect HAIs in hospitalized patients, no standardized surveillance methodology has yet been developed for the ambulatory care setting. Therefore, it is likely that many HAIs and other adverse events in these settings go undetected unless they affect large numbers of patients or cause significant morbidity. The risk of disease transmission in the outpatient setting varies according to the services provided and the populations served. For instance, the risk of transmission of infectious agents in an internal medicine practice that does not perform invasive procedures is lower than the risk of infection in a hemodialysis center, where the transmission of blood-borne pathogens has been well defined. Table 5–1 contains examples of outbreaks that have been reported in a variety of ambulatory care settings.[3–23]

Table 5–1   Examples of Outbreaks Reported in Ambulatory Care Settings

Outbreak	Setting	Associated With	Year Reported/ Reference
Burkholderia cepacia bloodstream infections	Hematology oncology clinic	Probable contamination of multi-dose medication vials due to lack of aseptic technique, including use of common needle and syringe to access multiple multidose vials	2007[3]
Pseudomonas aeruginosa infections following prostate biopsies	Urology clinic	Transrectal ultrasound (TRUS)-guided prostate biopsy with TRUS equipment that had not been adequately cleaned or properly sterilized; biopsy needle guide was soaked in high-level disinfectant and should have been sterilized; tap water rinse was used after disinfection	2005[4]
Skin reactions following mesotherapy injections	Outpatient treatment in private home	Unsafe injection practices by unlicensed practitioner; non-FDA-approved products	2005[5]
M. tuberculosis infection in personnel and patients in renal dialysis center	Renal dialysis center	Healthcare worker (HCW) with tuberculosis (TB); HCW had previous positive tuberculin skin test but never received treatment for TB infection.	2004[6]
Patient fatalities from Cyanobacteria toxins	Hemodialysis clinic	Phytoplankton from the dialysis clinic's water source	2001[7]
Pseudo-outbreak of *Aureobasidium* sp. lower respiratory tract infections	Outpatient bronchoscopy suite	Reuse of single-use plastic stopcocks between patients undergoing bronchoalveolar lavage	2000[8]
Sterile peritonitis among patients undergoing continuous cycling peritoneal dialysis	Dialysis center at a university hospital	Peritoneal dialysis solution from a single manufacturer; solution potentially contained an endotoxin; implicated lots were recalled	1998[9]

Table 5–1   (*Continued*)

Outbreak	Setting	Associated With	Year Reported/ Reference
Epidemic keratoconjunctivitis (EKC)	Eye care clinic	Lack of handwashing by personnel; inadequate decontamination of diagnostic lenses	1998[10]
Acremonium kiliense endophthalmitis	Ambulatory surgery center	Air contaminated by *A. kiliense* in ventilation system humidifier water	1996[11]
Pseudomonas putida pseudo-pneumonia	Pulmonary clinic	Bronchoscope contaminated by improper maintenance of automated bronchoscope washer	1996[12]
Pseudomonas aeruginosa urinary tract infections	Urodynamic suite	Improper reuse and disinfection of single-use urodynamic testing equipment	1996[13]
Pseudomonas (currently *Burkholderia*) *cepacia* bacteremia	Oncology clinic	Contaminated 500 ml bag of 5% dextrose solution used to prepare heparin flush solution over a 2-week period	1993[14]
Patient-to-patient transmission of HIV	Private surgeon's office	Unknown	1993[15]
Adenovirus type 8 EKC	Outpatient eye clinic	Inadequate handwashing by personnel; inadequate disinfection of instruments	1993[16]
Legionella pneumophila pneumonia	Outpatient clinic	Contaminated air conditioning unit	1990[17]
MDR-TB in healthcare workers and HIV infected patients	Outpatient HIV clinic and hospital	Human immunodeficiency virus (HIV)-infected patients with MDR-TB	1989[18]
Septic arthritis caused by *Serratia marcescens*	Physician's office	Injection site and multidose vials cleansed with cotton balls soaked in contaminated benzalkonium chloride antiseptic	1987[19]
Hepatitis B	Weight reduction clinic	Jet injector gun—nozzle tip contaminated with blood was difficult to disinfect	1986[20]
Hepatitis B	Dentist's office	Dentist was asymptomatic carrier of hepatitis B	1986[21]
Group A beta hemolytic streptococcus abscesses	Pediatrician's office	Contamination of multidose vial of diphtheria-tetanus-pertussis vaccine	1985[22]
Measles	Pediatrician's office	12-year-old boy with cough and rash was in office for 1 hour	1985[23]

FDA = Food and Drug Administration; MDR-TB = Multidrug-resistant tuberculosis

PHYSICIANS' OFFICES AND OUTPATIENT CLINICS

In a literature review, Goodman and Solomon characterized 23 reports of case clusters and outbreaks that occurred in general medical offices, clinics, and emergency departments from 1961 through 1990.[2]

- Thirteen episodes involved common source transmission in which the agent was transmitted by a contaminated medical device (e.g., *Salmonella* via an endoscope and hepatitis B via acupuncture needles) or by contaminated fluids (e.g., disinfectants, benzalkonium chloride antiseptic, multidose medication vials, and multidose vials of influenza or diphtheria-tetanus-pertussis vaccines); in 10 of these outbreaks the mode of transmission was via injection and the causative agents were *Mycobacterium chelonae*, group A beta-hemolytic streptococci, *Pseudomonas* (now *Burkholderia*) *cepacia*, *Serratia marcescens*, *Mycobacterium abscessus*, or *Mycobacterium fortuitum*.[19,20,24–34]

- Nine episodes involved organisms transmitted via the airborne or droplet route (*Mycobacterium tuberculosis*, measles, Epstein-Barr virus, and rubella).[18,23,35–41]

- One report documented person-to-person (staff-to-patient) transmission of epidemic keratoconjunctivitis caused by adenovirus type 8 in an emergency department.[42]

Outbreaks Associated with Products and Devices (Common Source Outbreaks)

Many common source outbreaks in outpatient clinics and private physicians' offices have been associated with the use of intrinsically or extrinsically contaminated fluids.[43–48] Intrinsic contamination (i.e., contamination of the product before it reaches the consumer) is rarely reported; however, extrinsic contamination (i.e., that which occurs during use or preparation of a product) is documented often. Many users are not aware that antiseptic and disinfectant solutions may be intrinsically contaminated or may become extrinsically contaminated during use.

Intrinsically Contaminated Products

Intrinsic contamination of povidone-iodine solutions has caused outbreaks and pseudo-outbreaks in healthcare settings.[45–47] The first report of intrinsic contamination of povidone-iodine was in 1981, when *Pseudomonas cepacia* pseudobacteremias in four New York City hospitals were associated with use of a povidone-iodine solution from a single manufacturer.[45]

Other fluids that are sold as sterile have also been found to be intrinsically contaminated. In 1998, 10 children who received outpatient therapy at a hospital-based hematology/oncology service developed sepsis caused by *Enterobacter cloacae*.[43] The source of the outbreak was traced to intrinsically contaminated prefilled saline syringes, and the manufacturer initiated a recall of the product.

These incidents illustrate the importance of promptly recognizing clusters and outbreaks of infection and other adverse events and the possibility that they are related to the use of a product. Infections or pseudo-infections believed to be due to intrinsic (not extrinsic or in-use) contamination of a product should be reported immediately to the healthcare organization's pharmacy, the manufacturer, and MedWatch, the US Food and Drug Administration's (FDA) Adverse Event Reporting Program. Reports can be submitted to the FDA by telephone at 1-800-FDA-1088 or by completing a form on the FDA's Web site at http://www.fda.gov/medwatch.

Extrinsically Contaminated Products

Extrinsically contaminated fluids that have been associated with outbreaks in the ambulatory care setting include vaccines,[22] benzalkonium chloride antiseptic,[19] 5% dextrose intravenous fluid,[14] and gentian violet skin-marking solution.[44] Benzalkonium chloride antiseptic has been responsible for many outbreaks and is not recommended for use in the healthcare setting because of the ease with which it may become contaminated during use.[19,48–51] One outbreak related to use of benzalkonium chloride involved 10 patients who developed *Serratia marcescens* joint infections after being treated by two orthopedic surgeons who shared an office.[19] All of the patients had received injections of methylprednisolone and lidocaine in the office. The reservoir of the organism was determined to be a canister of cotton balls soaking in benzalkonium chloride. Two previously used vials of methylprednisolone were also culture-positive for *S. marcescens*. The outbreak terminated when the physicians' office discontinued the use of the benzalkonium chloride solution. Facilities using this antiseptic should find an alternative product.

An outbreak of *Mycobacterium chelonae* postoperative surgical site infections (SSI) occurred in eight patients who had cosmetic plastic surgery in a dermatologist's office. The source of the organism was traced to a contaminated gentian violet solution used to demarcate the incision site.[44] The investigators concluded that only sterile skin-marking agents should be used in surgical procedures.

Contaminated Devices

Contaminated medical devices that have been associated with outbreaks in outpatient care settings include jet gun injectors,[20,34] bronchoscopes,[12] and urodynamic testing equipment.[13] There are several reports of outbreaks associated with the use of jet gun injectors. Thirty-one cases of hepatitis B occurred over a 23-month period in a weight reduction clinic where attendees received parenteral human chorionic gonadotrophin given by jet injection.[20] One factor that contributed to this outbreak was the design of the jet gun nozzle tip, which made it difficult to clean and disinfect once it became contaminated with blood. Another outbreak associated with a jet gun injector occurred in a podiatry practice where eight patients developed *Mycobacterium chelonae* foot infections after injection with lidocaine.[34] The source of the organism was a distilled water/quaternary ammonium disinfectant solution in which the jet injector was soaked between procedures. These two outbreaks emphasize the need to clean jet gun injectors carefully and to disinfect them appropriately with a high-level disinfectant and according to the manufacturer's instructions.

Control Measures for Preventing Product- and Device-Related Outbreaks

The following measures should be used to prevent the transmission of infection by contaminated products and devices:

- Personnel handling sterile fluids and medications must be instructed in and adhere to proper aseptic technique to prevent extrinsic (in-use) contamination of solutions.

- To prevent transmission of infectious agents by medical devices, reusable equipment must be cleaned thoroughly according to the manufacturer's directions to remove dirt and organic debris before disinfection or sterilization.

- Semicritical items that come in contact with mucous membranes or nonintact skin must be free of microbial contamination. If reusable, these items must be either sterilized or disinfected with a high-level disinfectant.[49] Examples of semicritical devices are bronchoscopes, gastrointestinal endoscopes, vaginal specula, and cervical diaphragm fitting rings. More information on disinfection and sterilization of medical devices can be found in the Resources section at the end of this chapter.

- An appropriate disinfectant should be chosen based on the composition and the use of the item being disinfected, and the disinfectant manufacturer's instructions for use should be followed.[49,52,53]

- Devices that enter tissues or the vascular system, such as surgical instruments, cardiac catheters, urinary catheters, and implants and needles, must be sterile. If these devices are reusable, they must be mechanically cleaned and then sterilized after each use and wrapped and stored properly so they are not contaminated by dirt or microorganisms.[53,54]

- Personnel should be instructed to read the labels on cleansers, antiseptics, and disinfectants and to carefully follow the directions. Care must be taken to ensure that these products are appropriately used[52,53]:
  1. Cleansers are solutions that are formulated to remove dirt and debris and should be used for cleaning soil from an item or surface. They will not inactivate microorganisms.
  2. Antiseptic solutions are formulated to inactivate microorganisms on skin and tissues. They should not be used as disinfectants to decontaminate devices and equipment because they will not be effective at destroying microbial pathogens present on these surfaces.
  3. Disinfectants are formulated to inactivate microorganisms on inanimate surfaces.

- Single-use items, especially needles and syringes, should be used only once and discarded.

- High-level disinfection and sterilization of medical devices and instruments should be done in accordance with standardized published practices and manufacturers' instructions.[53]

- Wherever high-level disinfection or sterilization of medical devices and instruments is performed there should be a quality assurance program that ensures compliance with standardized published protocols.

• Benzalkonium chloride solution should not be used as a skin antiseptic in the healthcare setting because it is easily contaminated and has been associated with numerous outbreaks.[51] An alternative product should be chosen.

Outbreaks associated with products and devices are also discussed in Chapter 3. Infection prevention and control personnel should be familiar with products and devices that have been associated with outbreaks in all types of healthcare settings, since many products and devices are used in a variety of settings.

Outbreaks Associated with Patient-to-Patient Transmission

In addition to common source transmission, pathogens may also be transmitted from patient-to-patient via direct contact or the airborne route.

Transmission via Direct Contact

Patient-to-patient transmission of human immunodeficiency virus (HIV) has been documented in a private surgical practice in Australia, although the mode of transmission was not identified.[15] Investigators concluded that a breach in infection control precautions was responsible for the transmission of HIV from an infected patient to four other patients who had minor surgery on the same day.

Hlady et al. reported a large outbreak of hepatitis B virus (HBV) transmitted to approximately 300 patients in a dermatology practice in Florida from 1985 through 1991.[55] The outbreak was detected when personnel at a county health department recognized that eight patients with acute hepatitis B infection reported between 1985 and 1991 had visited the same dermatologist prior to onset of their symptoms. An investigation revealed that the dermatologist routinely operated without gloves, did not wash his hands between patients, used a common needle that remained in a multidose vial to access medications (although he did use a separate syringe for each patient), and reused electrocautery tips without cleaning them between patients. Because the dermatologist was not found to be an HBV carrier, the investigators concluded that transmission occurred from patient-to-patient due to the physician's failure to use standard precautions or sterile surgical technique.

Transmission via Unsafe Injection Practices

The global burden of disease attributable to unsafe injection practices in healthcare settings is great. Contaminated injections caused an estimated 21 million infections due to HBV, 2 million infections due to hepatitis C virus (HCV), and 260,000 infections due to HIV in 2000.[56] Although many of these HAIs occurred in resource-poor countries where needle reuse is common owing to economic and supply constraints, outbreaks of blood-borne viruses and other infectious agents transmitted via injections also occurred in healthcare settings in developed nations.

Outbreaks associated with unsafe injection practices have occurred in a variety of outpatient healthcare settings, such as pain remediation clinics, acupuncture practices, physicians' offices, and hematology oncology clinics.[57–61]

In one outbreak, a physician notified the New York City Department of Health of seven patients who had acute HCV infection and had undergone procedures at the same private physician's office.[60] An investigation led to the identification of five more patients with acute HCV infection and a patient with chronic HCV infection who had been treated prior to the 12 acute cases. The health department notified over 2000 clinic patients that they had potentially been exposed to blood-borne pathogens and offered testing for HCV, HBV, and HIV. Over 1300 patients were screened and an additional seven patients who were likely infected at the clinic were detected. No clinic-related HBV or HIV infections were identified. A case-control study revealed that the most likely route of transmission was via contaminated multidose vials of anesthesia medication used in the clinic.[60]

Transmission of blood-borne pathogens by injections can be prevented if healthcare providers adhere to basic aseptic technique when preparing and administering parenteral medications, as outlined in Exhibit 5–1. The following measures are recommended in addition to those listed in Exhibit 5–1[61–64]:

- Both initial training and continuing education programs on basic aseptic technique and safe injection practices are provided for patient care personnel in ambulatory care settings.
- An infection prevention and control program that is tailored to the individual practice setting is implemented and includes the following:
  - Written protocols for preventing the transmission of infections in patients and personnel based on recognized standards and the requirements of accrediting and government agencies
  - Oversight of personnel who provide injections and prepare parenteral medications, including competency training, a system for reporting breaches in proper technique, and a mechanism for ensuring that reported breaches in technique are promptly addressed. Breaches that are reported but not promptly addressed have resulted in continuing transmission of blood-borne pathogens from patient to patient.[60]

Transmission via the Airborne Route

Measles and tuberculosis are two diseases spread via the airborne route that have caused outbreaks in ambulatory and acute care settings.

Measles. Measles is highly communicable from person to person via the airborne route, and transmission in medical settings has been well documented.[23,36,37,40,41] The virus that causes measles can remain airborne for prolonged periods. In an outbreak that occurred in a pediatrician's office, infection developed in three children who arrived at the office an hour or more after a child with measles had left.[41]

Measles is rarely seen in the United States due to a highly immunized population; however, measles is still endemic in many countries. Measles transmission in the United States is usually associated with an imported case. In

Exhibit 5–1   Infection Control and Safe Injection Practices to Prevent Patient-to-Patient Transmission of Blood-Borne Pathogens

Injection safety
- Use a sterile, single-use, disposable needle and syringe for each injection and discard intact in an appropriate sharps container after use.
- Use single-dose medication vials, prefilled syringes, and ampules when possible. Do not administer medications from single-dose vials to multiple patients or combine leftover contents for later use.
- If multiple-dose vials are used, restrict them to a centralized medication area or for single patient use. Never reenter a vial with a needle or syringe used on one patient if that vial will be used to withdraw medication for another patient. Store vials in accordance with manufacturer's recommendations and discard if sterility is compromised.
- Do not use bags or bottles of intravenous solution as a common source of supply for multiple patients.
- Use aseptic technique to avoid contamination of sterile injection equipment and medications.

Patient-care equipment
- Handle patient-care equipment that might be contaminated with blood in a way that prevents skin and mucous membrane exposures, contamination of clothing, and transfer of microorganisms to other patients and surfaces.
- Evaluate equipment and devices for potential cross-contamination of blood. Establish procedures for safe handling during and after use, including cleaning and disinfection or sterilization as indicated.

Work environment
- Dispose of used syringes and needles at the point of use in a sharps container that is puncture-resistant and leak-proof and that can be sealed before completely full.
- Maintain physical separation between clean and contaminated equipment and supplies.
- Prepare medications in areas physically separated from those with potential blood contamination.
- Use barriers to protect surfaces from blood contamination during blood sampling.
- Clean and disinfect blood-contaminated equipment and surfaces in accordance with recommended guidelines.

Hand hygiene and gloves
- Perform hand hygiene (i.e., hand washing with soap and water or use of an alcohol-based hand rub) before preparing and administering an injection, before and after donning gloves for performing blood sampling, after inadvertent blood contamination, and between patients.
- Wear gloves for procedures that might involve contact with blood and change gloves between patients.

Source: Modified from Centers for Disease Control and Prevention. Transmission of hepatitis B and C viruses in outpatient settings—New York, Oklahoma, and Nebraska, 2000–2002. *MMWR.* 2003; 52(38):904. http://www.cdc.gov/mmwr/preview/mmwrhtml/mm5238a1.htm. Accessed May 11, 2008.

2005, 66 confirmed cases of measles were reported to the Centers for Disease Control and Prevention (CDC) and 34 of these were from a single outbreak in Indiana associated with an unvaccinated 17 year old returning home to the United States from Romania.[65,66] Measles outbreaks can cause significant morbidity and disruption in the healthcare, community, and public health settings. In the Indiana outbreak, three persons were hospitalized, including a healthcare worker who required treatment in the intensive care unit.

Strategies for preventing transmission of measles in physicians' offices and other ambulatory healthcare settings include:

- Prompt recognition of patients with measles (measles should be considered in any patient, whether an adult or a child, who has fever and a rash)
- Separation of patients with known or suspected measles from other patients (this may be difficult due to ease of airborne spread and lack of adequate ventilation in many ambulatory care settings)
- Postexposure prophylaxis of potentially exposed contacts, such as patients, persons accompanying patients, and medical personnel
- Postexposure immunization of patients and personnel according to the recommendations of the Advisory Committee on Immunization Practices.[67,68]

Transmission of measles can be prevented if recommendations for immunization of children, adolescents, and adults are followed. Guidelines for preventing transmission of measles have been published by the CDC[69,70] and the American Academy of Pediatrics.[71] Measles outbreaks and prevention and control measures are discussed in detail in Chapter 3. Because the incidence of measles in the United States is low,[68] one case of measles should be considered an outbreak and should promptly be reported by telephone to the local health department so that measures to prevent further spread can be implemented as soon as possible. Appendix C contains a protocol for controlling an outbreak of measles in a healthcare facility, including a physician's office (Appendix C is available for download at this text's Web site: http://www.jbpub.com/catalog/9780763757793/).

Tuberculosis. Transmission of tuberculosis (TB) in the ambulatory care setting is well recognized.[18,35,72–74] Multiple outbreaks of TB infection and disease, including multidrug-resistant tuberculosis, occurred in the United States in the late 1980s and early 1990s. Several of these outbreaks involved patients and personnel in outpatient settings.[18,35,74] There are also reports of TB outbreaks among emergency room personnel[73,75] and among patients and staff at an outpatient methadone clinic[72] following exposure to patients with pulmonary TB.

The epidemiology and mode of transmission of *Mycobacterium tuberculosis* and control measures used to prevent the spread of TB are discussed in Chapter 7. Recommendations for preventing the spread of TB in the healthcare setting have been published by the CDC and include the following[76]:

- Prompt recognition of persons (patients and personnel) that have signs and symptoms suggestive of pulmonary TB

- Prompt isolation of persons with known or suspected pulmonary TB in a private room with negative airflow and air exhausted to the outside
- Prompt and appropriate diagnostic workup for persons with signs and symptoms of pulmonary TB (i.e., medical history and physical, chest radiograph, tuberculin skin testing, and smear and culture of sputum for acid-fast bacilli)
- Use of respiratory protection by personnel caring for a patient with known or suspected TB
- Prompt treatment of infected persons with antituberculosis medications

Patients who come to an ambulatory care facility with signs and symptoms suggestive of pulmonary TB should be instructed to wear a mask and should be separated from other patients until the diagnosis is confirmed or ruled out.

DENTAL SETTINGS

Outbreaks in dental settings have long been recognized.[1,21,77] Goodman and Solomon reviewed 13 reports of infectious disease transmission that occurred in dental practices between 1961 and 1990.[2] They noted the following:

- Nine were reports of transmission of HBV from an infected dentist or oral surgeon to patients.[21,77–84]
- One involved gingivostomatitis caused by herpes simplex transmitted by a dental hygienist with herpetic whitlow.[85]
- One investigated a presumed transmission of HIV from an infected dentist to his patients.[86]
- One involved oral abscesses caused by *Pseudomonas aeruginosa* from a contaminated dental unit water system.[87]
- One involved intraoral and pulmonary TB transmitted by a dentist with infectious pulmonary TB.[88]

Hepatitis B virus is the most common agent involved in reported outbreaks in the dental setting. Investigations of these HBV outbreaks found that HBV was transmitted directly from an infected dentist or oral surgeon to the patient(s).[21,77–84] There was no evidence in these reports of transmission from patient-to-patient via contaminated instruments or equipment. There have been no reported cases of dentist-to-patient HBV transmission in the United States since 1987.[89] This is a result of the widespread implementation of standard precautions in US dental practices and the increasing rates of HBV immunization in dental personnel and patients. However, in 2007 Redd et al. reported the first documented case of patient-to-patient transmission of HBV in a dental setting.[89] The investigation began following the report of a 60-year-old woman who developed acute hepatitis B but had none of the traditional risk factors. Using molecular epidemiologic techniques, the investigators determined that HBV transmission occurred between this patient and another patient with chronic HBV infection who had surgery less than 3 hours earlier in the same outpatient oral surgery center. The HBV isolates from the two patients were found to be identical using DNA sequencing. None of the dental practice staff had HBV infection and no lapse in infection control technique was found. Although the mode of transmission could not be determined, cross-contamination via an environmental surface soiled with the blood of the HBV-infected patient was suspected.

One of the most highly publicized events involving transmission of an infection from a healthcare provider to a patient was the 1990 report of HIV transmitted to a patient by a dentist with acquired immune deficiency syndrome.[90] Further investigation linked the Florida dentist to HIV infection in six of his patients[86,91,92]; however, the mode of transmission of HIV was not able to be determined.

Measures Used to Prevent Transmission of Infection in Dental Settings

Control measures for preventing transmission of infectious agents, including HIV, HBV, and other bloodborne pathogens, in the dental setting have been published by the CDC,[93,94] the American Dental Association[95,96] and the Organization for Safety and Asepsis Procedures.[97] These recommendations include:

- Development and implementation of a comprehensive, infection prevention and control program that includes personnel health policies and procedures and is specific for the particular dental setting[94]
- A mechanism for routinely evaluating the infection prevention and control program. Examples of methods for evaluating infection control programs can be found in Table 5–2.[94]
- Education and training of dental healthcare personnel at initial employment and periodically thereafter[94]
- Use of personal protective equipment, gloves, and standard precautions by personnel[93,94,96]
- Use of aseptic technique by personnel, including safe injection practices for parenteral medication[94]
- Use of appropriate hand hygiene practices[64,94,96]
- HBV immunization of susceptible dental personnel[67,94]
- Appropriate cleaning, disinfection, and sterilization of instruments and equipment including dental handpieces and other devices attached to air and water lines[94(Appendix A)] (Appendix A is available for download at this text's Web site: http://www.jbpub.com/catalog/9780763757793/)
- Use of mechanical, chemical, and biological monitors according to manufacturers' instructions to ensure the sterilization process[94]
- Decontamination of environmental surfaces using appropriate cleaning and disinfecting products[94(Appendix A)]
- Implementation of a program to ensure the quality of dental unit water and water lines[94,96,98]

Table 5–2   Examples of Methods for Evaluating Infection Control Programs

Program Element	Evaluation Activity
Appropriate immunization of dental healthcare personnel (DHCP)	Conduct annual review of personnel records to ensure up-to-date immunizations.
Assessment of occupational exposures to infectious agents	Report occupational exposures to infectious agents. Document the steps that occurred around the exposure and plan how such exposure can be prevented in the future.
Comprehensive postexposure management plan and medical follow-up program after occupational exposures to infectious agents	Ensure the postexposure management plan is clear, complete, and available at all times to all DHCP. All staff should understand the plan, which should include toll-free phone numbers for access to additional information.
Adherence to hand hygiene before and after patient care	Observe and document circumstances of appropriate or inappropriate handwashing. Review findings in a staff meeting.
Proper use of personal protective equipment to prevent occupational exposures to infectious agents	Observe and document the use of barrier precautions and careful handling of sharps. Review findings in a staff meeting.
Routine and appropriate sterilization of instruments using a biologic monitoring system	Monitor paper log of steam cycle and temperature strip with each sterilization load, and examine results of weekly biologic monitoring. Take appropriate action when failure of sterilization process is noted.
Evaluation and implementation of safer medical devices	Conduct an annual review of the exposure control plan and consider new developments in safer medical devices.
Compliance of water in routine dental procedures with current drinking US Environmental Protection Agency water standards (fewer than 500 CFU of heterotrophic water bacteria)	Monitor dental water quality as recommended by the equipment manufacturer, using commercial self-contained test kits, or commercial water-testing laboratories.
Proper handling and disposal of medical waste	Observe the safe disposal of regulated and nonregulated medical waste and take preventive measures if hazardous situations occur.
Healthcare-associated infections	Assess the unscheduled return of patients after procedures and evaluate them for an infectious process. A trend might require formal evaluation.

Source: Centers for Disease Control and Prevention. Guidelines for Infection Control in Dental Health-Care Settings, 2003. *MMWR*. 2003;52(RR-17):37. http://www.cdc.gov/oralhealth/infectioncontrol/guidelines/index.htm. Accessed May 11, 2008.

HEMODIALYSIS AND PERITONEAL DIALYSIS CENTERS

Numerous outbreaks have been reported in hemodialysis and peritoneal dialysis centers. Many of the infectious disease-related outbreaks have been caused by the HBV, although HCV, HIV, *Mycobacterium tuberculosis*, and a variety of bacteria and bacterial endotoxins have also been responsible.[99–119] Numerous noninfectious disease outbreaks have been reported,[120–127] including anaphylactoid reactions associated with improperly processed hemodialyzers,[120] hypotension associated with improperly installed filters in a water treatment system,[122] sterile peritonitis resulting from chemical agents used in peritoneal dialysis and intrinsic endotoxin contamination of peritoneal dialysis solution,[9,125] and reactions to toxins in hemodialysis water systems and fluids.[7,124] Table 5–3 contains examples of outbreaks reported in dialysis centers.

Table 5–3   Examples of Outbreaks Reported in Dialysis Centers

Outbreak	Comments/Associated With	Year Reported/ Reference
Tuberculosis	Exposure to hemodialysis technician with pulmonary tuberculosis	2004[6]
Sterile (culture-negative) peritonitis following peritoneal dialysis	Use of dialysate containing icodextrin; such reactions could be due to a substance contaminating the icodextrin or to hypersensitivity to icodextrin	2003[126]
Vascular access site infections	Malfunctioning catheters from a single manufacturer; manufacturer later recalled catheter	2002[119]
Acute illness and hospitalization shortly following hemodialysis	Cases occurred on a single day in the same outpatient dialysis center; most likely due to parenteral exposure to volatile sulfur-containing compounds from the water near the reverse osmosis (RO) unit; improperly maintained RO membrane allowed sulfur-reducing bacteria to grow and produce toxic levels of disulfides; resulted in 16 patients hospitalized and 2 deaths	2002[124]
Pyrogenic reactions and *Serratia liquefaciens* bloodstream infections	Extrinsic (in-use) contamination of medication (epoetin alfa) due to repeated use of single-use vials to obtain multiple doses and pooling of residual epoetin alpha from single-use vials for later use	2001[115]
Acute liver failure causing morbidity and mortality	Parenteral exposure to cyanotoxins from phytoplankton in water source used by dialysis center	1998[127] 2001[7]

Table 5–3   (*Continued*)

Outbreak	Comments/Associated With	Year Reported/ Reference
Hemolysis following hemodialysis	Blood tubing sets produced by a single manufacturer had a narrow aperture that caused mechanical lysis of red blood cells	1998[123]
Bacterial bloodstream infections—Canada, United States, Israel	Contamination of the waste drain ports in the same model of hemodialysis machine	1998[113] 1999[114]
Bloodstream infections caused by multiple pathogens	Contamination of newly installed attachment used to drain spent priming saline in hemodialysis system	1998[112]
Hepatitis B virus (HBV) infection, Texas	Lack of separation of patients with chronic HBV infection from HBV-negative patients; lack of review of monthly HBsAg* results; lack of use of standard precautions; poor compliance with recommendations for HBV prevention	1996[99]
Human immuno-deficiency virus (HIV) infection	Reusable needle used on patient with HIV improperly processed with benzalkonium chloride by soaking in a common pan with needles used on other patients	1995[108]
Anaphylactoid reactions	Reuse of hollow-fiber hemodialyzers repro-cessed with automated reprocessing system	1992[120]
Bacteremia with gram-negative organisms and *Enterococcus casseliflavus*	Venous blood tubing cross-contaminated with ultrafiltrate waste	1992[109]
Hepatitis C virus infection	No common source or person-to-person mode of transmission documented; probable cause was lack of adequate infection prevention and control precautions	1992[103]
Hypotension	Ultrafilters preserved in sodium azide were not rinsed prior to installation in dialysis center water treatment system; dialysis water became contaminated with sodium diazide	1990[122]
Hepatitis B virus infection	Failure to isolate patient with chronic HBV; shared equipment and staff	1989[100]
Hepatitis B virus infection	Associated with shared multidose vial used by patient with chronic HBV	1983[101]

*HBsAg= hepatitis B surface antigen

Transmission of HBV in hemodialysis centers has long been recognized.[100] Several factors help to promote the transmission of HBV in the dialysis setting:

- HBV may be present in high titers ($\geq 10^9$ virus particles per milliliter) in the blood and body fluids of infected patients.[99]
- HBV can survive for a prolonged period in the environment.[128]
- Equipment and surfaces in dialysis settings can easily become contaminated with blood.[128]

The majority of outbreaks of hepatitis B infection in hemodialysis facilities are associated with lack of adherence to recommended infection prevention and control practices for preventing the transmission of blood-borne pathogens. The following factors have contributed to HBV outbreaks:[99,128]

- Failure to use separate rooms for hemodialyzing patients with chronic HBV infection
- Cross-contamination due to failure to use dedicated machines, medications, supplies, and staff for patients with chronic hepatitis B infection
- Lack of adherence to standard precautions
- Deficiencies in cleaning and disinfection procedures for equipment and environmental surfaces
- Failure to restrict sharing of medications and supplies between patients.

Patient-to-patient transmission of HCV in hemodialysis centers has been documented, but the exact mode for transmission has not been elucidated. Possible modes of transmission include carriage on the hands of healthcare workers and contamination of the hemodialysis machine.[104,105,107]

Measures Used to Prevent Transmission of Infection in Dialysis Centers

Recommendations and guidelines for preventing the transmission of infection in dialysis settings have been published by the CDC and the National Kidney Foundation.[99,128–131] The Association for the Advancement of Medical Instrumentation (AAMI) provides standards for dialysis water purity and water distribution and storage systems,[132] and the CDC Guidelines for Environmental Infection Control in Health-care Facilities provides an overview of dialysis water quality and dialysate.[49] The International Society for Peritoneal Dialysis provides treatment and infection prevention guidelines for peritoneal dialysis.[133] The CDC recommendations are outlined in Exhibit 5–2.

Recommendations for preventing the transmission of blood-borne pathogens in hemodialysis centers include the following:

- Implementation of a comprehensive infection surveillance, prevention, and control program specifically designed for the hemodialysis setting that includes the elements shown in Exhibit 5–3
- Use of standard precautions by personnel

Exhibit 5–2   Recommended Infection Control Practices for Hemodialysis Units at a Glance

Infection Control Precautions for All Patients

- Wear disposable gloves when caring for the patient or touching the patient's equipment at the dialysis station; remove gloves and wash hands between each patient or station.
- Items taken into the dialysis station should either be disposed of, dedicated for use only on a single patient, or cleaned and disinfected before being taken to a common clean area or used on another patient.
  - Nondisposable items that cannot be cleaned and disinfected (e.g., adhesive tape, cloth-covered blood pressure cuffs) should be dedicated for use only on a single patient.
  - Unused medications (including multiple dose vials containing diluents) or supplies (e.g., syringes, alcohol swabs) taken to the patient's station should be used only for that patient and should not be returned to a common clean area or used on other patients.
- When multiple dose medication vials are used (including vials containing diluents), prepare individual patient doses in a clean (centralized) area away from dialysis stations and deliver separately to each patient. Do not carry multiple dose medication vials from station to station.
- Do not use common medication carts to deliver medications to patients. Do not carry medication vials, syringes, alcohol swabs, or supplies in pockets. If trays are used to deliver medications to individual patients, they must be cleaned between patients.
- Clean areas should be clearly designated for the preparation, handling, and storage of medications and unused supplies and equipment. Clean areas should be clearly separated from contaminated areas where used supplies and equipment are handled. Do not handle and store medications or clean supplies in the same or an adjacent area to where used equipment or blood samples are handled.
- Use external venous and arterial pressure transducer filters/protectors for each patient treatment to prevent blood contamination of the dialysis machines' pressure monitors. Change filters/protectors between each patient treatment, and do not reuse them. Internal transducer filters do not need to be changed routinely between patients.
- Clean and disinfect the dialysis station (e.g., chairs, beds, tables, machines) between patients.
  - Give special attention to cleaning control panels on the dialysis machines and other surfaces that are frequently touched and potentially contaminated with patients' blood.
  - Discard all fluid, and clean and disinfect all surfaces and containers associated with the prime waste (including buckets attached to the machines).
- For dialyzers and blood tubing that will be reprocessed, cap dialyzer ports and clamp tubing. Place all used dialyzers and tubing in leak-proof containers for transport from station to reprocessing or disposal area.

Hepatitis B Vaccination

- Vaccinate all susceptible patients against hepatitis B.
- Test for anti-HBs 1–2 months after last dose.
  - If anti-HBs is <10 mIU/mL, consider patient susceptible, revaccinate with an additional three doses, and retest for anti-HBs.
  - If anti-HBs is >10 mIU/mL, consider patient immune, and retest annually.
  - Give booster dose of vaccine if anti-HBs declines to <10 mIU/mL and continue to retest annually.

Continued

Exhibit 5–2   (*Continued*)

Management of HBsAg-Positive Patients
- Follow infection control practices for hemodialysis units for all patients.
- Dialyze HBsAg-positive patients in a separate room using separate machines, equipment, instruments, and supplies.
- Staff members caring for HBsAg-positive patients should not care for HBV-susceptible patients at the same time (e.g., during the same shift or during patient changeover).

Source: Centers for Disease Control and Prevention. Recommendations for preventing transmission of infections among chronic hemodialysis patients. *MMWR.* 2001;50(RR-05):20–21. http://www.cdc.gov/mmwr/PDF/rr/rr5005.pdf or http://www.cdc.gov/mmwr/preview/mmwrhtml/rr5005a1.htm. Accessed May 11, 2008.

Schedule for Routine Testing for Hepatitis B Virus (HBV) and Hepatitis C Virus (HCV) Infections

Patient Status	On Admission	Monthly	Semiannual	Annual
All patients	HBsAg,* Anti-HBc* (total), Anti-HBs,* Anti-HCV, ALT†			
HBV-susceptible, including nonresponders to vaccine		HBsAg		
Anti-HBs positive (>10 mIU/mL), anti-HBc negative				Anti-HBs
Anti-HBs and anti-HBc positive	No additional HBV testing needed			
Anti-HCV negative	ALT		Anti-HCV	

* Results of HBV testing should be known before the patient begins dialysis.
† HBsAg=hepatitis B surface antigen; anti-HBc=antibody to hepatitis B core antigen; anti-HBs=antibody to hepatitis B surface antigen; anti-HCV=antibody to hepatitis C virus; ALT=alanine aminotransferase.

- Requirement for monthly testing of serum specimens from all susceptible patients for hepatitis B surface antigen (HbsAg) and prompt review of the results of this testing
- Hepatitis B immunization of susceptible hemodialysis patients
- Isolation of HbsAg-positive patients by room, machines, instruments, medications, supplies, and staff
- Avoidance of sharing instruments, medications, and supplies between patients
- Preparation of multidose medication vials in a clean centralized area away from areas used for patient care, laboratory work, or waste disposal

Exhibit 5–3 Components of a Comprehensive Infection Control Program to Prevent Transmission of Infections Among Chronic Hemodialysis Patients

- Infection control practices for hemodialysis units:
  - Infection control precautions specifically designed to prevent transmission of blood-borne viruses and pathogenic bacteria among patients
  - Routine serologic testing for hepatitis B virus and hepatitis C virus infections
  - Vaccination of susceptible patients against hepatitis B
  - Isolation of patients who test positive for hepatitis B surface antigen
- Surveillance for infections and other adverse events
- Infection control training and education

Source: Centers for Disease Control and Prevention. Recommendations for preventing transmission of infections among chronic hemodialysis patients. *MMWR.* 2001;50(RR-05):18. http://www.cdc.gov/mmwr/preview/mmwrhtml/rr5005a1.htm. Accessed April 11, 2008.

- Implementation of routine cleaning and disinfection protocols for equipment and environmental surfaces
- Separation of areas used to store clean supplies and handle contaminated items
- Storage of blood specimens in designated areas away from medication preparation or clean supply areas
- A program for monitoring and maintenance of water treatment systems in hemodialysis centers in accordance with recognized standards[128,132]
- A surveillance program that monitors dialysis-related infections and other adverse events and reports results to the center's staff and management[134]

For additional information on infection prevention and control practices in the dialysis setting, the reader is referred to Chapter 3 in this text and to the resources and recommended reading sections at the end of this chapter.

OPHTHALMOLOGY OFFICES AND CLINICS

Many reports of outbreaks of healthcare-associated epidemic keratoconjunctivitis (EKC) have been published.[1,2,10,16,135–149] Goodman and Solomon reviewed 11 reports of infectious disease outbreaks in ophthalmology offices and eye clinics[2]: 10 were outbreaks of EKC caused by adenovirus transmitted by inadequately disinfected equipment (frequently a tonometer) and/or by poor hand hygiene practices by physicians and other healthcare personnel,[137–146] and one episode was a cluster of cases of *Mycobacterium chelonei* keratitis associated with invasive procedures in which a contaminated solution was the likely source of the organism.[147]

Adenovirus can survive for prolonged periods on instruments and environmental surfaces. Person-to-person transmission of adenovirus can occur via direct contact with an infected person or with infective secretions, such as those on the hands of a healthcare worker or contaminated instruments or medications. In a report of an outbreak involving 63 patients at a large university medical center ophthalmology clinic, the CDC noted that exposure to a particular healthcare worker or exposure to pneumotonometry were risk factors for acquiring EKC.[148] Contaminated ocular devices, particularly tonometers, are frequently implicated in healthcare-associated outbreaks. Since tonometers vary in design, it is important that methods used for cleaning and disinfecting or sterilizing these instruments allow for adequate disinfection and sterilization of the instrument's tip and adjacent parts after each patient use.[148–150]

Measures Used to Prevent Spread of Epidemic Keratoconjunctivitis

Recommendations for preventing the spread of infection and for controlling EKC outbreaks in ophthalmology practices have been published by the American Academy of Ophthalmology (AAO) (available for download from the AAO Web site),[150] the CDC,[148] Buehler et al.,[138] Montessori et al.,[10] and Gottsch et al.[151] Prevention and control measures to limit the spread of adenovirus and other infectious agents in ophthalmology practices include the following:

- Proper hand hygiene practices both before and after examining patients[64]
- Appropriate cleaning and disinfection or sterilization protocols for the types of equipment used[148,150]
- Implementation of routine protocols for cleaning and disinfection or sterilization of equipment after each patient
- Triage of patients with signs and symptoms of conjunctivitis (e.g., eye discharge or redness)
- Meticulous administration of eye drops to avoid contaminating the dropper and the medication
- Careful cleaning and disinfection of environmental surfaces[49]
- Use of gloves for contact with infective eye secretions (e.g., when a patient has clinical signs and symptoms of conjunctivitis and during an EKC outbreak)
- Restriction of personnel with conjunctivitis from direct contact with patients (for up to 14 days for personnel with viral conjunctivitis)[148]

The CDC recommends the following regarding tonometer tips:

[They] be cleaned with soap and water or with another cleansing agent suggested by the manufacturer and disinfected by soaking for at least 10 minutes in a solution containing 500–5000 ppm chlorine (e.g., a 1:100–1:10 dilution of household bleach) or in any commercial germicidal solution that is registered with the Environmental Protection Agency as a "sterilant" and is compatible with the tonometer. The soaking time in commercial germicides necessary to achieve high-level disinfection (which includes inactivation of adenovirus type 8 and bacteria that are pathogenic to the eye) varies by type and concentration of solution and should be indicated by the germicide manufacturer on the product label.[148(p600)]

When using any commercially available cleaner or disinfectant, it is important to read carefully the indications for use and to follow the directions on the label.

GASTROINTESTINAL ENDOSCOPY AND BRONCHOSCOPY PROCEDURE SUITES

Numerous outbreaks associated with bronchoscopy and gastrointestinal endoscopic procedures have been reported in inpatient and outpatient settings. Most of these were caused by failure to adequately clean and disinfect endoscopes or by contamination of automated endoscope processors. Outbreaks related to endoscopic procedures, including prevention and control measures, are discussed in Chapter 3.

AMBULATORY SURGERY CENTERS

According to the National Survey of Ambulatory Surgery conducted by the National Center for Health Statistics, an estimated 71.9 million procedures were performed on 39.9 million discharges from hospitals and freestanding ambulatory surgery centers during 1996: 40.4 million procedures were for inpatients and 31.5 million were for ambulatory patients.[152] An estimated 17.5 million (84%) of the ambulatory surgery visits were in hospital-based outpatient surgery departments, and 3.3 million (16%) occurred in freestanding centers. This survey was repeated in 2006; however, the results were not available as of April 2008.[153]

Despite the large number of procedures performed in ambulatory surgery centers, there are few reports of outbreaks in these settings. A review of textbooks and references related to ambulatory surgery and a search of the MEDLINE database from1985 through March 2008 revealed reports of outbreaks that were associated with cataract surgery, podiatric surgery, and contaminated betamethasone injections in an ambulatory surgery center, in addition to several reports noted earlier in this chapter.[44]

Cataract extraction is one of the most common surgeries performed in the United States.[154] Cataract surgery is performed in freestanding ambulatory surgery centers and hospital inpatient and outpatient surgery departments. Outbreaks of toxic anterior segment syndrome (TASS) associated with cataract surgery have been reported in all of these settings.[154–157] TASS, an acute, noninfectious inflammation of the anterior segment of the eye, has been associated with the following

> (1) contaminants on surgical instruments, resulting from improper or insufficient cleaning; (2) products introduced into the eye during surgery, such as irrigating solutions or ophthalmic medications; or (3) other substances that enter the eye during or after surgery, such as topical ointments or talc from surgical gloves.[154]

An outbreak of *Acremonium kiliense* endophthalmitis occurred following cataract surgery in four patients in an ambulatory surgical center.[11] An epidemiologic study discovered that the infected patients had surgery either on the first operative day of the week or soon after the operating room opened. Cultures of perioperative medications and environmental samples were negative for *A. kiliense* except for water from a grossly contaminated humidifier reservoir in the heating, ventilation, and air-conditioning (HVAC) system. Further investigation revealed that the HVAC system was routinely turned off after the last case on Thursday and switched back on when surgery resumed the following Tuesday. The investigators concluded that the HVAC system was contaminated by the humidifier water, and agitation of the system probably dislodged fungal spores when the system was turned on. The spores were then carried on air currents into the operating room. No further cases occurred after the HVAC system was left running 7 days a week and the humidifier was removed.

An outbreak of *Proteus mirabilis* surgical site infections occurred in patients who underwent outpatient podiatric surgery.[158] An investigation traced the source to inadequately sterilized bone drills. The cluster of infections was recognized in part because it was caused by an uncommon strain of *P. mirabilis*.

An outbreak of *Serratia marcescens* infections occurred in 2001 in 11 patients who had procedures in a hospital-affiliated ambulatory surgery center (five cases with meningitis, one with septic arthritis, and five with epidural abscess).[159] An investigation revealed that all of the patients had received epidural or joint injections with contaminated betamethasone that had been compounded at a local pharmacy. This appears to be the first reported outbreak of infections associated with improper pharmacy compounding.[159]

Preventing Infections in Ambulatory Surgery Settings

In 2007 the American Society of Cataract and Refractive Surgery and the American Society of Ophthalmic Registered Nurses published recommended practices for cleaning and sterilizing intraocular surgical instruments.[160] To prevent infections and other adverse events associated with improperly processed intraocular surgical instruments, infection control professionals (ICPs) should refer to these guidelines when developing infection prevention programs for cataract surgery centers.

The CDC published guidelines for preventing surgical site infections in ambulatory, same-day, and outpatient operating rooms as well as conventional inpatient operating rooms,[161] and these should be used when developing infection surveillance, prevention, and control programs for the ambulatory surgery setting.

Because the incidence of SSIs associated with the types of procedures performed in outpatient surgery centers is low, many ambulatory surgical centers do not routinely conduct surveillance for SSIs. Therefore, it is likely that clusters and outbreaks of infection in this setting are not detected unless they are caused by an unusual organism or result in significant morbidity or mortality. As more procedures are moved from the inpatient to the outpatient setting, surveillance programs for HAIs and other adverse events in ambulatory surgery settings should be implemented to detect adverse events in these settings so that risk factors and preventive measures can be identified.[161–163] The surveillance program should include the use of standardized data collection methods and definitions for SSIs, stratification of SSI rates according to risk factors associated with SSIs, and data feedback to perioperative and performance improvement personnel.

Outbreaks occurring in inpatient surgical settings are discussed in Chapter 3.

THE CHANGING FACE OF HEALTH CARE

In the past few decades the majority of health care in the United States has transitioned from the acute care hospital setting to outpatient and ambulatory care, long-term care, and home care settings.[164] Many ICPs have expanded their infection surveillance, prevention, and control programs to include these settings. As discussed in this chapter, guidelines for developing infection surveillance, prevention, and control programs in ambulatory care settings have been published by individuals, professional organizations, and government agencies, and there are many resources on professional and government agency Web sites.

Information on developing and implementing surveillance programs in a variety of healthcare settings, including ambulatory care, can be found in Chapter 2.

In a study conducted by the Association for Professionals in Infection Control and Epidemiology on the status of infection surveillance, prevention, and control programs in the United States from 1992 through 1996, the number of facilities performing surveillance for HAIs in outpatient settings increased by 44.0%, from 100 to 144.[165] However, surveillance programs for ambulatory care settings are not as well developed as those for acute care settings, and the epidemiology of HAIs in the outpatient setting has not been well characterized. The CDC National Healthcare Safety Network will be expanding to include data on HAIs associated with outpatient care.[166] This should help to characterize the epidemiology of HAIs in ambulatory care settings.

CONCLUSIONS

Risk Factors Associated with Infectious Disease Outbreaks in the Ambulatory Care Setting

Many outbreaks in ambulatory care settings occur because (1) the responsibility for implementing an infection surveillance, prevention, and control program is often not assigned to a specific individual, and (2) personnel working in outpatient care settings are frequently not familiar with basic infection control practices.

Based on the reports of the outbreaks discussed in this chapter, one can identify the following risk factors as causing or contributing to infectious disease outbreaks in the ambulatory care setting:

- Inadequate cleaning, disinfection, sterilization, and storage of instruments and equipment
- Inappropriate use of barrier precautions, such as gloves, by healthcare personnel

- Inadequate hand hygiene practices by healthcare workers
- Failure to use aseptic technique
- Failure to use appropriate isolation precautions for patients who have, or are suspected of having, an infection that can be transmitted to others
- Lack of temporary work restriction of infected healthcare personnel
- Lack of familiarity with established infection prevention and control practices on the part of ambulatory care personnel

Measures Used to Prevent Transmission of Infectious Agents in the Ambulatory Care Setting

The specific measures that should be implemented to prevent the transmission of infectious agents in each outpatient practice setting will depend on the types of patients, the procedures and treatments performed, and the equipment and devices that are used.

To prevent the transmission of infection to patients and personnel, each ambulatory care setting should have an infection surveillance, prevention, and control program that addresses the following:

- Assignment of responsibility for coordinating and implementing the program to specific individuals
- Processes for identifying the types of patients and procedures performed and the risk for infection and other adverse events
- Infection prevention and control policies and procedures that are specific for the healthcare setting
- Protocols for implementing standard precautions[70,93]
- Identification of the types of reusable devices and instruments used and determination of whether they must be disinfected or sterilized[49,53]
- Protocols for cleaning and disinfection or sterilization of reusable devices and instruments in accordance with the manufacturer's instructions and the recommendations of relevant organizations, such as the Association of periOperative Registered Nurses,[167] the AAO,[149] the American Dental Association,[98] and the AAMI[168]
- Protocols for monitoring the effectiveness of the sterilization process, wherever a sterilizer is used[167,168]
- Protocols for identifying and isolating persons known to have, or suspected of having, a transmissible infection[70,71,76]
- Protocols for restricting infected personnel from direct patient contact[69]
- Policies for the immunization of healthcare workers[67]
- Protocols for handling multidose medication vials
- Education and training of ambulatory care personnel, upon hire and periodically thereafter, on basic infection prevention and control practices such as standard precautions; triage and isolation of infected patients; separation of clean and dirty items; the use of aseptic technique; and cleaning, disinfection, and sterilization practices, as appropriate for the setting.

REFERENCES

1. Herwaldt LA, Smith LA, Carter CD. Infection control in the outpatient setting. *Infect Control Hosp Epidemiol.* 1998;19:41–74.

2. Goodman RA, Solomon SL. Transmission of infectious diseases in outpatient health care settings. *JAMA.* 1991;265:2377–2381.

3. Abe K, Tobin M, Sunenshine R, et al. Outbreak of *Burkholderia cepacia* bloodstream infection at an outpatient hematology and oncology practice. *Infect Control Hosp Epidemiol.* 2007; 28:1311–1313.

4. Centers for Disease Control and Prevention. *Pseudomonas aeruginosa* infections associated with transrectal ultrasound-guided prostate biopsies—Georgia, 2005. *MMWR.* 2006; 55: 776–777.

5. Centers for Disease Control and Prevention. Outbreak of mesotherapy-associated skin reactions—District of Columbia Area, January–February 2005. *MMWR.* 2005; 54(44);1127–1130.

6. Centers for Disease Control and Prevention. Tuberculosis transmission in a renal dialysis center—Nevada, 2003. *MMWR.* 2004;53(37):873–875.

7. Carmichael WW, Azevedo SMFO, An JS, et al. Human fatalities from cyanobacteria: chemical and biological evidence for cyanotoxins. *Environ Health Perspect.* 2001;109:663–668. http://ehpnet1.niehs.nih.gov/docs/2001/109p663-668carmichael/abstract.html. Accessed April 4, 2008.

8. Wilson SJ, Evert RJ, Kirkland KB, Sexton DJ. A pseudo-outbreak of *Aureobasidium* species lower respiratory tract infections caused by reuse of single-use stopcocks during bronchoscopy. *Infect Control Hosp Epidemiol.* 2000;21(7):470–472.

9. Mangram AJ, Archibald LK, Hupert M et al. Outbreak of sterile peritonitis among continuous cycling peritoneal dialysis patients. *Kidney Int.* 1998;54:1367–1371. http://www.nature.com/ki/journal/v54/n4/full/4490374a.html. Accessed April 14, 2008.

10. Montessori V, Scharf S, Holland S, Werker DH, Roberts FJ, Bryce E. Epidemic keratoconjunctivitis outbreak at a tertiary referral eye care clinic. *Am J Infect Control.* 1998;26: 399–405.

11. Fridkin SK, Kremer FB, Bland LA, Padhye A, McNeil MM, Jarvis WR. *Acremonium kiliense endophthalmitis* that occurred after cataract extraction in an ambulatory surgical center and was traced to an environmental reservoir. *Clin Infect Dis.* 1996;22:222–227.

12. Umphrey J, Raad I, Tarrand J, Hill LA. Bronchoscopes as a contamination source of *Pseudomonas putida. Infect Control Hosp Epidemiol.* 1996;17(suppl):P42. Abstract M2.

13. Climo M, Pastor A, Wong E. Outbreak of *P. aeruginosa* infections related to contaminated urodynamic testing equipment. *Infect Control Hosp Epidemiol.* 1996;17(suppl):P48. Abstract M58.

14. Pegues DA, Carson LA, Anderson RI, et al. Outbreak of *Pseudomonas cepacia* bacteremia in oncology patients. *Clin Infect Dis.* 1993;16:407–411.

15. Chant K, Lowe D, Rubin G, et al. Patient-to-patient transmission of HIV in private surgical consulting rooms [letter]. *Lancet.* 1993;342:1548–1549.

16. Jernigan JA, Lowry BS, Hayden FG, et al. Adenovirus type 8 epidemic keratoconjunctivitis in an eye clinic: risk factors and control. *J Infect Dis.* 1993;167:1307–1313.

17. O'Mahoney MC, Stanwell-Smith RE, Tillett HE, et al. The Stafford outbreak of Legionnaires' disease. *Epidemiol Infect.* 1990;104:361–380.

18. Centers for Disease Control. Nosocomial transmission of multidrug-resistant tuberculosis to health care workers and HIV-infected patients in an urban hospital—Florida. *MMWR.* 1990;39:718–722.

19. Nakashima AK, McCarthy MA, Martone WJ, Anderson RL. Epidemic septic arthritis caused by *Serratia marcescens* and associated with a benzalkonium chloride antiseptic. *J Clin Microbiol.* 1987;25:1014–1018.

20. Centers for Disease Control. Hepatitis B associated with jet gun injection. *MMWR.* 1986; 35:373–376.

21. Shaw F Jr, Barrett CL, Hamm R, et al. Lethal outbreak of hepatitis B in a dental practice. *JAMA.* 1986;255:3260–3264.

22. Stetler HC, Garbe PL, Dwyer DM, et al. Outbreaks of group A streptococcal abscesses following diphtheria-tetanus toxoid-pertussis vaccination. *Pediatr.* 1985;75:299–303.

23. Bloch AB, Orenstein WA, Ewing WM, et al. Measles outbreak in a pediatric practice: airborne transmission in an office setting. *Pediatr.* 1985;75:676–683.

24. Beecham HJ, Cohen ML, Parkin WE. *Salmonella typhimurium* transmission by fiberoptic upper gastrointestinal endoscopy. *JAMA.* 1979;241:1013–1015.

25. Borghans JGA, Stanford JL. *Mycobacterium chelonei* in abscesses after injection of diphtheria-pertussis-tetanus-polio vaccine. *Am Rev Respir Dis.* 1973;107:1–8.

26. Edell TA. *Serratia marcescens* abscesses in soft tissue associated with intramuscular methylprednisolone injections. In: Program and Abstracts of the 28th Annual Epidemic Intelligence Service Conference; April 2–6, 1979; Atlanta, GA.

27. Georgia Department of Human Resources. Abscesses in an allergy practice due to *Mycobacterium chelonae. Ga Epidemiol Rep.* April 1990.

28. Greaves WL, Hinman AR, Facklam RR, et al. Streptococcal abscesses following diphtheria-tetanus toxoid-pertussis vaccination. *Pediatr Infect Dis J.* 1982;1:388–390.

29. Inman PM, Beck A, Brown AE, Stanford JL. Outbreak of injection abscesses due to *Mycobacterium* abscessus. *Arch Dermatol.* 1969;100:141–147.

30. Kobler E, Schmuziger P, Hartmann G. Hepatitis nach Akupunktur. *Schweizerische Medizinische Woschenschrift.* 1979;109:1828–1829.

31. Kothari T, Reyes MP, Brooks N, Brown WJ, Lerner AM. *Pseudomonas cepacia* septic arthritis due to intra-articular injections of methylprednisolone. *Can Med Assoc J.* 1977;116:1230–1235.

32. Lowry PW, Jarvis WR, Oberle AD, et al. *Mycobacterium chelonae* causing otitis media in an ear, nose, and throat practice. *N Engl J Med.* 1968;319:978–982.

33. Owen M, Smith A, Coultras J. Granulomatous lesions occurring at site of injections of vaccines and antibiotics. *South Med J.* 1963;56:949–952.

34. Wenger JD, Spika JS, Smithwick RW, et al. Outbreak of *Mycobacterium chelonae* infection associated with use of jet injectors. *JAMA.* 1990;264:373–376.

35. Centers for Disease Control. *Mycobacterium tuberculosis* transmission in a health clinic–Florida, 1988. *MMWR.* 1989;38:256–258, 263–264.

36. Centers for Disease Control. Measles—Washington, 1990. *MMWR.* 1990;39:473–476.

37. Davis RM, Orenstein WA, Frank JA Jr. Transmission of measles in medical settings, 1980 through 1984. *JAMA.* 1986;255:1295–1298.

38. Ginsburg CM, Henle G, Henle W. An outbreak of infectious mononucleosis among the personnel of an outpatient clinic. *Am J Epidemiol.* 1976;104:571–575.

39. Greaves WL, Orenstein WA, Stetler HC, et al. Prevention of rubella transmission in medical facilities. *JAMA.* 1982;248:861–864.

40. Istre GR, McKee PA, West GR, et al. Measles spread in medical settings: an important focus of disease transmission? *Pediatr.* 1987;79:356–358.

41. Remington PL, Hall WN, Davis IH, Herald A, Gunn RA. Airborne transmission of measles in a physician's office. *JAMA.* 1985;253:1574–1577.

42. Richmond S, Burman R, Crosdale E, et al. A large outbreak of keratoconjunctivitis due to adenovirus type 8. *J Hygiene.* 1984;93:285–291.

43. Centers for Disease Control and Prevention. *Enterobacter cloacae* bloodstream infections associated with contaminated prefilled saline syringes—California, November 1998. *MMWR.* 1998;47:959–960.

44. Safranek TJ, Jarvis WR, Carson LA, et al. *Mycobacterium chelonae* wound infections after plastic surgery employing contaminated gentian violet skin-marking solution. *N Engl J Med.* 1987;317:197–201.

45. Berkelman RL, Lewin S, Allen JR, et al. Pseudobacteremia attributed to contamination of povidone-iodine with *Pseudomonas cepacia. Ann Intern Med.* 1981;95:32–36.

46. Panlilio AL, Beck-Sague CM, Siegel JD, et al. Infections and pseudoinfections due to povidone-iodine solution contaminated with *Pseudomonas cepacia*. *Clin Inf Dis*. 1992;14:1078–1083.

47. Parrott PL, Terry PM, Whitworth EN, et al. *Pseudomonas aeruginosa* peritonitis associated with contaminated poloxamer-iodine solution. *Lancet*. 1982;2:683–685.

48. Sautter RL, Mattman LH, Legaspi RC. *Serratia marcescens* meningitis associated with a contaminated benzalkonium chloride solution. *Infect Control*. 1984;5:223–225.

49. Sehulster LM, Chinn RYW, Arduino MJ, et al. Guidelines for environmental infection control in health-care facilities, 2003. Recommendations of CDC and the Healthcare Infection Control Practices Advisory Committee (HICPAC). *MMWR*. 2003;52(RR-10):1–42. http://www.cdc.gov/ncidod/dhqp/gl_environinfection.html. Accessed May 11, 2008.

50. Dixon RE, Kaslow RA, Mackel DC, Fulkerson CC, Mallinson GF. Aqueous quaternary ammonium antiseptics and disinfectants: use and misuse. *JAMA*. 1976;236:2415–2417.

51. Donowitz LG. Benzalkonium chloride is still in use. *Infect Control Hosp Epidemiol*. 1991;12:186–187.

52. McDonnell G, Russell AD. Antiseptics and disinfectants: activity, action, and resistance. *Clin Microbiol Rev*. 1999;12(1):147–179. http://cmr.asm.org/cgi/content/full/12/1/147. Accessed April 14, 2008.

53. Rutala WA, Weber DJ. Disinfection and sterilization in health care facilities: what clinicians need to know. *Clin Infect Dis*. 2004;39(5):702–709. http://www.journals.uchicago.edu/doi/abs/10.1086/423182. Accessed April 5, 2008.

54. Centers for Disease Control and Prevention. Notice to readers: medical equipment malfunctions associated with inappropriate use of cleaning and disinfecting liquids—United States, 2007. *MMWR*. 2008;57(06):152. http://www.cdc.gov/mmwR/preview/mmwrhtml/mm5706a6.htm. Accessed April 14, 2008.

55. Hlady WG, Hopkins RS, Ogilby TE, Allen ST. Patient-to-patient transmission of hepatitis B in a dermatology practice. *Am J Public Health*. 1993;83:1689–1693.

56. Hauri AM, Armstrong GL, Hutin YJF. The global burden of disease attributable to contaminated injections given in health care settings. *Inte J STD & AIDS*. 2004;15(1):7–16.

57. Comstock RD, Malknee S, Fox JL, et al. A large nosocomial outbreak of hepatitis C and hepatitis C among patients receiving pain remediation treatments. *Infect Control Hosp Epidemiol*. 2004;25:576–583.

58. Walsh B, Maguire H, Carrington D. Outbreak of hepatitis B in an acupuncture clinic. *Commun Dis Public Health*. 1999;2(2):137–140.

59. DeOliveira AM, White K, Leschinsky DP, et al. An outbreak of hepatitis C virus infections among outpatients at a hematology/oncology clinic. *Ann Intern Med*. 2005;142:898–902.

60. Centers for Disease Control and Prevention. Transmission of hepatitis B and C viruses in outpatient settings—New York, Oklahoma, and Nebraska, 2000–2002. *MMWR*. 2003;52(38):901–906. http://www.cdc.gov/mmwr/preview/mmwrhtml/mm5238a1.htm. Accessed April 5, 2008.

61. Williams IT, Perz JF, Bell BP. Viral hepatitis transmission in ambulatory health care settings. *Clin Infect Dis*. 2004;38:1592–1598. http://www.journals.uchicago.edu/doi/full/10.1086/420935. Accessed April 11, 2008.

62. Chiarello LA. Prevention of patient to patient transmission of bloodborne viruses. *Sem Infect Contr*. 2001;1:44–48.

63. Centers for Disease Control and Prevention. O'Grady NP, Alexander M, Dellinger EP, et al. Guidelines for the prevention of intravascular catheter-related infections. *MMWR*. 2002;51(No. RR-10). http://www.cdc.gov/mmwr/preview/mmwrhtml/rr5110a1.htm. Accessed April 5, 2008.

64. Centers for Disease Control and Prevention. Guideline for hand hygiene in health-care settings. Recommendations of the Healthcare Infection Control Practices Advisory Committee and the HICPAC/SHEA/APIC/IDSA Hand Hygiene Task Force. *MMWR*. 2002;51(No. RR-16). http://www.cdc.gov/mmwr/preview/mmwrhtml/rr5116a1.htm. Accessed April 5, 2008.

65. Centers for Disease Control and Prevention. Import-associated measles outbreak—Indiana, May–June 2005. *MMWR*. 2005;54(42):1073–1075. http://www.cdc.gov/mmwr/preview/mmwrhtml/mm5442a1.htm. Accessed April 5, 2008.

66. Parker AA, Staggs W, Dayan GH, et al. Implications of a 2005 measles outbreak in Indiana for sustained elimination of measles in the United States. *N Engl J Med*. 2006;355(5):447–455. http://content.nejm.org/cgi/content/abstract/355/5/447. Accessed April 5, 2008.

67. Centers for Disease Control and Prevention. Immunization of health-care workers: recommendations of the Advisory Committee on Immunization Practices (ACIP) and the Hospital Infection Control Practices Advisory Committee (HICPAC). *MMWR*. 1997;6(RR-18): 1–42. http://www.cdc.gov/mmwr/preview/mmwrhtml/00050577.htm. Accessed April 6, 2008.

68. Centers for Disease Control and Prevention. Measles, mumps, and rubella—vaccine use and strategies for elimination of measles, rubella, and congenital rubella syndrome and control of mumps: recommendations of the Advisory Committee on Immunization Practices (ACIP). *MMWR*. 1998;47(RR-08):1–57. http://www.cdc.gov/MMWR/preview/MMWRhtml/00053391.htm. Accessed April 6, 2008.

69. Centers for Disease Control and Prevention. Guideline for infection control in health care personnel, 1998. *Am J Infect Control*. 1998;26:289–354. http://www.cdc.gov/ncidod/dhqp/gl_hcpersonnel.html. Accessed April 6, 2008.

70. Siegel JD, Rhinehart E, Jackson M, Chiarello L, and the Healthcare Infection Control Practices Advisory Committee. Guideline for isolation precautions: preventing transmission of infectious agents in healthcare settings, June 2007. http://www.cdc.gov/ncidod/dhqp/gl_isolation.html. Accessed April 6, 2008.

71. American Academy of Pediatrics. Measles. In: Peter G, ed. *2006 Red Book: Report of the Committee on Infectious Diseases*. 24th ed. Elk Grove Village, IL: American Academy of Pediatrics; 2006.

72. Conover C, Ridzon R, Valway S, et al. Outbreak of multidrug-resistant tuberculosis at a methadone treatment program. *Int J Tuberc Lung Dis*. 2001;5(1):59–64.

73. Griffith DE, Hardeman JL, Zhang Y, Wallace RJ, Mazurek GH. Tuberculosis outbreak among healthcare workers in a community hospital. *Am J Respir Crit Care Med*. 1995;152: 808–811.

74. Couldwell DL, Dore GJ, Harkness JL, et al. Nosocomial outbreak of tuberculosis in an outpatient HIV treatment room. *AIDS*. 1996;10:521–525.

75. Sokolove PE, Mackey D, Wiles J, Lewis RJ. Exposure of emergency department personnel to tuberculosis: PPD testing during an epidemic in the community. *Ann Emerg Med*. 1994;24:418–421.

76. Centers for Disease Control and Prevention. Guidelines for preventing the transmission of *Mycobacterium tuberculosis* in health-care settings, 2005. *MMWR*. 2005;54(RR-17):1–141. http://www.cdc.gov/mmwr/preview/mmwrhtml/rr5417a1.htm. Accessed April 14, 2008.

77. Ahtone JL, Goodman RA. Hepatitis B and dental personnel: transmission to patients and prevention issues. *J Am Dent Assoc*. 1983;106:219–222.

78. Centers for Disease Control. Outbreak of hepatitis B associated with an oral surgeon—New Hampshire. *MMWR*. 1987;36:132–133.

79. Goodman RA, Ahtone JL, Flinton RJ. Hepatitis B transmission from dental personnel to patients: unfinished business. *Ann Intern Med*. 1982;96:119.

80. Goodwin D. An oral surgeon-related hepatitis B outbreak. *Calif Morbid*. April 16, 1976.

81. Hadler SC, Sorley DL, Acree KH, et al. An outbreak of hepatitis B in a dental practice. *Ann Intern Med*. 1981;95:133–138.

82. Levin ML, Maddrey WC, Wanda JR, Mendeloff AI. Hepatitis B transmission by dentists. *JAMA*. 1974;228:1139–1140.

83. Reingold AL, Kane MA, Murphy BL, et al. Transmission of hepatitis B by an oral surgeon. *J Infect Dis*. 1982;145:262–268.

84. Rimland D, Parkin WE, Miller GB Jr, Schrack WD. Hepatitis B outbreak traced to an oral surgeon. *N Engl J Med*. 1977;296:953–958.

85. Manzella JP, McConville JH, Valenti W, et al. An outbreak of herpes simplex virus type I gingivostomatitis in a dental hygiene practice. *JAMA*. 1984;252:2019–2022.

86. Centers for Disease Control. Update: transmission of HIV infection during an invasive dental procedure. *MMWR*. 1991;40:21–27, 33.

87. Martin MV. The significance of the bacterial contamination of dental unit water systems. *Br Dent J.* 1987;183:152–154.

88. Smith WHR, Mason KD, Davies D, Onions JP. Intraoral and pulmonary tuberculosis following dental treatment. *Lancet.* 1982;1:842–844.

89. Redd JT, Baumbach J, Kohn W, Nainan O, Khristova M, Williams I. Patient-to-patient transmission of hepatitis B virus associated with oral surgery. *J Infect Dis.* 2007;95:1311–1314. http://www.journals.uchicago.edu/doi/pdf/10.1086/513435. Accessed April 11, 2008.

90. Centers for Disease Control. Possible transmission of human immunodeficiency virus to a patient during an invasive dental procedure. *MMWR.* 1990;39:489–493.

91. Ciesielski CA, Marianos DW, Ou CY, et al. Transmission of human immunodeficiency virus to a patient during an invasive dental procedure. *MMWR.* 1990;39:489–493.

92. Ciesielski CA, Marianos DW, Schochetman G, Witte JJ, Jaffe J. The 1990 Florida dental investigations: the press and the science. *Ann Intern Med.* 1994;121:886–888.

93. Centers for Disease Control. Update: universal precautions for prevention of transmission of human immunodeficiency virus, and other bloodborne pathogens in health-care settings. *MMWR.* 1988;37:377–382, 387–388.

94. Centers for Disease Control and Prevention. Guidelines for infection control in dental health-care settings—2003. *MMWR.* 2003;52(No. RR-17) http://www.cdc.gov/oralhealth/infectioncontrol/guidelines/index.htm. Accessed April 11, 2008.

95. DePaola LG. Managing the care of patients infected with bloodborne diseases. *J Am Dent Assoc.* 2003;134:350–358. http://jada.ada.org/cgi/content/full/134/3/350. Accessed April 11, 2008.

96. Kohn WG, Harte JA, Malvitz DM, et al. Guidelines for infection control in dental health care settings—2003. *J Am Dent Assoc.* 2004;135;33–47. http://jada.ada.org. Accessed April 11, 2008.

97. Organization for Safety and Asepsis Procedures (OSAP). From Policy to Practice: OSAP's Interactive Guide to the CDC Guidelines. http://osaplms.ts.karta.com. Accessed April 11, 2008.

98. American Dental Association. ADA statement on dental unit waterlines. July 2004. http://www.ada.org/prof/resources/positions/statements/lines.asp. Accessed April 11, 2008.

99. Centers for Disease Control and Prevention. Outbreaks of hepatitis B virus infection among hemodialysis patients—California, Nebraska, and Texas, 1994. *MMWR.* 1996;45:285–289. http://www.cdc.gov/mmwr/preview/mmwrhtml/00040762.htm. Accessed April 11, 2008.

100. Niu MT, Penberthy LT, Alter MJ, Armstrong CW, Miller GB, Hadler SC. Hemodialysis-associated hepatitis B: report of an outbreak. *Dial Transplantation.* 1989;18:542–555.

101. Alter MJ, Ahtone J, Maynard JE. Hepatitis B virus transmission associated with a multiple-dose vial in a hemodialysis unit. *Ann Intern Med.* 1983;99:330–333.

102. Favero MS, Tokars JI, Arduino MJ, Alter MJ. Nosocomial infections associated with hemodialysis. In: Mayhall CG, ed. *Hospital Epidemiology and Infection Control.* 2nd ed. Philadelphia, PA: Lippincott, Williams & Wilkins; 1999:897–917.

103. Niu MT, Alter MJ, Kristensen C, Margolis HS. Outbreak of hemodialysis-associated non-A, non-B hepatitis and correlation with antibody to hepatitis C virus. *Am J Kidney Dis.* 1992;19:345–352.

104. Katsoulidou A, Paraskevis D, Kalapothaki V, et al. Molecular epidemiology of a hepatitis C outbreak in a hemodialysis unit. *Nephrol Dial Transplant.* 1999;14:1188–1194. http://ndt.oxfordjournals.org/cgi/reprint/14/5/1188. Accessed April 14, 2008.

105. Savey A, Simon F, Izopet J, Lepoutre A, Fabry J, Desenclos JC. A large outbreak of hepatitis C virus infections at a hemodialysis center. *Infect Control Hosp Epidemiol.* 2005;26:752–760.

106. Ansadli F, Bruzzone B, DeFlorentiis D, et al. An outbreak of hepatitis C virus in a haemodialysis unit: molecular evidence of patient-to-patient transmission. *Ann Ig.* 2003;15(5):6856–6891.

107. Delarocque-Astagneau E, Baffoy N, Thiers V, et al. Outbreak of hepatitis C infection in a hemodialysis unit: potential transmission by the hemodialysis machine? *Infect Control Hosp Epidemiol.* 2002;23:328–334.

108. Velandi M, Fridkin SK, Cardenas V, et al. Transmission of HIV in dialysis centre. *Lancet.* 1995;345:1417–1422.

109. Longfeld RN, Wortham WG, Fletcher LL, Nauscheutz WF. Clustered bacteremias in a hemodialysis unit: cross-contamination of blood tubing from ultrafiltrate waste. *Infect Control Hosp Epidemiol.* 1992;13:160–164.

110. Flaherty JP, Garcia-Houchins S, Chudy R, Arnow PM. An outbreak of gram-negative bacteremia traced to contaminated O-rings and reprocessed dialysers. *Ann Intern Med.* 1993;119:1072–1078.

111. Beck-Sague CM, Jarvis WR, Bland LA, Arduino MJ, Aguero SM, Verosic G. Outbreak of gram-negative bacteremia and pyrogenic reactions in a hemodialysis center. *Am J Nephrol.* 1990;10:397–403.

112. Arnow PM, Garcia-Houchins S, Neagle MB, Bova JL, Dillon JJ, Chou T. An outbreak of bloodstream infections arising from hemodialysis equipment. *J Infect Dis.* 1998;178:783–791.

113. Centers for Disease Control and Prevention. Outbreaks of gram-negative bacterial bloodstream infections traced to probable contamination of hemodialysis machines—Canada, 1995 United States, 1997; and Israel, 1997. *MMWR.* 1998;47(03);55–58. http://www.cdc.gov/mmwr/preview/mmwrhtml/00051244.htm. Accessed April 11, 2008.

114. Wang SA, Levine RB, Carson L, et al. An outbreak of gram-negative bacteremia in waste drain ports in hemodialysis patients traced to hemodialysis waste drain ports. *Infect Control Hosp Epidemiol.* 1999;20:746–751.

115. Grohskopf LA, Roth VR, Feikin DR, et al. *Serratia liquefaciens* bloodstream infections from contamination of epoetin alfa at a hemodialysis center. *N Engl J Med.* 2001;344(20):1491–1497. http://content.nejm.org/cgi/reprint/344/20/1491.pdf. Accessed April 12, 2008.

116. Jochimsen EM, Frenette C, Delorme M, et al. A cluster of bloodstream infections and pyrogenic reactions among hemodialysis patients traced to dialysis machine waste-handling option units. *Am J Nephrol.* 1998;18(6):485–489.

117. Price CS, Hacek D, Noskin GA, Peterson LR. An outbreak of bloodstream infections in an outpatient hemodialysis center. *Infect Control Hosp Epidemiol.* 2002;23:725–729.

118. Tuberculosis transmission in a renal dialysis center—Nevada, 2003. *MMWR.* 2004;53(37): 873–875. http://www.cdc.gov/mmwR/preview/mmwrhtml/mm5337a4.htm. Accessed April 11, 2008.

119. Hannah EL, Stevenson KB, Lowder CA, et al. Outbreak of hemodialysis vascular access site infections related to malfunctioning permanent tunneled catheters: making the case for active surveillance. *Infect Control Hosp Epidemiol.* 2002;23:538–541.

120. Pegues DA, Beck-Sague CM, Woolleen SW, et al. Anaphylactoid reactions associated with reuse of hollow-fiber hemodialyzers and ACE inhibitors. *Kidney Int.* 1992;42:1232–1237.

121. Centers for Disease Control. Update: acute allergic reactions associated with reprocessed hemodialyzers—United States, 1989–1990. *MMWR.* 1991;40:147, 153–154.

122. Gordon SM, Drachman J, Bland LA, Reid MH, Favero M, Jarvis WR. Epidemic hypotension in a dialysis center caused by sodium azide. *Kidney Int.* 1990;37:110–115.

123. Centers for Disease Control and Prevention. Multistate outbreak of hemolysis in hemodialysis patients—Nebraska and Maryland, 1998. *MMWR.* 1998;47(23);483–484. http://www.cdc.gov/mmwr/preview/mmwrhtml/00053608.htm. Accessed April 11, 2008.

124. Selenic D, Alvarado-Ramy F, Arduino M, et al. Epidemic parenteral exposure to volatile sulfur-containing compounds at a hemodialysis center. *Infect Control Hosp Epidemiol.* 2004;25(3):256–261.

125. Martin J, Sansone G, Cirugeda A, Sanchez-Tomero JA, Munoz C, Selgas R. Severe peritoneal mononucleosis associated with icodextrin use in continuous ambulatory peritoneal dialysis. *Adv Perit Dial.* 2003;19:191–194.

126. Boer WH, Vos PF, Fieren MW. Culture-negative peritonitis associated with the use of icodextrin-containing dialysate in twelve patients treated with peritoneal dialysis. *Perit Dial Int.* 2003;23(1):33–38.

127. Pouria S, Andrade A, Barbosa J, et al. Fatal microcystin intoxication in haemodialysis unit in Caruaru, Brazil. *Lancet.* 1998;352:21–26.

128. Centers for Disease Control and Prevention. Recommendations for preventing transmission of infections among chronic hemodialysis patients. *MMWR*. 2001;50(RR-05):1–43. http://www.cdc.gov/mmwr/preview/mmwrhtml/rr5005a1.htm. Accessed April 11, 2008.

129. Centers for Disease Control and Prevention. Guidelines for the prevention of intravascular catheter-related infections. *MMWR*. 2002;51(No.RR-10):1–34. http://www.cdc.gov/mmwr/PDF/rr/rr5110.pdf. Accessed April 11, 2008.

130. Centers for Disease Control and Prevention. Guidelines for Vaccinating Kidney Dialysis Patients and Patients with Chronic Kidney Disease. June 2006. http://www.cdc.gov/vaccines/pubs/downloads/b_dialysis_guide.pdf. Accessed April 11, 2008.

131. National Kidney Foundation. Dialysis outcomes quality initiative: clinical practice guidelines. *Am J Kidney Dis*. 1997;30:S137–S240.

132. Association for the Advancement of Medical Instrumentation. Dialysis. Arlington, VA: AAMI. 2007. http://www.aami.org/publications/standards/dialysis.html. Accessed April 12, 2008.

133. Piraino B, Bailie GR, Bernardini J, et al. Peritoneal dialysis-related infections recommendations: 2005 Update. *Perit Dial Int*. 2005;25:107–131. http://www.ispd.org/treatment_guidelines.html. Accessed April 13, 2008.

134. Klevens RM, Edwards JR, Andrus ML, et al. Dialysis Surveillance Report: National Healthcare Safety Network (NHSN)—data summary for 2006. *Semin Dial*. 2008;21(1):24–48.

135. Cheung D, Bremner J, Chan JT. Epidemic kerato-conjunctivitis—do outbreaks have to be epidemic? *Eye*. 2003;17(3):356–363.

136. Viney KA, Petsoglou C, Doyle BK. Bug breakfast in the bulletin: epidemic keratoconjunctivitis: an outbreak in New South Wales. *NSW Public Health Bull*. 2006;17(11–12):180. http://www.health.nsw.gov.au/public-health/phb/HTML2006/novdec06html/article6p180.html. Accessed April 13, 2008.

137. Engelmann I, Madishc I, Pommer H, Heim A. An outbreak of epidemic keratoconjunctivitis caused by a new intermediate adenovirus 22/H8 identified by molecular typing. *Clin Infect Dis*. 2006;43(7):e64–36. http://www.journals.uchicago.edu/doi/abs/10.1086/507533. Accessed April 13, 2008.

138. Buehler JW, Finton RF, Goodman RA, et al. Epidemic keratoconjunctivitis: report of an outbreak in an ophthalmology practice and recommendations for prevention. *Infect Control Hosp Epidemiol*. 1984;5:390–394.

139. Keenlyside RA, Hierholzer JC, D'Angelo LJ. Keratoconjunctivitis associated with adenovirus type 37: an extended outbreak in an ophthalmologist's office. *J Infect Dis*. 1983;147:191–198.

140. Koo D, Bouvier B, Wesley M, et al. Epidemic keratoconjunctivitis in a university medical center ophthalmology clinic: need for re-evaluation of the design and disinfection of instruments. *Infect Control Hosp Epidemiol*. 1989;10:547–552.

141. Murrah WF. Epidemic keratoconjunctivitis. *Am J Ophthalmol*. 1988;20:36–38.

142. Nagington J, Sutehall GM, Whipp P. Tonometer disinfection and viruses. *Br J Ophthalmol*. 1983;67:674–676.

143. Warren D, Nelson KE, Farrar JA, et al. A large outbreak of epidemic keratoconjunctivitis: problems in controlling nosocomial spread. *J Infect Dis*. 1989;160:938–943.

144. Wegman DH, Guinee VF, Millian SJ. Epidemic keratoconjunctivitis. *Am J Public Health*. 1970;60:1230–1237.

145. Darougar S, Grey RHB, Thaker U, McSwiggan DA. Clinical and epidemiological features of adenovirus keratoconjunctivitis in London. *Br J Ophthalmol*. 1985;67:1–7.

146. Vastine DW, West CE, Yamashiroya H, et al. Simultaneous nosocomial and community outbreak of epidemic keratoconjunctivitis with types 8 and 19 adenovirus. *Trans Am Acad Ophthalmol Otolaryngol*. 1976;81:826–840.

147. Newman PE, Goodman RA, Waring GO, et al. A cluster of cases of *Mycobacterium chelonei keratitis* associated with outpatient office procedures. *Am J Ophthalmol*. 1984;97:344–348.

148. Centers for Disease Control. Epidemic keratoconjunctivitis in an ophthalmology clinic–California. *MMWR*. 1990;39:598–601. http://www.cdc.gov/mmwr/preview/mmwrhtml/00001741.htm. Accessed April 13, 2008.

149. D'Angelo LJ, Hierholzer JC, Holman RC, Smith JD. Epidemic keratoconjunctivitis caused by adenovirus type 8: epidemiologic and laboratory aspects of a large outbreak. *Am J Epidemiol.* 1981;113:44–49.

150. American Academy of Ophthalmology. Clinical statement. Minimizing transmission of blood-borne pathogens and surface infectious agents in ophthalmic offices and operating rooms. San Francisco: American Academy of Ophthalmology; 2002. http://one.aao.org/CE/PracticeGuidelines/ClinicalStatements_Content.aspx?cid=bfa87dce-adc9-4450-94a2-e49493154238. Accessed April 13, 2008.

151. Gottsch JD, Froggatt W III, Smith DM, et al. Prevention and control of epidemic keratoconjunctivitis in a teaching eye institute. *Ophthalmic Epidemiol.* 1999;6(1):29–39.

152. Owings MF, Kozak LJ. Ambulatory and inpatient procedures in the United States, 1996. National Center for Health Statistics. *Vital Health Stat.* 1998;13(139). http://www.cdc.gov/nchs/data/series/sr_13/sr13_139.pdf. Accessed April 13, 2008.

153. National Center for Health Statistics. National hospital discharge and ambulatory surgery data. http://www.cdc.gov/nchs/nsas.htm#new. Accessed April 13, 2008.

154. Centers for Disease Control and Prevention. Toxic anterior segment syndrome after cataract surgery—Maine, 2006. *MMWR.* 2007;56(25):629–630. http://www.cdc.gov/mmwr/preview/mmwrhtml/mm5625a2.htm. Accessed April 13, 2008.

155. Hellinger WC, Hasan SA, Bacalis LP, et al. Outbreak of toxic anterior segment syndrome following cataract surgery associated with impurities in autoclave steam moisture. *Infect Control Hosp Epidemiol.* 2006;27:294–298.

156. Unal M, Yucel I, Akar Y, Oner A, Altin M. Outbreak of toxic anterior segment syndrome associated with glutaraldehyde after cataract surgery. *J Cataract Refract Surg.* 2006;32:1696–701.

157. Werner L, Sher JH, Taylor JR, et al. Toxic anterior segment syndrome and possible association with ointment in the anterior chamber following cataract surgery. *J Cataract Refract Surg.* 2006;32:227–235.

158. Rutala WA, Weber DJ, Thomann CA. Outbreak of wound infections following podiatric surgery due to contaminated bone drills. *Foot Ankle.* 1987;7:350–354.

159. Civen R, Vugia DJ, Alexander R, et al. Outbreak of *Serratia marcescens* infections following injection of betamethasone compounded at a community pharmacy. *Clin Infect Dis.* 2006;43(7):831–837. http://www.journals.uchicago.edu/doi/abs/10.1086/507336. Accessed April 13, 2008.

160. American Society of Cataract and Refractive Surgery, American Society of Ophthalmic Registered Nurses. Recommended practices for cleaning and sterilizing intraocular surgical instruments. Fairfax, VA: American Society of Cataract and Refractive Surgery; 2007. http://www.ascrs.com/upload/asornspecialtaskforcereport.pdf. Accessed April 14, 2008.

161. Mangram AJ, Horan TC, Pearson ML, Silver LC, Jarvis WR. Guideline for Prevention of Surgical Site Infection, 1999. Centers for Disease Control and Prevention (CDC) Hospital Infection Control Practices Advisory Committee. http://www.ascrs.com/upload/asornspecialtaskforcereport.pdf. Accessed April 14, 2008.

162. Manian FA. Surveillance of surgical site infections in alternative settings: exploring the current options. *Am J Infect Control.* 1997;25:102–105.

163. Manian FA, Meyer L. Comprehensive surveillance of surgical wound infections in outpatient and inpatient surgery. *Infect Control Hosp Epidemiol.* 1990;11:515–520.

164. Jarvis WR. Infection control and changing health-care delivery systems. *Emerg Infect Dis.* 2001;7:170–173.

165. Nguyen GT, Proctor SE, Sinkowitz-Cochran RL, Garrett DO, Jarvis WR, and the Association for Professionals in Infection Control and Epidemiology. Status of infection surveillance and control programs in the United States, 1992–1996. *Am J Infect Control.* 2000;28(6):392–400.

166. Edwards JR, Peterson KD, Andrus ML, et al. National Healthcare Safety Network (NHSN) Report, data summary for 2006, issued June 2007. *Am J Infect Control.* 2007;35:290–301. http://www.cdc.gov/ncidod/dhqp/pdf/nhsn/2006_NHSN_Report.pdf. Accessed April 13, 2008.

167. Association of PeriOperative Registered Nurses (AORN). *Perioperative Standards and Recommended Practices*. 2008 ed. Denver, CO: AORN; 2008. http://www.aorn.org/AORNStore. Accessed April 13, 2008.

168. Association for the Advancement of Medical Instrumentation. Sterilization in health care facilities, 2006–2007. Arlington, VA: AAMI. 2006. http://www.aami.org.

SUGGESTED READINGS AND RESOURCES

Suggested Readings

Garcia-Houchins S. Dialysis. In: *APIC Text of Infection Control and Epidemiology*. Washington, DC: Association for Professionals in Infection Control and Epidemiology. 2005:49-1–49-17.

Goodman RA, Solomon SL. Transmission of infectious diseases in outpatient health care settings. *JAMA*. 1991;265:2377–2381.

Herwaldt LA, Smith SD, Carter CD. Infection control in the outpatient setting. *Infect Control Hosp Epidemiol*. 1998;19:41–74.

Additional Information on Outbreaks and Infection Prevention and Control in Ambulatory Care Settings

For comprehensive reviews of outbreaks that have been reported in a variety of outpatient settings, including the infection control deficiencies that contributed to their occurrence and measures that can be used to prevent them, the reader is referred to the articles by Goodman and Solomon[1] and by Herwaldt, Smith, and Carter.[2]

Resources

The following national agencies and organizations have guidelines, position papers, or standards that can be used for developing infection surveillance, prevention and control programs in the ambulatory care setting.

American Academy of Ophthalmology: Resources, guidelines, and training courses on infection prevention and control. http://www.aao.org.

American Academy of Pediatrics: *2006 Red Book: Report of the Committee on Infectious Diseases*. Peter G, ed. 24th ed. Elk Grove Village, IL: American Academy of Pediatrics; 2006. http://www.aap.org.

American Dental Association: Resources and publications http://www.ada.org.

Association for the Advancement of Medical Instrumentation. Standards for dialysis water quality, storage, and distribution and standards for disinfection and sterilization in health care settings. www.aami.org.

Association of Perioperative Registered Nurses: Standards for operating rooms and cleaning, disinfection and sterilization of equipment. www.aorn.org.

CDC Home page: www.cdc.gov. The *Morbidity and Mortality Weekly Report* (*MMWR*) and most of the CDC guidelines noted in this chapter can be downloaded from this Web site.

CDC Recommended Infection Control Guidelines for Dentistry. Information on dental infection control issues as well as consensus evidence-based recommendations. See also the slide set and accompanying speaker notes. http://www.cdc.gov/oralhealth/. Accessed April 14, 2008.

CDC. General recommendations on immunization: recommendations of the Advisory Committee on Immunization Practices (ACIP). *MMWR*. 2006;55(No. RR-15).

CDC. Prevention of varicella: recommendations of the Advisory Committee on Immunization Practices (ACIP). *MMWR*. 2007;56(No. RR-4).

CDC Infection Control in Health Care Settings website: http://www.cdc.gov/ncidod/dhqp/.

CDC Dialysis-Associated Infections: infection prevention and control guidelines and links to outbreak reports and surveillance data. http://www.cdc.gov/ncidod/dhqp/dpac_dialysis_pc.html. Accessed April 11, 2008.

DisinfectionandSterilization.org: Guidelines and resources on cleaning, disinfection and sterilization in health care settings. http://disinfectionandsterilization.org/.

Food and Drug Administration (FDA) Adverse Event Reporting System. MedWatch—The FDA Safety Information and Adverse Event Reporting System. http://www.fda.gov/medwatch/.

General vaccine and immunization information: http://www.cdc.gov/vaccines/default.htm.

Immunization schedules, recommendations and guidelines, and information for Health Care Workers: http://www.cdc.gov/vaccines/recs/schedules/default.htm. Accessed April 6, 2008.

Organization for Safety and Asepsis Procedures: provides resources on infection control for the dental community. http://www.osap.org/index.cfm.

CHAPTER 6

Pseudo-Outbreaks Reported in Healthcare Settings

Kathleen Meehan Arias

> Simple people . . . are very quick to see the live facts which are going on about them.
>
> —Oliver Wendell Holmes

INTRODUCTION

Healthcare-associated pseudo-outbreaks, or pseudoepidemics, have long been recognized in the healthcare setting.[1–5] As used in this chapter, a pseudo-outbreak is defined as a real clustering of false infections or an artefactual clustering of real infections. Twenty-nine (11%) of the 265 nosocomial epidemics investigated by the Hospital Infections Program of the Centers for Disease Control and Prevention (CDC) between 1956 and 1979 were actually pseudo-outbreaks.[3] A review of those pseudo-outbreaks found that the majority were traced to errors in collecting, handling, or processing specimens.[3] The processing errors that occurred in the laboratory were most frequently associated with a change in personnel, technique, or culture media.

Table 6–1 lists examples of pseudo-outbreaks that have been reported in healthcare settings.[6–33]

In addition to errors in collecting and processing specimens, healthcare-associated pseudo-outbreaks have been traced to intrinsically contaminated iodine solutions[6,12,34] and organisms in hospital tap water.[28,29] Pseudo-outbreaks have also resulted from the improper categorization of an infection or other condition as being nosocomial rather than community aquired.[1,23,30]

Pseudoepidemics have been associated with a variety of microorganisms (bacteria, viruses, and fungi) and frequently involve blood cultures and respiratory tract specimens. False-positive cultures of blood or other normally sterile sites are more likely to be recognized because infections at these sites are closely monitored by clinicians and infection prevention and control personnel. For instance, in one report vancomycin-resistant *Enterococcus* (VRE) was isolated from sterile body sites collected from five patients over a 3-day period. Because this was an increase in the number of cases of VRE, an epidemiologic investigation was conducted. When a review of the patients' records showed that none had signs or symptoms of VRE infection, specimen contamination and a pseudo-outbreak were suspected.[34] Further investigation led to the conclusion that cross-contamination in the laboratory occurred when a technician was processing the patients' cultures along with a stored isolate of VRE that had been retained for analysis. Comparison of the stored and patient isolates

Table 6–1   Examples of Pseudo-Outbreaks Reported in Healthcare Settings

Pseudo-Outbreak	Associated With	Year Reported/ Reference
Ochrobactrum anthropi in blood cultures from inpatients and outpatients	Improper specimen collection allowed cross-contamination of blood cultures at time of collection from nonsterile erythrocyte sedimentation rate blood collection tubes	2007[6]
Acinetobacter lwoffii in a variety of specimens from five inpatient units	Introduction of new automated laboratory system for identifying gram-negative organisms	2007[7]
Hepatitis B virus infection in pregnant woman undergoing routine screening	Cross-contamination in lab following introduction and use of semiautomatic cap remover for blood collection tubes	2006[8]
Increase in several types of healthcare-associated infections (HAIs)	Failure to use appropriate criteria to diagnose and classify HAIs	2007[9]
Chlamydia trachomatis in state residential facility	False-positive test results for possible genital infections	2002[10]
Mycobacterium chelonae and *Methylobacterium mesophilicum* in bronchoscopy specimens	Automated washers contaminated with biofilm that rendered them resistant to decontamination; washers contaminated endoscopes and bronchoscopes	2001[11]
Pseudomonas putida in outpatient ENT clinic	Intrinsically contaminated antifog solution	2000[12]
Mycobacterium tuberculosis	Specimen cross-contamination due to faulty ventilation in the laboratory	1998[13]
Cluster of *Alcaligenes xylosoxidans*	Contaminated saline used in laboratory as diluent in processing specimens	1998[14]
M. chelonae respiratory tract pseudoinfections	Contaminated multidose lidocaine sprayers	1997[15]
Respiratory tract infections with *Acinetobacter* species	Laboratory errors in processing respiratory specimens	1997[16]
PPD skin-test conversions	Use of 250 tuberculin units (TU) of PPD instead of 5 TU	1997[17]
Multidrug-resistant *Pseudomonas aeruginosa* in a hematology oncology unit	Improper stool collection technique	1997[18]
Multidrug-resistant *Mycobacterium tuberculosis*	False-positive cultures due to inadequate cleaning and disinfection of bronchoscope	1997[19]
Pseudomonas (now *Burkholderia*) *cepacia* pseudobacteremia	Contaminated blood gas analyzer	1996[20]

Table 6–1   *(Continued)*

Pseudo-Outbreak	Associated With	Year Reported/ Reference
Rhodotorula rubra	Improper disinfection and drying of bronchoscopes	1995 [21]
Nontuberculous mycobacteria	Contaminated probe on automated lab instrument	1995 [22]
Cluster of methicillin-resistant *Staphylococcus aureus*	Cluster suggesting nosocomial infection found to be coincidental	1995 [23]
Pseudomonas aeruginosa orthopedic infections	Contaminated saline used in laboratory as diluent in processing specimens	1994 [24]
Enterobacter cloacae pseudobacteremia	Laboratory contamination during use of a new blood culturing system	1993 [25]
Mycobacterium xenopi	Specimen contamination by potable water containing *M. xenopi*	1993 [26]
Respiratory tract infections caused by nontuberculous mycobacteria	Contaminated bronchoscope cleaning machine and laboratory contamination of an antimicrobial solution	1992 [27]
Copepod pseudo-outbreak in stool specimens	Copepods in hospital tap water	1992 [28]
Pseudocontamination of hospital drinking water	Presence of nonpathogenic freshwater organisms	1992 [29]
Senile hemangioma in a nursing home	Incorrect perception that lesions had recent and rapid onset	1991 [30]
Pseudobacteremia with enterococcus and *Staphylococcus aureus*	Contaminated radiometric blood culture device	1987 [31]
Influenza A	Cross-contamination in the laboratory	1984 [32]
Pseudomonas (now *Burkholderia*) *cepacia* pseudobacteremia	Povidone iodine intrinsically contaminated at manufacturing plant	1981 [33]

ENT = ears, nose, throat; PPD = purified protein derivative

showed similar susceptibility patterns and pulsed-field gel electrophoresis demonstrated that they were a single strain.

Many pseudoepidemics are the result of contamination of clinical specimens or cultures. Specimens may be contaminated at the time of collection, during transport, or during processing in the laboratory. An example of a pseudo-outbreak that resulted from specimen contamination at the point of collection was reported by Verweij et al.,[18] who investigated a cluster of multidrug-resistant *Pseudomonas aeruginosa* involving 10 neutropenic patients in a hematology unit. The epidemic strain was isolated from surveillance stool cultures. An epidemiologic investigation revealed that healthcare workers had collected the surveillance stool cultures by sampling feces that were in the toilet and were therefore contaminated by the toilet water. Isolates of *P. aeruginosa* from the stool samples in the outbreak and from the toilet water were shown to be identical by genotyping. The "outbreak" subsided when personnel were instructed how properly to collect stool specimens for culture.

Common causes of pseudo-outbreaks include the following:

- Errors in specimen collection or processing[6,14,16,18,24,26,35-37]
- Cross-contamination in the laboratory[13,20,23,31,32,34,38]
- Contaminated equipment, medical devices, or solutions[12,15,19,21,27,33,39-42]
- Failure to recognize that patients' infections are community acquired rather than nosocomial[1,23]
- Failure to use appropriate criteria to diagnose healthcare-associated infection (HAI)[9,43]
- Failure to recognize that an organism causing an outbreak or cluster may actually be several unrelated strains[44]
- Contaminated tap water and ice[28,29,45-48]

PSEUDO-OUTBREAKS INVOLVING *MYCOBACTERIUM* SPECIES

There are multiple reports in the literature of clusters and pseudoepidemics involving *Mycobacterium tuberculosis* and nontuberculous mycobacteria (NTM).[49] The majority of the reported pseudo-outbreaks have been caused by laboratory errors,[13,22,50-52] false-positive tuberculin skin tests,[17] and contaminated bronchoscopes.[19,27,41,42]

Pseudo-Outbreaks of *Mycobacterium tuberculosis*

Pseudo-outbreaks of tuberculosis (TB) have been associated with false-positive *M. tuberculosis* cultures resulting from laboratory errors. Opportunities for laboratory contamination occur during the many steps involved in processing specimens and the prolonged incubation period necessary for isolating *M. tuberculosis* from culture. Laboratory contamination of TB specimens and cultures has been shown to occur during the initial specimen processing, incubation, reading or sampling of the cultures, and susceptibility testing. Cross-contamination has been attributed to a faulty exhaust hood and to instrument or reagent contamination, resulting in carry-over of mycobacteria from one specimen to another, and to the inadvertent inoculation of one patient's culture into another patient's culture during subculturing.[50,53-57] In addition, contamination with low numbers of mycobacteria that may not have been detected in the past is now more easily recognized with newer, more sensitive laboratory equipment and methodologies.[51]

To avoid the misdiagnosis of TB, false-positive *M. tuberculosis* cultures should be suspected under the following conditions:

- A single positive culture occurs in a patient who has multiple negative smears for acid-fast bacilli (AFB).

- A patient's signs, symptoms, and clinical presentation are not consistent with TB.
- Another AFB smear-positive and culture-positive specimen was processed the same day as the suspect specimen.
- Only a few colonies are present on solid growth media or the time for detection in a broth medium is prolonged.
- Molecular typing, such as DNA fingerprinting, shows the suspect isolate is identical to that of a likely source of contamination.
- The patient with the suspect isolate cannot be epidemiologically linked to the patient with the putative source isolate.

Measures that can be used to identify clusters and minimize cross-contamination and the occurrence of false-positive cultures have been published by Small et al.[57] and by Tokars et al.[58]

A pseudo-outbreak of TB that was not associated with laboratory contamination occurred among the staff of a county residence for retarded adults (RRA) in New York in 1995.[17] An unexpected cluster of tuberculin skin test conversions among the staff of the residence prompted the county nursing service to conduct an extensive contact investigation to identify the source of infection. Persons with a positive tuberculin skin test were evaluated for signs and symptoms of TB and received a chest radiograph. Five staff members of the RRA were placed on isoniazid (INH) prophylaxis. The investigation resulted in a considerable amount of anxiety in the staff and the community. Over 100 community members were screened with a tuberculin skin test, either as part of the contact investigation or on community members' request because of concern that they were infected. No potential source of infection among staff or clients of the residence or any of their contacts was found. When the state health department was asked to assist in the investigation, its review of the results of the county's findings led to a suspicion that the purified protein derivative (PPD) solution may have been defective or the techniques used to apply or to read the test may have been inappropriate. A careful review of the tuberculin skin-testing program at the residence revealed that the staff of the facility had been tested with 250 TU (tuberculin units) of PPD rather than with the 5 TU that is recommended for a TB skin-testing program. The newly PPD-positive staff were retested with 5 TU of PPD and were found to be negative, so INH prophylaxis was discontinued. The estimated cost of the investigation was at least $15,000. This included "administration and management salaries, nursing time, staff time for retesting, reading, medical visits, employee overtime for TB training, 5 days of 24-hour RRA coverage for the resident who was hospitalized for bronchoscopy, liver-function tests, prescriptions, eight chest radiographs, and other administrative costs" for the county RRA and costs of the investigation that the local health unit and state health department incurred.[17(p573)]

Pseudo-outbreaks of TB have resulted in (1) individuals being misdiagnosed with a disease that carries considerable stigma; (2) extensive contact investigations of personnel, family members, friends, and other contacts of patients with an incorrect diagnosis; (3) needless hospitalization, including airborne (or respiratory) isolation; (4) unnecessary bronchoscopy to confirm the diagnosis;

(5) unwarranted treatment and prophylaxis with antituberculous medications; (6) excessive costs to health departments and healthcare facilities; (7) widespread anxiety and fear of contagion in those affected; and (8) adverse publicity for the facility involved.

Pseudo-Outbreaks of Nontuberculous Mycobacteria

There are many reports in the literature of clusters and pseudo-outbreaks involving NTM, such as *Mycobacterium chelonei, M. xenopi, M. marinum, M. abscessus, M. scrofulaceum, M. terrae, M. gordonae, M. fortuitum,* and *M. avium-intracellulare*.[49] NTM pseudoepidemics have been associated with laboratory processing errors[38,59–61] and with contamination of laboratory reagents,[27] specimens,[26,62,63] probes on laboratory instruments,[22] multidose lidocaine sprayers,[15] potable water,[26,45,46] and bronchoscopes and bronchoscope cleaner/disinfectors.[11,27,41,42] In three of these reported outbreak investigations, patients with false-positive NTM cultures were started on antituberculous therapy while identification of the AFB organism was pending—even though the patients had no apparent mycobacterial disease.[22,26,27]

NTM are commonly found in municipal water supplies. In a 1983 survey of 115 dialysis centers in the United States, NTMs were found in the water supplied to 95 (83%) of the centers.[64] Therefore, whenever NTMs are isolated from clinical specimens, the clinician must carefully evaluate the patient's clinical picture to determine if the isolate is causing infection or is a contaminant that was introduced into the specimen during collection (e.g., by a contaminated bronchoscope or by NTMs in the water that may have been used to rinse the patient's mouth) or during specimen processing in the laboratory. When a cluster or an increase in the number of isolates of NTM occurs, a clinical and epidemiologic investigation should be conducted to determine if a true outbreak or a pseudo-outbreak is occurring. The clinical investigation should consist of a review of the medical history and records of each of the patients from whom an NTM is isolated and a determination of whether the organism is causing an infection or is likely to be a contaminant. The epidemiologic investigation should evaluate potential sources for the organisms. If the organisms are judged to be contaminants, then specimen collection and processing methods need to be reviewed and observed. If the organisms are causing disease, then the source may be contaminated water, ice, or solutions used by the patients, or a contaminated medical device such as a bronchoscope.

In one report, a perceived increase in the number of respiratory tract infections caused by AFB prompted an investigation that found that 16 of 46 bronchoscopies yielded specimens that were positive for AFB.[27] Two of the 16 patients were diagnosed with a mycobacterial infection—an acquired immune deficiency syndrome patient with *Mycobacterium avium-intracellulare* infection and another patient with cavitary tuberculosis. In four patients only the smears were AFB-positive—the cultures were negative. NTMs (*M. chelonei* and *M. gordonae*) were isolated from the cultures of the other 10 patients; however, none of these had clinical evidence of mycobacterial disease. Despite the lack of evidence for disease, four of the patients were treated with antituberculous medication pending culture results. The investigation led to the discovery of two sources for the NTMs: a contaminated water tank in an automated endoscope washer/disinfector and an antimicrobial culture media additive that was contaminated with *M. gordonae.*

PSEUDO-OUTBREAKS OF NONINFECTIOUS ETIOLOGY

Not all pseudo-outbreaks are of an infectious nature. Pseudoepidemics of senile hemangioma have been reported in hospitalized patients and nursing home residents.[30,65,66] One reported pseudo-outbreak occurred in an 800-bed long-term care facility. It began when a healthcare worker noticed that an elderly resident of a psychogeriatric ward had numerous skin lesions.[30] Since the lesions had not been previously noticed, the ward staff considered them to be of recent onset. Because the lesions were presumed to be of infectious etiology, the staff examined the other residents on the ward and found all 34 of them to have similar lesions. The day after the lesions were noticed on the first resident, a dermatologist diagnosed the lesions on another resident as senile hemangioma. Because the nursing staff were convinced that the lesions had occurred suddenly and had spread among the residents, the public health department and an infectious disease specialist were consulted on day 3 of the outbreak. Based on the lack of clinical and laboratory evidence that either an infectious agent or an environmental toxin was involved, the investigators concluded that the lesions were senile hemangioma. Despite the fact that the investigation was completed by day 4 of the reported outbreak, caregivers (many of whom had little medical training) "were suspicious and fearful of exposure to a pathogen as yet undiscovered by medical science,"[30(p521)] and continued to be skeptical of the diagnosis. Some of the staff, especially those who were pregnant, requested work schedule revisions. The estimated cost to the long-term care facility for the pseudoepidemic was $10,000. Pseudoepidemics of senile hemangioma have occurred mainly because of the misperception that the lesions had a recent and rapid onset. These pseudo-outbreaks are difficult to control because the caregivers involved must accept the conclusion that the lesions were present long before they were noticed.

RECOGNIZING A PSEUDO-OUTBREAK

It is important that pseudo-outbreaks be recognized promptly because they frequently result in unnecessary diagnostic and treatment procedures, consume valuable infection control and laboratory resources, and cause undue concern of patients, their families, and healthcare staff. Pseudo-outbreaks may be difficult to recognize and may occur for a prolonged period before they are detected.[63] Typically, a pseudo-outbreak is recognized when an unusual organism is isolated from several patients, when there is a sudden increase in the number of isolates of a common pathogen, or when a common pathogen is isolated from several patients who have no signs and symptoms of infection.[61]

Laboratory staff, infection prevention and control personnel, and clinicians should routinely review culture results for evidence of clusters or unusual organisms so that outbreaks and pseudo-outbreaks may be quickly recognized. Frequently, the identity of an organism causing a cluster of pseudoinfections, or the types of specimens from which it is isolated, will provide a clue to the source of the organism. In one report, the sudden occurrence of positive cultures of normally sterile bone allograft specimens prompted an epidemiologic investigation.[67] The grafts grew *Pseudomonas cepacia* (now *Burkholderia cepacia*) and *Commomonas acidovorans*. Since these organisms grow well in an aqueous habitat, a water source was suspected. An investigation revealed that a single laboratory technologist had processed all four of the bone allografts that grew gram-negative organisms. A review of her work practices revealed that she had allowed the test tubes containing the bone to float in a sonicator water bath rather than securing them in a test tube rack or beaker. Cultures from the water bath grew the same organisms that were isolated from the bone specimens. The bacterial isolates from the bone allografts had the same antibiogram as those from the water bath, and pulsed-field gel electrophoresis indicated they were the same strains.[67]

Pseudomonas and *Burkholderia* species multiply readily in aqueous solutions and often have been implicated in pseudo-outbreaks. Studies have identified *Pseudomonas* spp. in postoperative pseudoinfections associated with a contaminated bottle of sterile saline that was used in the laboratory to process tissue specimens[24] and with outbreaks of bacteremia, peritonitis, and pseudoinfections that were associated with intrinsically contaminated iodine solutions.[33,39,68] Pseudobacteremia attributed to intrinsic contamination of povidone-iodine was reported by Berkelman et al. in 1981.[33] Their investigation was prompted by a New York hospital that reported to the Hospital Infections Branch at the CDC the occurrence of 17 blood cultures positive for *Pseudomonas cepacia* over a 3-month period. A review of the cases revealed that none of the 14 patients had clinical evidence of gram-negative bacteremia. Despite the fact that none of the patients had clinical signs and symptoms of gram-negative sepsis, four of the patients received antimicrobial therapy for possible bacteremia based on the culture results. A telephone survey of other hospitals in the New York City area uncovered three additional hospitals that were experiencing pseudobacteremias with *P. cepacia*. *P. cepacia* was eventually recovered from 52 patients in four hospitals over a 7-month period. An extensive epidemiologic investigation implicated 10% povidone-iodine solution from one manufacturer as the source of the contamination. The povidone-iodine was used at all four hospitals as a skin preparation for collection of blood cultures. *P. cepacia* was also isolated from an abdominal wound that had been packed with povidone-iodine–soaked dressings and from a sputum culture of a patient whose tracheostomy site was cleansed with the implicated povidone-iodine solution.[33]

VERIFYING THE DIAGNOSIS AND VERIFYING THE EXISTENCE OF AN OUTBREAK

The first two steps in the investigation of any potential outbreak are: (1) verify the diagnosis, and (2) verify the existence of an outbreak. Failure to follow these two very important steps before continuing an outbreak investigation may lead the investigator on the proverbial wild goose chase. At the beginning of an outbreak investigation, it is necessary to verify the diagnosis of any reported or suspected cases before proceeding, to avoid wasting time investigating an outbreak that may not exist.

For example, infection control professionals (ICPs) in acute and long-term care settings occasionally receive calls from personnel reporting an outbreak of methicillin-resistant *Staphylococcus aureus* (MRSA) on a particular healthcare unit. When such a call occurs, the ICP should first ask for the names of the patients or residents that the healthcare worker believes are involved in the reported outbreak and then should promptly review the patients' culture reports and medical records. This quick review may reveal that some of the MRSA isolates are actually methicillin-resistant *Staphylococcus epidermidis* or that several of the patients or residents were already culture-positive for MRSA when admitted to the unit. If this is the case, these findings should be promptly reported to the healthcare worker who expressed concern in order to prevent rumors and fears that the facility is experiencing an outbreak. If clinical features appear to be inconsistent with laboratory results, a pseudoinfection should be suspected. If a cluster or increase in the number of pseudoinfections is detected, then a pseudo-outbreak should be suspected. In this case, the investigator should carefully analyze each step in specimen collection and processing.

Surveillance artefact is a frequent cause of pseudoepidemics, so it is important to verify that an outbreak exists (i.e., that there is an increase in the expected number of healthcare-associated cases).[1] Surveillance artefact may occur due to (1) failure to properly distinguish community-acquired infections from HAIs, (2) a coincidental occurrence of unrelated cases, or (3) a change in the facility's method of conducting surveillance.

Bannatyne et al. reported the results of their investigation of an apparent cluster of three MRSA cases in a hospital with a low incidence of MRSA.[23] A review of the culture reports revealed that the three isolates, which appeared over a 16-day period, had different antibiotic susceptibility patterns. Further investigation into the patients' medical histories revealed that two of the patients had prior positive MRSA cultures when at other institutions. Although the three isolates exhibited temporal and geographic clustering, the investigators were able to hypothesize that the organisms were unrelated. When the organisms were typed, they were found to be different phage types, thus confirming the hypothesis that the strains were not related.[23]

Molecular techniques for identifying and characterizing microorganisms have greatly facilitated the understanding of the epidemiology of HAIs and outbreaks.[69,70] Personnel responsible for investigating a pseudo-outbreak should consider using molecular testing of isolates in combination with an epidemiologic investigation to identify and confirm the likely source of a pseudoepidemic. As with any laboratory test, care must be taken when evaluating typing results because these results must be combined with a careful epidemiologic study in order to confirm the transmission of a single strain or multiple strains of an organism. Molecular techniques used for characterizing a variety of pathogens implicated in outbreaks and pseudo-outbreaks are discussed in Chapter 11.

PREVENTING PSEUDO-OUTBREAKS

Pseudo-outbreaks can be prevented when laboratory personnel implement and adhere to protocols that reduce the risk of specimen contamination and when clinicians, laboratory personnel, and ICPs (1) quickly recognize the occurrence of false-positive cultures, (2) are alert to the occurrence of clusters or an increased number of infections/pseudoinfections, (3) use objective criteria for diagnosing the presence of an infection, and (4) use appropriate criteria for categorizing an infection as healthcare or community associated.

SUMMARY

Outbreak investigations generally require a large time commitment on the part of the investigators, many of whom are pulled away from their normal job duties. Outbreaks result in a great deal of anxiety and fear in personnel, patients, residents, visitors, and the community. They cause disruption in the lives of patients, residents, and personnel and in the provision of healthcare services. In addition, pseudoinfections or a pseudo-outbreak may result in unnecessary treatment or prophylaxis of patients, residents, or staff and the loss of confidence in medical personnel and the laboratory. To avoid these adverse effects, it is important that pseudoinfections and artefactual clusters of real infections be recognized and acted upon promptly.

REFERENCES

1. Weinstein RA, Stamm WE. Pseudoepidemics in hospital. *Lancet.* 1977;2:862–864.
2. Kusek JW. Nosocomial pseudoepidemics and pseudoinfections: an increasing problem. *Am J Infect Control.* 1981;9:70–75.
3. Stamm WE, Weinstein RA, Dixon RE. Comparison of endemic and epidemic nosocomial infections. *Am J Med.* 1981;70:393–397.
4. Jarvis WR. Nosocomial outbreaks: the Centers for Disease Control's Hospital Infections Program experience, 1980–1990. *Am J Med.* 1991;91(suppl 3B):101S–106S.
5. Herwaldt LA, Smith SD, Carter CD. Infection control in the outpatient setting. *Infect Control Hosp Epidemiol.* 1998;19:41–74.
6. Labarca JA, Garcia P, Balcells ME, et al. Pseudo-outbreak of *Ochrobactrum anthropi* bacteremia related to cross-contamination from erythrocyte sedimentation tubes. *Infect Control Hosp Epidemiol.* 2007;28(6):763–765.
7. Apisarnthanarak A, Kiratisin P, Thongphubeth K, Yuakyen C, Mundy LM. Pseudo-outbreak of *Acinetobacter Iwoffii* infection in a tertiary care center in Thailand. *Infect Control Hosp Epidemiol.* 2007;28(5):637–639.
8. Diederen BM, Verhulst C, van't Veen A, van Keulen PH, Kluytmans JA. Pseudo-outbreak of hepatitis B virus infection associated with contamination of a semiautomatic cap remover. *Infect Control Hosp Epidemiol.* 2006;27(11):1258–1260.
9. Calfee DP, Kornblum J, Jenkins SG. Pseudo-outbreak of *Bordetella bronchiseptica* infection associated with contaminated rabbit blood used as a broth culture supplement. *Infect Control Hosp Epidemiol.* 2007;28(6):758–760.

10. Gust DA, Wang SA, Black CM, et al. A pseudo-outbreak of *Chlamydia trachomatis* in a state residential facility: implications for diagnostic testing. *J Infect Dis.* 2002;185(6):841–844.

11. Kressel AB, Kidd F. Pseudo-outbreak of *Mycobacterium chelonae* and *Methylobacterium mesophilicum* caused by contamination of an automated endoscopy washer. *Infect Control Hosp Epidemiol.* 2001;22(7):414–418.

12. Romney M, Sherlock C, Stephens G, Clarke A. Pseudo-outbreak of *Pseudomonas putida* in a hospital outpatient clinic originating from a contaminated commercial anti-fog solution—Vancouver, British Columbia. *Can Commun Dis Rep.* November 1, 2000;26(21):183–184.

13. Segal-Maurer S, Kreiswirth BN, Burns JM, et al. *Mycobacterium tuberculosis* specimen contamination revisited: the role of laboratory environmental control in a pseudo-outbreak. *Infect Control Hosp Epidemiol.* 1998;19:101–105.

14. Gravowitz EV, Keenholtz SL. A pseudoepidemic of *Alcaligenes xylosoxidans* attributable to contaminated saline. *Am J Infect Control.* 1998;26:146–148.

15. Cox R, deBorja K, Bach MC. A pseudo-outbreak of *Mycobacterium chelonae* infections related to bronchoscopy. *Infect Control Hosp Epidemiol.* 1997;18:136–137.

16. Sule O, Ludlam HA, Walker CW, Brown DFJ, Kauffman ME. A pseudo-outbreak of respiratory infection with *Acinetobacter* species. *Infect Control Hosp Epidemiol.* 1997;18:510–512.

17. Grabau JC, Burrows DJ, Kern ML. A pseudo-outbreak of purified protein derivative skin-test conversions caused by inappropriate testing materials. *Infect Control Hosp Epidemiol.* 1997;18:571–574.

18. Verweij PE, Bilj D, Melchers W, et al. Pseudo-outbreak of multiresistant *Pseudomonas aeruginosa* in a hematology unit. *Infect Control Hosp Epidemiol.* 1997;18:128–131.

19. Agerton T, Valway S, Gore B, et al. Transmission of a highly drug-resistant strain (strain W1) of *Mycobacterium tuberculosis*. *JAMA.* 1997;278:1073–1077.

20. Gravel-Topper D, Sample ML, Oxley C, Toye B, Woods DE, Garber GE. Three-year outbreak of pseudobacteremia with *Burkholderia cepacia* traced to a contaminated blood gas analyzer. *Infect Control Hosp Epidemiol.* 1996;17:737–740.

21. Hagan ME, Klotz SA, Bartholomew W, Potter L, Nelson M. A pseudoepidemic of *Rhodotorula rubra*: a marker for microbial contamination of the bronchoscope. *Infect Control Hosp Epidemiol.* 1995;16:727–728.

22. Mehta JB, Kefri M, Soike DR. Pseudoepidemic of nontuberculous mycobacteria in a community hospital. *Infect Control Hosp Epidemiol.* 1995:16:633–634.

23. Bannatyne RM, Wells BA, MacMillan SA, Thibault MC. A cluster of MRSA—the little outbreak that wasn't. *Infect Control Hosp Epidemiol.* 1995;16:380.

24. Forman W, Axelrod P, St John K, et al. Investigation of a pseudo-outbreak of orthopedic infections caused by *Pseudomonas aeruginosa*. *Infect Control Hosp Epidemiol.* 1994;15:652–657.

25. Pearson ML, Pegues DA, Carson LA, et al. Cluster of *Enterobacter cloacae* pseudobacteremias associated with use of an agar slant blood culturing system. *J Clin Microbiol.* 1993;31:2599–2603.

26. Sniadack DH, Ostroff SM, Karlix MA, et al. A nosocomial pseudo-outbreak of *Mycobacterium xenopi* due to a contaminated potable water supply: lessons in prevention. *Infect Control Hosp Epidemiol.* 1993;14:636–641.

27. Gubler JG, Salfinger M, von Graevenitz A. Pseudoepidemic of nontuberculous mycobacteria due to a contaminated bronchoscope cleaning machine: report of an outbreak and review of the literature. *Chest.* 1992;101:1245–1249.

28. Van Horn KG, Tatz JS, Li KI, Newman L, Wormser GP. Copepods associated with a perirectal abscess and copepod pseudo-outbreak in stools for ova and parasite examinations. *Diagn Microbiol Infect Dis.* 1992;15:561–565.

29. Klotz SA, Normand RE, Kalinsky RG. "Through a drinking glass and what was found there": pseudocontamination of a hospital's drinking water. *Infect Control Hosp Epidemiol.* 1992; 13:477–481.

30. Poulin C, Schlech WF. A pseudo-outbreak in a nursing home. *Infect Control Hosp Epidemiol.* 1991;12:521–522.

31. Bradley SF, Wilson KH, Rosloniec MA, Kauffman CA. Recurrent pseudobacteremias traced to a radiometric blood culture device. *Infect Control.* 1987;8:281–283.

32. Budnick LD, Moll ME, Hull HF, Mann JM, Kendal AP. A pseudo-outbreak of influenza A associated with use of laboratory stock strain. *Am J Public Health.* 1984;76:607–609.

33. Berkelman RL, Lewin S, Allen JR, et al. Pseudobacteremia attributed to contamination of povidone-iodine with *Pseudomonas cepacia*. *Ann Intern Med.* 1981;95:32–36.

34. Grinbaum RS, Guimarães T, Kusano E, Hosino N, Sader H, Cereda RF. A pseudo-outbreak of vancomycin-resistant *Enterococcus faecium*. *Infect Control Hosp Epidemiol.* 2003;24:461–464.

35. Medeiros EAS, Lott TJ, Lopes Colombo A, et al. Evidence for a pseudo-outbreak of *Candida guilliermondii* fungemia in a University Hospital in Brazil. *J Clin Micro.* 2007;45:942–947. http://jcm.asm.org/cgi/content/full/45/3/942?view=long&pmid=17229862#R21. Accessed March 20, 2008.

36. Ender PT, Durning SJ, Woelk WK, et al. Pseudo-outbreak of methicillin-resistant *Staphylococcus aureus*. *Mayo Clin Proc.* 1999;74(9):885–889.

37. Park YS, Kim SY, Park SY, et al. Pseudo-outbreak of *Stenotrophomonas maltophilia* bacteremia in a general ward. *Am J Infect Control.* 2008;36:29–32.

38. Oda GV, DeVries MM, Yakrus MA. Pseudo-outbreak of *Mycobacterium scrofulaceum* linked to cross-contamination with a laboratory reference strain. *Infect Control Hosp Epidemiol.* 2001;22(10):649–651. [Erratum in: *Infect Control Hosp Epidemiol.* 2001;22(12):785.]

39. Panlilio AL, Beck-Sague CM, Siegel JD, et al. Infections and pseudoinfections due to povidone-iodine solution contaminated with *Pseudomonas cepacia*. *Clin Infect Dis.* 1991;14:1078–1083.

40. Silva CV, Magalhães VD, Pereira CR, Kawagoe JY, Ikura C, Ganc AJ. Pseudo-outbreak of *Pseudomonas aeruginosa* and *Serratia marcescens* related to bronchoscopes. *Infect Control Hosp Epidemiol.* 2003;24(3):195–197.

41. Fraser VJ, Jones M, Murray P, Medoff G, Zhang Y, Wallace RJ. Contamination of fiberoptic bronchoscopes with *Mycobacterium chelonae* linked to an automated bronchoscope disinfection machine. *Am Rev Respir Dis.* 1992;145:853–855.

42. Maloney S, Welbel S, Daves B, et al. *Mycobacterium abscessus* pseudoinfection traced to an automated endoscope washer: utility of epidemiologic and laboratory investigation. *J Infect Dis.* 1994;169:1166–1169.

43. Ehrenkranz NJ, Richter EI, Phillips PM, Shultz JM. An apparent excess of operative site infections: analyses to evaluate false-positive diagnosis. *Infect Control Hosp Epidemiol.* 1995;16:712–716.

44. Bonten MJM, Gaillard CA, van Tiel FH, van der Geest S, Stobberingh EE. A typical case of cross-acquisition: the importance of genotypic characterization of bacterial strains. *Infect Control Hosp Epidemiol.* 1995;16:415–416.

45. El Sahly HM, Septimus E, Soini H, et al. *Mycobacterium simiae* pseudo-outbreak resulting from a contaminated hospital water supply in Houston, Texas. *Clin Infect Dis.* 2002;35(7):802–807.

46. Labombardi VJ, O'Brien AM, Kislak JW. Pseudo-outbreak of *Mycobacterium fortuitum* due to contaminated ice machines. *Am J Infect Control.* 2002;30(3):184–186.

47. Gebo KA, Srinivasan A, Perl TM, Ross T, Groth A, Merz WG. Pseudo-outbreak of *Mycobacterium fortuitum* on a human immunodeficiency virus ward: transient respiratory tract colonization from a contaminated ice machine. *Clin Infect Dis.* 2002;35(1):32–38.

48. Lalande V, Barbut F, Varnerot A, et al. Pseudo-outbreak of *Mycobacterium gordonae* associated with water from refrigerated fountains. *J Hosp Infect.* 2001;48(1):76–79.

49. Phillips MS, von Reyn CF. Nosocomial infections due to nontuberculous mycobacteria. *Clin Infect Dis.* 2001;33(8):1363–1374.

50. Centers for Disease Control and Prevention. Multiple misdiagnoses of tuberculosis resulting from laboratory error—Wisconsin, 1996. *MMWR.* 1997;46:797–801.

51. Nivin B, Fujiwara PI, Hannifin J, Kreiswirth BN. Cross-contamination with *Mycobacterium tuberculosis*: an epidemiological and laboratory investigation. *Infect Control Hosp Epidemiol.* 1998;19:500–503.

52. Cronin W, Rodriguez E, Valway S, et al. Pseudo-outbreak of tuberculosis in an acute-care general hospital: epidemiology and clinical implications. *Infect Control Hosp Epidemiol.* 1998;19:345–347.

53. Braden CR, Templeton GL, Stead WW, Bates JH, Cave MD, Valway SE. Retrospective detection of laboratory cross-contamination of *Mycobacterium tuberculosis* cultures with use of DNA fingerprint analysis. *Clin Infect Dis.* 1997;24:34–40.

54. Burman WJ, Stone BL, Reeves RR, et al. The incidence of false-positive cultures for *Mycobacterium tuberculosis*. *Am J Respir Crit Care Med.* 1997;155:321–326.

55. Dunlap NE, Harris RH, Benjamin WH Jr, Harden JW, Hafner D. Laboratory contamination of *Mycobacterium tuberculosis* cultures. *Am J Respir Crit Care Med.* 1995;152:1702–1704.

56. Nitta AT, Davidson PT, De Koning ML, Kilman RJ. Misdiagnosis of multidrug-resistant *Mycobacterium tuberculosis* possibly due to laboratory-related errors. *JAMA.* 1996;276: 1980–1983.

57. Small PM, McClenny NB, Singh SP, Schoolnik GK, Tompkins LS, Mickelsen PA. Molecular strain typing of *Mycobacterium tuberculosis* to confirm cross-contamination in the mycobacteriology laboratory and modification of procedures to minimize occurrence of false-positive cultures. *J Clin Microbiol.* 1993;31:1677–1682.

58. Tokars JI, Rudnick JR, Kroc K, et al. US hospital mycobacteriology laboratories: status and comparison with state public health department laboratories. *J Clin Microbiol.* 1996;34:680–685.

59. Goodman RA, Smith JD, Kubica GP, Dougherty EM, Sikes RK. Nosocomial mycobacterial pseudoinfection in a Georgia hospital. *Infect Control.* 1984;5:573–576.

60. Jacobson E, Gurevich I, Schoch P, Cunha BA. Pseudoepidemic of nontuberculous mycobacteria in a community hospital. *Infect Control Hosp Epidemiol.* 1996;17:348.

61. Bearman G, Vaamonde C, Larone D, Drusin L, Zuccotti G. Pseudo-outbreak of multidrug-resistant *Mycobacterium tuberculosis* associated with presumed laboratory processing contamination. *Infect Control Hosp Epidemiol.* 2002;23:620–622.

62. Bennett SN, Peterson DE, Johnson DR, Hall WN, Robinson-Dunn B, Dietrich S. Bronchoscopy-associated *Mycobacterium xenopi* pseudoinfections. *Am J Resp Crit Care Med.* 1994;150:245–250.

63. Bettiker RL, Axelrod PI, Fekete T, et al. Delayed recognition of a pseudo-outbreak of *Mycobacterium terrae*. *Am J Infect Control.* 2006;34:343–347.

64. Carson LA, Bland LA, Cusick LB, et al. Prevalence of nontuberculous mycobacteria in water supplies of hemodialysis centers. *Appl Environ Microbiol.* 1988;54:3122–3125.

65. Seville RH, Rao PS, Hutchinson DN, Birchall G. Outbreak of Campbell de Morgan spots. *BMJ.* 1970;1:408–409.

66. Honish A, Grimsrud K, Miedzinski L, Gold E, Cherry R. Outbreak of Campbell de Morgan spots in a nursing home—Alberta. *Can Dis Wkly Rep.* 1988;14:211–212.

67. Mermel LA, Josephson SL, Giorgio C. A pseudo-epidemic involving bone allografts. *Infect Control Hosp Epidemiol.* 1994;15:757–758.

68. Parrott PL, Terry PM, Whitworth EN, et al. *Pseudomonas aeruginosa* peritonitis associated with contaminated poloxamer-iodine solution. *Lancet.* 1982;2:683–685.

69. Jarvis WR. Usefulness of molecular epidemiology for outbreak investigations. *Infect Control Hosp Epidemiol.* 1994;15:500–503.

70. Singh A, Goering R, Simjee S, Foley SL, Zervosi MJ. Application of molecular techniques to the study of hospital infection. *Clin Microbiol Rev.* 2006;19:512–530.

CHAPTER 7

Organisms and Diseases Associated with Outbreaks in a Variety of Healthcare Settings

Kathleen Meehan Arias

> *A mighty creature is the germ.*
>
> —Ogden Nash[1]

INTRODUCTION

The outbreaks discussed in this book have been categorized into the healthcare setting in which they have most frequently been reported (i.e., acute, long-term, or ambulatory care). It is evident, however, that many agents and disease syndromes, such as gastroenteritis and respiratory illness, have been associated with endemic and epidemic infections in more than one type of healthcare setting. Organisms such as methicillin-resistant *Staphylococcus aureus* (MRSA), vancomycin-resistant *Enterococcus* (VRE) species, *Mycobacterium tuberculosis*, norovirus, *Sarcoptes scabiei*, and *Clostridium difficile* frequently cause healthcare-associated outbreaks in hospitals and long-term care (LTC) facilities. *M. tuberculosis* has also been responsible for outbreaks in ambulatory care settings such as clinics and emergency rooms. Endemic and epidemic gastrointestinal diseases can occur in many settings and can affect patients, residents, personnel, and visitors. It is important to note that because of the absence of routinely available laboratory tests for some organisms, the etiology of healthcare-associated epidemics and clusters of infectious gastroenteritis is not always determined, especially if the causative agent is viral.

The purpose of this chapter is to review outbreaks that have been caused by MRSA, VRE, *M. tuberculosis*, *C. difficile*, influenza virus, norovirus, *Sarcoptes scabiei*, and several other parasites, and to outline control measures that have been used to prevent and interrupt these outbreaks. Since outbreaks of gastrointestinal illness frequently occur in a variety of healthcare settings, they will also be discussed.

ORGANISMS ASSOCIATED WITH NOSOCOMIAL OUTBREAKS IN A VARIETY OF HEALTHCARE SETTINGS

Methicillin-Resistant *Staphylococcus aureus* in the Acute Care Setting

Epidemiology

MRSA emerged as an important clinical problem shortly after the introduction of methicillin.[2] The rise in the proportion of hospital-associated infections caused by *S. aureus* resistant to the beta-lactam antibiotics has been documented by nosocomial infection surveillance systems in many countries.[3–8] The first hospital outbreaks of MRSA in the United States occurred in the late 1960s, and multiple outbreaks have been reported worldwide.[9–17] Initially associated with large tertiary care hospitals, MRSA has become endemic in many institutions and is now the most common multidrug-resistant pathogen seen in US hospitals.[18] Once considered to be strictly healthcare-associated, distinct strains that are transmitted in the community and differ genetically from those that have been traditionally considered healthcare-associated have been isolated from persons with no prior history of hospitalization.[19] Community-acquired strains of MRSA have caused outbreaks in diverse populations, such as sports teams, children in day care centers, inmates in prison, and students.[20–27] Not surprisingly, strains that initially were associated with community-acquired infections have also been responsible for outbreaks in healthcare facilities.[27–30]

Risk factors for acquiring MRSA include previous hospitalization or nursing home stay, length of stay, prior antibiotic therapy, diabetes, an open wound, admission to a critical care or burn unit, surgery, and proximity to a patient with MRSA.[14,19,25,31,32] Colonization often precedes infection, and one study estimated that 30–60% of colonized patients will develop a MRSA infection.[33] It is well recognized that patients may remain colonized for many months.[12,19,31] Prolonged colonization of hospital personnel also may occur— one study found that several healthcare workers carried MRSA in their nares for 3 or more months.[34] Several studies have demonstrated that MRSA can survive for long periods on environmental surfaces, and the rooms of patients with MRSA can become substantially contaminated.[35]

Mode of Transmission

In the acute care setting, the major mode of transmission of MRSA is via hands that become contaminated by contact with colonized or infected persons, or devices, items, or environmental surfaces contaminated with MRSA.[25,30] Direct contact involves body surface-to-body surface contact, such as occurs when a healthcare worker turns a patient. Although transient contamination of healthcare worker's hands is considered to be the primary mode of transmission from person to person, infected and colonized personnel have served as reservoirs in common-source outbreaks.[25,27] A physician with a prolonged upper respiratory tract infection and MRSA colonization was the likely source for an outbreak in a surgical intensive care unit,[36] nasal carriers were implicated in an outbreak in a burn unit,[28] and another outbreak was associated with a healthcare worker who had chronic otitis externa.[37] Hospital personnel, especially house staff who rotate between facilities, have been found to spread MRSA from hospital to hospital and may be responsible for introducing the organism into a facility.[38,39]

A colonized healthcare worker was identified as the index case in a widespread outbreak associated with a single clone of MRSA that occurred over a 2-year period in several healthcare facilities in Australia.[40] Colonized and infected patients, such as neonates that are transferred from one hospital to another, can also serve as a method for interinstitutional spread and introducing MRSA into a facility.[41]

Control Measures

Guidelines for preventing the endemic and epidemic transmission of MRSA in the acute care setting have been published by the Centers for Disease Control and Prevention (CDC),[25,42] professional organizations,[43–44] many state health departments,[45] and other public health agencies. Guidelines for preventing, managing, and controlling a MRSA outbreak can be found in the CDC's *Management of Multidrug-Resistant Organisms in Healthcare Settings, 2006.*[25] There is no single set of evidence-based practices for interrupting a MRSA outbreak in a healthcare setting. However, published reports demonstrate that MRSA outbreaks can be interrupted by using a combination of interventions that include the following:

- Hand hygiene (i.e., washing hands with plain or antimicrobial soap or disinfecting hands with a waterless antiseptic hand rub)[41,44]
- Laboratory-based surveillance (i.e., the review of positive cultures) to identify infected and colonized cases[25]
- Surveillance cultures to detect colonized and infected patients[25]
- Surveillance cultures to detect colonized and infected personnel—only if a thorough epidemiologic investigation links a specific healthcare worker to a cluster of cases (i.e., a common-source outbreak is suspected)[25]
- Contact precautions and use of barriers for infected and colonized patients[25,41]
- Cohorting of patients and staff [25]
- Education of healthcare personnel, patients, and visitors regarding preventing the spread of the organism[25,41]
- Treatment of infected patients, residents, or personnel
- Decolonization of personnel, patients, and residents in certain situations[25,42]

Hand hygiene. Appropriate hand hygiene, regardless of the use of gloves, is essential to control the person-to-person transmission of MRSA.[25,42,46] Hand hygiene may be accomplished either by washing hands with plain or antimicrobial soap or disinfecting hands with a waterless antiseptic hand rub (usually alcohol based). When soap and water are used, regardless of the type of soap, personnel should be instructed to vigorously rub and clean all surfaces of the hands and to wash their wrists and forearms. If the hands are not visibly soiled, antiseptic hand rubs are generally recommended over the handwashing because hand rubs have better antimicrobial activity and are more convenient to use.[25]

Laboratory-based surveillance to identify cases. Ongoing surveillance is an essential element of any infection prevention and control program and is necessary to establish an endemic or baseline rate of MRSA in order to be able to recognize outbreaks and clusters.[25] Routine surveillance for MRSA is generally conducted by regularly reviewing laboratory reports for *S. aureus* isolates that are resistant to methicillin (or nafcillin, oxacillin, etc., depending on which antibiotic is reported by the microbiology laboratory). It should be noted that many patients who are colonized or infected will not be detected by routine cultures obtained for clinical indications. Once MRSA is identified, criteria must be used to determine if the organism is colonizing or infecting the patient and if an infection is community or hospital associated. Many hospitals use the criteria developed for the National Healthcare Safety Network /National Nosocomial Infections Surveillance (NNIS) system to categorize a nosocomial infection.[47,48] However, because patients may be colonized with MRSA for prolonged time periods, it is often difficult to determine if MRSA isolated from a hospitalized patient was present but undetected at the time of admission or was acquired in the hospital. Some infections, by definition, will be categorized as nosocomial or healthcare-associated even though the causative agent may have been part of the patient's flora at admission. If an outbreak is suspected, laboratory records should be reviewed retrospectively and prospectively to identify both infected and colonized patients and a line list of healthcare-associated cases should be maintained as discussed in Chapter 8. Both colonized and infected cases should be identified in order to determine the extent of an outbreak.

Active surveillance testing of patients. Because many patients may be colonized, with no overt signs or symptoms of infection, surveillance cultures are recommended during an outbreak investigation to detect colonization and to determine the extent of transmission of the organism.[11,12,25,40,49] Since many distinct strains of MRSA may be found in an institution,[11,12,16,40] surveillance cultures should not be done to detect transmission as a result of an outbreak unless the MRSA isolates are subjected to a discriminatory molecular typing test to provide evidence of strain relatedness. This is especially important if an outbreak is suspected in an area that has a high endemic rate of MRSA. Methods for selecting appropriate culture sites, screening tests, and procedures for collecting specimens are discussed in Chapter 11.

Surveillance cultures of personnel. Because most outbreaks are caused by transmission of MRSA from patient-to-patient on the hands of personnel, many clusters and outbreaks can be terminated by implementing contact precautions and reeducating all personnel on the importance and use of routine infection prevention and control measures, such as standard precautions and proper hand hygiene techniques. Generally, culturing of personnel is not recommended unless (1) initial control measures, such as contact isolation and the use of barriers and hand hygiene, fail to terminate the spread of the organism and (2) a thorough epidemiologic investigation links personnel to a cluster of cases (i.e., a common-source outbreak is suspected).[25,49] Common-source outbreaks are often associated with a personnel carrier and should be suspected if an increase in MRSA cases occurs abruptly, such as when several cases appear in a short time period on a single unit, or when several postoperative wound infections occur in a short time period. When conducting surveillance cultures, it should be remembered that at any given time 20–90% of personnel may be nasal carriers of *S. aureus*, and fewer than 10% of healthy carriers disperse the organism into the air.[50] In addition, personnel who are found to be colonized are not necessarily the source of an outbreak because they may have become colonized by contact with the true source or by contact with colonized or infected patients. Because many strains of MRSA may be circulating in a facility, surveillance cultures should not be done unless all of the MRSA isolates from both personnel and patients involved in an outbreak or cluster are subjected to a discriminatory molecular typing test to confirm that they are the same strain.

Contact precautions and use of barriers. Although much is known about the epidemiology and the mode of transmission of MRSA, opinions vary considerably on the use and effectiveness of contact isolation precautions and the use of barriers such as gloves, gowns, and/or masks.[11,12, 25,51–54] Most authorities recommend the use of some type of contact isolation and barrier precautions to restrict transmission, especially to control an outbreak. The Healthcare Infection Control Practices Advisory Committee (HICPAC) *Guideline for Isolation Precautions, 2007,*[42] and the HICPAC *Management of Multidrug-Resistant Organisms in Healthcare Settings, 2006,*[25] recommend that gloves and gowns be worn when entering the room of a patient on contact precautions. One carefully conducted study found that contact isolation was effective in controlling the epidemic spread of MRSA in a neonatal intensive care unit.[55] Each hospital must identify which measures are appropriate for its specific situation.[53]

Education of healthcare workers. Educational programs on the epidemiology and mode of transmission of MRSA and the importance of contact precautions and hand hygiene should be provided for all members of the healthcare team, including physicians.[25] An educational program that actively involved staff surgeons and house staff was effective at limiting the spread of MRSA in one hospital.[56]

Treatment of infected or colonized patients. Patients who are either infected or colonized with MRSA may serve as reservoirs. Most patients with infection will be treated with antimicrobials; however, the use of antibiotics to eliminate colonization in patients must be approached with caution because many decolonization regimens have been found to promote the development of resistant organisms.[25,57,58] Before providing treatment or prophylaxis to patients, a physician with expertise in infectious diseases should be consulted.

Treatment of infected or colonized personnel. When an outbreak or cluster is detected, the investigator should search for personnel with obvious signs and symptoms of infection or skin breakdown. Personnel with infections should be treated; however, eradication of nasal carriage in personnel is recommended only when there is convincing epidemiologic evidence that a culture-positive healthcare worker is the source of the epidemic strain.[25,36,57] Before providing treatment or prophylaxis to personnel, a physician with expertise in infectious diseases should be consulted. Restricting the activities of culture-positive personnel is controversial. If a colonized healthcare worker is epidemiologically linked to cases, the worker should be restricted from patient care until carriage has been eradicated.[25]

If a healthcare worker is treated for decolonization, repeat cultures should be done to confirm that the carrier state has been eradicated. Since antimicrobial agents used for decolonizing carriers may promote resistant strains of MRSA, only those personnel who are epidemiologically linked to disease transmission should be treated. Discussions of regimens used for eradicating staphylococcal carriage in healthcare workers have been published elsewhere.[25,50,58]

MRSA in the Long-Term Care Setting

Epidemiology

Although the first outbreak of MRSA involving nursing home residents was reported in 1970, reports about the occurrence and epidemiology of MRSA in LTC facilities were scarce until the late 1980s.[59–67] Outbreaks of MRSA have now been reported from a variety of LTC settings worldwide.[17] The global increase in colonization and infection caused by MRSA in acute care institutions has been paralleled by a similar increase in the LTC setting.[68–72] Studies have shown colonization rates for MRSA among residents in LTC facilities ranging from 5% to 82%[62,65,67,68,70–74]: one found from 4.9% to 15.6% on each of eight culture surveys collected over a 15-month period,[72] one detected 8.8% of patients colonized at least once over a 1-year period,[68] and a prevalence survey conducted during an outbreak in a Veterans Affairs nursing home indicated that 34% of the 114 patients were colonized.[61] Several studies have documented colonization of residents at the time of admission to the facility,[61,67,70,73,75] and several have found that residents may be persistently colonized for months to years.[69] A study by Hsu noted that although a few nursing home residents had persistent colonization, most showed only a temporary or intermittent carriage.[73] The transfer of residents and patients between acute care hospitals and LTC facilities plays a role in maintaining reservoirs of MRSA in each setting.[60,62,73,74]

Risk factors for acquiring MRSA colonization in the LTC setting include previous hospitalization, poor functional status, presence of a decubitus ulcer or other wound, underlying diseases and medical conditions that jeopardize skin integrity, use of invasive devices that disrupt the skin barrier (such as gastrostomy tubes), and prior antimicrobial therapy.[61,66,69,73] Risk factors for infection include colonization with MRSA, a debilitated state requiring skilled nursing care, and hemodialysis.[63,65,76] A 1991 report of a 3-year prospective cohort study of 197 patients in a long-term care Veterans Administration Center found that colonization predicted infection, carriage persisted for a median of 118 days, and 8/32 (25%) patients with persistent carriage ultimately developed an MRSA infection.[65] Many of these residents had poor functional status and required hemodialysis. In other studies, reported rates of infection varied according to the population studied and ranged from 6% to 25% of patients who were colonized with MRSA.[61,65,66,69,70] The risk for serious infection with MRSA appears to be low for most residents of LTC facilities.[61,66,76,77]

Mode of Transmission

The major reservoir of MRSA in the LTC setting is colonized and infected residents. The primary mode of transmission is direct contact between residents or from resident to resident via transient carriage on the hands of personnel.[76] Transmission from one roommate to another appears to occur infrequently and occurs most often in residents who require extensive nursing care.[66] Although MRSA has been isolated from environmental surfaces, there is little evidence that the environment plays a major role in the transmission of MRSA.[66] Studies documenting the existence of several strains of MRSA in a facility support the hypothesis that MRSA is introduced and reintroduced into a facility from multiple sources.[68,72]

Control Measures

Recommendations for preventing the endemic and epidemic transmission of MRSA in the LTC setting have been published by the American Hospital Association,[78] Mulligan et al.,[76] Kauffman et al.,[63] and Bradley.[69] Many health departments and government agencies worldwide have developed guidelines for the detection, prevention, and control of MRSA outbreaks in LTC facilities and have posted these documents on their Web sites. Measures used to control a MRSA outbreak in the LTC setting include the following:

- Hand hygiene (i.e., washing hands with plain or antimicrobial soap or disinfecting hands with a waterless antiseptic hand rub)[42,46]
- Laboratory-based surveillance (i.e., the review of positive cultures) to identify infected and colonized cases[25]
- Surveillance cultures to detect colonized and infected patients/residents[25]
- Surveillance cultures to detect infected and colonized personnel—only if a thorough epidemiologic investigation links a specific healthcare worker to a cluster of cases (i.e., a common-source outbreak is suspected)[25]
- Contact precautions and use of barriers for infected and colonized patients/residents[25,42]
- Cohorting of patients/residents and staff[25]
- Education of healthcare personnel, residents/patients, and visitors regarding preventing the spread of the organism[25,42]
- Treatment of infected residents/patients and personnel
- Decolonization of personnel and residents/patients in certain situations[25,42]

Hand hygiene. Appropriate hand hygiene, regardless of the use of gloves, is essential to control the person-to-person transmission of MRSA.[25,42,46] Hand hygiene may be accomplished either by washing hands with plain or antimicrobial soap or disinfecting hands with a waterless antiseptic hand rub (usually alcohol based). When soap and water are used, regardless of the type of soap, personnel should be instructed to vigorously rub and clean all surfaces of the hands and to wash their wrists and forearms. If the hands are not visibly soiled, antiseptic hand rubs are generally recommended over the handwashing because hand rubs have better antimicrobial activity and are more convenient to use.[25]

Laboratory-based surveillance to identify cases. An ongoing surveillance program is necessary to establish the endemic, or baseline, level of MRSA in a LTC setting in order to recognize an outbreak or cluster of cases. Laboratory-based surveillance (i.e., the ongoing review of positive cultures of residents) should be routinely conducted in the LTC setting, even though it is generally less effective for detecting MRSA than in the acute care setting because cultures are less frequently collected. Criteria must be used to determine if a resident is colonized or infected and if the MRSA isolated was acquired in the facility (nosocomial) or elsewhere. Although there is no single widely accepted set of criteria for use in the LTC setting, many facilities use the nosocomial infection definitions developed by McGeer et al.[79] Surveillance for cases is a critical component of any outbreak investigation because it helps in defining the extent of the problem, the likely mode of transmission, and a possible source. Once an outbreak is suspected, a linelisting of nosocomial cases, both colonized and infected, should be constructed as discussed in Chapter 8.

Active surveillance testing of residents. Studies have shown that many residents of LTC facilities are colonized with MRSA. Although routine collection of surveillance cultures may not be a cost-effective use of limited infection control resources in an LTC facility,[60] if an outbreak is suspected, surveillance cultures of the nares and wounds are recommended to determine the extent of spread.[25] Since many distinct strains of MRSA may be found, MRSA isolates should be subjected to a discriminatory molecular typing test to provide evidence of strain relatedness. This is especially important if an outbreak is suspected in a facility with a high endemic rate of MRSA. Methods for collecting specimens and typing organisms are discussed in Chapter 11.

Surveillance cultures of personnel. Surveillance cultures of personnel in an LTC facility are rarely warranted because the primary mode of transmission is via transient carriage of MRSA on the hands of healthcare workers. Personnel should not be cultured unless there is epidemiologic evidence that links the cases to a specific healthcare worker.[25] The MRSA isolates from both personnel and residents involved should be subjected to a discriminatory molecular typing test to confirm that they are the same strain. Although personnel involved in an outbreak situation may be culture-positive for the epidemic strain, they are not necessarily the source of the outbreak—they may have become colonized by contact with infected or colonized residents.

Cohorting. The practice of cohorting during an outbreak (i.e., either separating those who are infected or colonized with MRSA from those who are not, or placing colonized/infected residents in the same room) has been shown to limit the spread of MRSA in a skilled nursing facility;[62] however, it is difficult to cohort residents in an LTC facility in which residents are encouraged to socialize at meals and during daily activities.

Contact precautions and use of barriers. Just as it has been debated in the acute care setting, the routine use of contact precautions[25,42] and barriers such as gloves, gowns, and masks to limit transmission of endemic MRSA in the LTC setting has been debated.[61,80] The debate notwithstanding, contact isolation has been shown to be useful in preventing the spread of MRSA in outbreak situations.[59,62] Each facility must identify which isolation precautions and types of specific barriers are appropriate for its particular setting.

Treatment of infected or colonized residents and patients. Treatment of infected residents and patients is generally recommended;[58] however, decolonization to eliminate carriage for the purpose of preventing either infection in a colonized resident or transmission to others has not been found to be a very effective infection control measure and can lead to development of resistant organisms.[68,77,81,82] Some investigators have reported recurrent colonization after completion of therapy.[82,83] Many LTC facilities have attempted to use antimicrobials to eradicate MRSA from their resident population; however, this has met with mixed success, possibly because of the reintroduction of the organism into the facility through the admission of colonized residents.[62,64,72,82] Before providing treatment or prophylaxis to residents or patients, a physician with expertise in infectious diseases should be consulted.

Treatment of colonized or infected personnel. When an outbreak or cluster is detected, the investigator should search for personnel with obvious signs and symptoms of infection or skin breakdown. Healthcare personnel who have a staphylococcal infection should be treated; however, it is not necessary to treat a healthcare worker who is colonized and asymptomatic unless he or she has been epidemiologically implicated as the source of an outbreak.[25] Before providing treatment or prophylaxis to personnel, a physician with expertise in infectious diseases should be consulted. If a healthcare worker is treated for decolonization, repeat cultures should be done to confirm that the carrier state has been eradicated. Because antimicrobial agents used for decolonizing carriers may promote resistant strains of MRSA, only those personnel who are epidemiologically linked to disease transmission should be treated. Discussions of regimens used for eradicating staphylococcal carriage in healthcare workers have been published elsewhere.[25,50,58]

Education of healthcare workers. Educational programs on hand hygiene, the mode of transmission of MRSA, and the importance of contact precautions should be provided frequently for caregivers in an LTC facility.[25,42,46]

Most LTC facilities have limited infection prevention and control resources. Because LTC facilities have diverse resident populations and different rates of MRSA colonization and infection, both endemic and epidemic control measures must be tailored to meet the needs and resources of the partic- ular setting.

Vancomycin-Resistant *Enterococcus* in the Acute Care Setting

Epidemiology

VRE was first recognized in Europe in the late 1980s and is now a major human pathogen worldwide.[84,85] The incidence of hospital-associated infections due to VRE increased dramatically in the United States between 1989 and 1993.[86] Since then, multiple hospital outbreaks have been reported worldwide, and most of these have occurred among critically ill patients in intensive care units and immunosuppressed patients on oncology or transplant units.[87-95] The first community-acquired cases in the United States were reported from New York City in 1993.[96] Although transmission in the community is fairly common in Europe, it appears to occur rarely in the United States where the major reservoir is infected and colonized patients.[97,98]

There are at least 17 species of enterococci—*Entercoccus faecium* and *Enterococcus faecalis* are the two most commonly encountered in clinical isolates, and *E. faecium* is inherently more resistant to antibiotics than *E. faecalis*. Some outbreaks of VRE appear to involve genetically unrelated strains. This may be because transposons contain the genetic determinants of resistance and transposons can spread easily between different strains of enterococci.[99] The enterococci are less virulent than *Staphylococcus aureus*, usually cause urinary tract infections, and occasionally cause endocarditis and bacteremia. Most serious enterococcal infections have been reported in severely compromised patients.[100–103]

Risk factors for developing VRE infection or colonization include severe underlying disease, intra-abdominal surgery, multiple-antibiotic therapy, vancomycin therapy, enteral feeding, history of major trauma, proximity to an unisolated VRE patient, sigmoidoscopy and colonoscopy, indwelling urinary or central vascular catheter, and prolonged hospital stay.[94,100,103–105]

Mode of Transmission

Although the majority of infections are believed to arise from a patient's endogenous flora, VRE can be spread from person to person by direct contact or indirectly via contaminated equipment or environmental surfaces[43,87,91,104,105] and transient carriage on healthcare workers' hands.[106] Studies demonstrate that the environment surrounding a patient with VRE can become substantially contaminated with VRE, and these organisms can be found on the hands of personnel who touch these surfaces.[107,108] Since the enterococci are normal inhabitants of the lower intestinal tract, patients may carry VRE asymptomatically in their stool, and rectal colonization may persist for months.[99,109,110] The epidemiology of VRE has not been clearly elucidated; however, since VRE can remain viable on inanimate surfaces for prolonged periods,[91,105-108,110–113] and outbreaks have been associated with use of electronic thermometers,[104] fomites can play a role in the transmission of VRE.

Control Measures

Guidelines for preventing the spread of VRE in acute care hospitals have been developed by the CDC's HICPAC,[25,42,103] and the Society for Healthcare Epidemiology of America (SHEA).[43] Many health departments and public health agencies worldwide have developed guidelines for preventing and controlling the transmission of VRE and other multidrug resistant organisms, and these guidelines are frequently posted on the agency's Web site. One of the primary recommendations for preventing the spread of VRE is to establish an antimicrobial stewardship program that limits use of vancomycin, which has consistently been reported as a major risk factor for colonization and infection with VRE.[25,103] There is also concern that excessive use of vancomycin will promote the development of vancomycin-resistant *Staphylococcus aureus* (VRSA). A few studies have been done on the efficacy of control measures used to prevent transmission of VRE. The use of contact isolation precautions, including gloves, gowns, and a private room, were found useful in limiting the spread of VRE in the acute care setting.[91] Infection control measures used to interrupt an outbreak of VRE in a cancer center included intense environmental cleaning, surveillance cultures of patients, contact isolation, cohorting of patients and staff, use of dedicated patient-care equipment, and staff education programs.[93]

The following measures are recommended to control outbreaks of VRE in the acute care setting[25,42,43,46]:

- Hand hygiene[46]
- Laboratory-based surveillance (i.e., the review of positive cultures) to identify cases
- Surveillance cultures of patients[25,43]
- Education of personnel[42,43]
- Contact precautions, including gloves and gowns, for infected and colonized patients[25]
- Cleaning and disinfection of equipment[25,43]
- Cleaning and disinfection of the environment[25,43]

Hand hygiene. Proper hand hygiene, regardless of the use of gloves, is essential to control the person-to-person transmission of VRE.[46] Because *E. faecium* has been isolated from hands after they were washed with plain soap, it is best to use an antimicrobial soap or a waterless antiseptic agent when caring for patients with VRE.[114]

Laboratory-based surveillance to identify cases. Ongoing surveillance should be conducted so that baseline endemic rates can be determined and potential outbreaks and clusters can be identified quickly. Routine surveillance for VRE is generally conducted by prospective review of laboratory reports for isolates of *Enterococcus* species that are resistant to vancomycin. As is the case with MRSA, not all patients who are colonized or infected will be detected by routine cultures obtained for clinical indications. Once VRE is identified, criteria must be used to determine if the organism is colonizing or infecting the patient and if an infection is community or hospital associated.[47,48] The laboratory should routinely notify patient care and infection control personnel when VRE is isolated so that contact isolation precautions can be implemented promptly. If an outbreak is suspected, laboratory records should be reviewed retrospectively and prospectively to identify both infected and colonized patients, and a line list of hospital-associated (nosocomial) cases should be maintained as discussed in Chapter 8. Both colonized and infected cases should be identified in order to determine the extent of the outbreak.

Surveillance cultures of patients. Point-prevalence culture surveys of patients on high-risk wards have been shown to be useful during VRE outbreaks to identify cases not detected by clinical cultures.[91,103] In an outbreak situation, VRE isolates from infected and colonized patients should be identified to the species level, and antimicrobial sensitivity testing should be done to help determine if the organisms may be epidemiologically related. VRE isolates may also be sent to a reference laboratory for strain typing by genotypic methods, as discussed in Chapter 11.

Education of personnel. Personnel involved in caring for patients with VRE should be given information on the extent of the VRE problem, the epidemiology and mode of transmission of VRE, and the importance of adhering to proper infection control practices with an emphasis on hand hygiene, standard precautions, isolation precautions, and equipment and environmental cleanliness.[25,42,43,46,103]

Contact precautions for infected and colonized patients. Aggressive infection control measures and strict compliance by hospital personnel are needed to limit the nosocomial spread of VRE and are specified in the HICPAC and SHEA guidelines[25,42,46]:

1. Infected and colonized patients should be placed in a single room or in the same room as other patients with VRE.
2. Gloves and a gown should be worn when entering the room because extensive environmental contamination with VRE has been documented in several studies.[43,87,91,110,112,113]
4. Gloves and gowns should be removed before leaving the patient's room.[25]
5. Hands should be washed with an antiseptic soap or cleaned with a waterless antiseptic agent before leaving the patient's room.
6. Noncritical items, such as stethoscopes, sphygmomanometers, and rectal thermometers, should be dedicated to use on patients with VRE; if this is not practical, these items should be cleaned and disinfected before use on other patients.
7. Stool or rectal cultures should be obtained on the roommates of newly identified cases to determine their colonization status and the need for isolation precautions.

If these measures are not effective at limiting nosocomial transmission of VRE, consideration should be given to cohorting patient care personnel to minimize contact of staff with VRE-positive and VRE-negative patients,[88,91,105] personnel should be reeducated on the importance of implementing and adhering to control measures, and verification should be obtained that equipment and environmental surfaces are being adequately cleaned and disinfected. Since personnel carriers have rarely been implicated in the transmission of VRE,[106] culturing of personnel is not generally recommended unless a careful epidemiologic study shows a link between a healthcare worker and cases.

Cleaning and disinfection of equipment and the environment. Because patient care equipment and the environment can play a role in the transmission of VRE, personnel responsible for cleaning and disinfecting patient care equipment and environmental surfaces should be instructed to adhere to hospital procedures. A system for monitoring adherence to cleaning and disinfection protocols should be implemented.[43]

VRE in the Long-Term Care Setting

Epidemiology

There are few published studies that describe the epidemiology of VRE and other multidrug-resistant organisms in LTC facilities. Brennen et al. conducted a 30-month study of vancomycin-resistant *E. faecium* (VREF) in a 400-bed LTC Veterans Administration facility and found 36 patients colonized with VREF.[115] The investigators noted the following: some patients had protracted carriage of VREF; 24 of the 36 patients had VREF at time of transfer from an acute care facility; the risk of VREF infection was low in the population studied; and patient-to-patient transmission of VREF was infrequent when contact precautions were used. Bonilla et al. studied VRE colonization of patients in the medical, intensive care, and LTC units of a Veterans Affairs Medical Center between December 1994 and August 1996.[110] They found that patients in the LTC unit were more likely to be colonized than those in the acute care units; seven different strain types were present; transmission from roommate to roommate was uncommon; environmental contamination with VRE was found in both the long-term and acute care settings; VRE was isolated from the hands of healthcare workers in both settings but personnel in the LTC unit were more likely to have VRE on their hands; and the hands of two healthcare workers remained culture-positive after washing.[110] Prevalence rates of colonization with VRE in LTC facilities range from 1.7% to 6%.[75,116–118] Studies and clinical experience show that patients and residents in both acute care and LTC facilities may be colonized with more than one type of resistant organism, such as MRSA and VRE.[115,117–120]

Previous hospitalization in an acute care facility is a major risk factor for VRE colonization in an LTC facility resident.[109,115] Other risk factors include prior use of antibiotics and the presence of a decubitis ulcer.[118,121] Colonization of wounds and asymptomatic rectal carriage occurs often among patients in acute and LTC settings and may persist for months.[91,104,109,117,122] Most studies of the epidemiology of VRE in LTC facilities were conducted in nursing homes and skilled care facilities, and residents were found to be colonized but not infected. During a 3-month study conducted in a 355-bed LTC facility with a ventilator unit and a subacute care unit, Pacio et al. detected 27 colonized residents, and 6 of these developed a symptomatic urinary tract infection.[75] Although colonization is common, VRE does not appear to be a frequent cause of infection in residents of nursing homes and skilled care facilities,[100,109,115,120,122] and the author was unable to find any published reports of outbreaks of VRE infection in an LTC facility.

The epidemiology of VRE is similar to that of MRSA in that both organisms were initially associated with outbreaks in the acute care setting and both have become endemic in many acute care and LTC facilities. Both VRE and MRSA can be introduced into an acute care or an LTC facility by the transfer of colonized or infected patients and residents who serve as reservoirs for transmission between these two settings.[121,123]

Mode of Transmission

The majority of VRE infections are believed to arise from a person's endogenous flora. The mode of transmission in the LTC setting has not been well studied. In the acute care setting, VRE can be spread from person to person by direct contact or indirectly via contaminated equipment or environmental surfaces[87,104,113] or by transient carriage on healthcare workers' hands.[106] Although extensive environmental contamination with VRE can occur in the LTC setting, especially when a patient has diarrhea or is incontinent, the role of the environment in the transmission of VRE is not clear. Nevertheless, enhanced environmental cleaning has been advocated by many to control the spread of multidrug-resistant organisms.[124] Studies of VRE carriage on the hands of healthcare personnel in the LTC setting are rare; however, Mody et al. found a 9% VRE hand colonization rate in one LTC facility during a study of the use of a new alcohol-based hand rub.[125]

Control Measures

The Long-Term Care Committee of SHEA developed a position paper that outlines the epidemiology and modes of transmission of VRE and provides guidelines for the control of VRE in the LTC setting.[100] The CDC HICPAC guidelines for isolation precautions and guidelines for managing multidrug-resistant organisms also provide recommendations for preventing the transmission of VRE in LTC settings.[25,42] In addition to the SHEA and HICPAC guidelines, many health departments have developed guidelines for controlling the spread of VRE and other multi-drug-resistant organisms in LTC facilities and have posted these on their Web sites.

The following measures, which have been explained in the section on control of VRE in the acute care setting, are recommended to control outbreaks of VRE in the LTC setting:

- An active surveillance program to identify cases (persons colonized or infected with VRE) that includes laboratory-based surveillance (i.e., the review of positive cultures)
- Surveillance cultures of residents if an outbreak is suspected
- Education of personnel at time of hire and periodically thereafter
- Contact isolation and barrier precautions for infected and colonized residents
- Implementation of protocols for cleaning and disinfection of equipment
- Implementation of protocols for cleaning and disinfection of the environment.

Staphylococcus aureus with Reduced Susceptibility to Vancomycin

Only a few isolated infections with *S. aureus* with reduced susceptibility to vancomycin (VRSA and vancomycin-intermediate *S. aureus*, or VISA) have been reported.[126–133] VISA was initially documented in a patient in Japan in 1996,[126] and the first clinical case in the United States occurred in 2002.[127] Subsequent infections have been reported from Asia, Europe, and the United States.[128–133] Because *S. aureus* is one of the most common causes of community-

and hospital-associated infection and is easily transmitted from person to person, the emergence of VRSA will pose serious infection control and public health consequences.[133] Guidelines to prevent the spread of *S. aureus* with reduced susceptibility to vancomycin have been developed by the CDC, and these should be used for reference when developing protocols to prevent the spread of VRSA/VISA.[134]

The following is a summary of measures recommended to prevent transmission of VRSA/VISA[134,135]:

- The laboratory should immediately notify infection prevention and control personnel, the clinical unit, and the attending physician of any *S. aureus* isolates with intermediate or total resistance to vancomycin.
- The patient should be placed in a single room, and contact precautions should be strictly enforced.[25,42,134]
- The number of persons entering the room should be limited to essential personnel—specific healthcare workers should be dedicated to provide one-on-one care whenever possible.
- Infection control personnel should initiate an epidemiologic investigation in conjunction with the state and local health departments and the CDC.
- A written plan for treatment and follow-up of the patient and a contact investigation, including surveillance cultures, should be developed in collaboration with local health departments, healthcare providers, and the CDC.[134]
- Compliance with contact precautions and good hand hygiene should be monitored and strictly enforced.[42,46]
- All personnel involved in direct patient care should be informed of the epidemiologic implications of VRSA/VISA and of the infection control precautions needed to contain it.
- The patient should be restricted to the isolation room except for essential medical purposes.
- Horizontal surfaces in the patient's immediate vicinity should be cleaned daily with a quaternary ammonium compound.
- Dedicated equipment, such as stethoscopes, thermometers, and blood pressure cuffs, should be used for the patient.
- All equipment, such as electrocardiogram and portable X-ray machines, should be disinfected as soon as tests are complete.
- If transfer is necessary, the receiving unit or institution should be informed of the patient's VRSA/VISA status.
- The health department and the CDC should be consulted prior to transferring or discharging the patient.

The occurrence of one case of *S. aureus* with reduced susceptibility to vancomycin (VRSA or VISA) should be considered an outbreak, and infection control measures, including placement of the patient in a private room, implementation of contact isolation precautions, and notification of the local or state health department, should be implemented immediately.

Mycobacterium tuberculosis in Acute Care and Ambulatory Care Settings

Epidemiology

Outbreaks and nosocomial transmission of *Mycobacterium tuberculosis* have long been recognized in the hospital setting.[136-156] Outbreaks have been associated with exposure to an infectious patient or healthcare worker and to cough-inducing and aerosol-producing procedures performed on infectious patients. A hospital outbreak that occurred in Texas in 1983–1984 resulted from exposure in the emergency room to a patient with unrecognized severe cavity tuberculosis (TB).[140] Six employees developed active TB, and an immunocompromised patient was also believed to have developed TB as a result of exposure to the patient. In 2003 a foreign-born nurse who worked in a nursery and maternity unit was diagnosed with acid-fast bacillus (AFB) smear-positive (infectious) tuberculosis.[156] The nurse had been diagnosed with latent TB infection (LTBI) 11 years earlier following a positive tuberculin skin test (TST) done for preemployment screening at the hospital. She declined treatment for LTBI at that time. An investigation revealed that she had likely been infectious for 3 months prior to diagnosis and had potentially exposed 32 co-workers, 613 infants in the newborn nursery, and 900 patients on the maternity unit. Despite extensive efforts to reach potentially exposed persons, only 227 (37%) of the infant contacts and 216 (24%) of the maternity unit contacts could be located and evaluated. Nineteen maternity unit patients with prior negative TST results and four infants were found to have a positive TST. Twenty-five of the 32 potentially exposed co-workers (78%) had documentation of a prior positive TST result and none had taken treatment for LTBI. None of the co-workers had symptoms of TB, and all were offered LTBI treatment; however, all declined. The remaining seven co-workers had negative TST results.

While many reported nosocomial outbreaks in hospitals have been associated with the close contact of patients and personnel to a person with unrecognized infectious TB, several epidemics have been associated with diagnostic and therapeutic procedures such as bronchoscopy,[138] endotracheal intubation and suctioning,[139] irrigation of an open abscess,[141] autopsy,[142-144] and sputum induction and aerosol treatments.[146] An outbreak in a Florida primary care health clinic was associated with sputum induction and aerosolized treatment of a patient with human immunodeficiency virus (HIV) infection.[145] This outbreak most likely could have been avoided if cough-inducing procedures such as aerosolized pentamidine and sputum induction had been carried out using either local exhaust ventilation, such as a booth or special enclosure, or a room meeting the ventilation requirements for TB isolation.[157] An outbreak in a drug treatment center was associated with a client with unrecognized pulmonary disease even though the client had a history of TB when admitted to the facility. Because the treatment center had no health screening program in place, no precautions were taken to prevent the transmission of *M. tuberculosis* from the new client.[151]

In New York an outbreak of multidrug-resistant tuberculosis (MDR-TB) in a hospital occurred despite that fact that the source patient was suspected of having pulmonary TB, was promptly placed in an isolation room, and personnel followed the hospital's TB protocol.[152] An investigation revealed that the ventilation system in some of the isolation rooms was not at negative pressure in relation to the corridor.

Since 1993, the overall incidence of tuberculosis in the United States has been declining, and in 2006 it reached the lowest number and rate of reported TB cases since measurement began in 1953.[158] However, the number of healthcare workers in the United States that are from foreign countries where TB is endemic is growing, and this growth is expected to continue to fill healthcare workers shortages.[159] Since many foreign-born healthcare workers with positive TST results do not receive treatment for LTBI, the potential for the development of TB disease in healthcare workers may increase.[156]

Mycobacterium tuberculosis in Long-Term Care Settings

Epidemiology

The endemic and epidemic transmission of *M. tuberculosis* among residents in LTC settings has long been recognized.[160–170] A study conducted by the CDC in 1984–1985 found that elderly nursing home residents were at greater risk for TB than elderly persons living in the community.[171] Outbreaks of TB in nursing homes have affected both residents and staff.[161,165–168,172] In one outbreak a highly infectious resident with unrecognized cavitary TB infected 30% (49/161) of previously TST-negative residents, eight of whom developed pulmonary TB, and 15% (21/138) of tuberculin-negative employees, one of whom developed TB.[161] The outbreak investigation revealed that the resident was an outgoing man who participated in social activities at the nursing home and who had probably been infectious for close to a year. In most of the outbreaks reported in the literature, the source for nosocomial transmission in LTC facilities is a resident with unrecognized pulmonary TB.

Ijaz et al. reported an outbreak whose source was determined to be a nursing home patient with unrecognized pulmonary TB that resulted in transmission to residents and personnel in two nursing homes and a hospital, including a nurse in the hospital who developed a tuberculous cervical abscess and a nursing home employee and a visitor that developed pulmonary TB.[172]

Multidrug-Resistant and Extensively Drug-Resistant *Mycobacterium tuberculosis*

Although drug resistance in *Mycobacterium tuberculosis* has been noted since shortly after the introduction of antituberculosis drugs, during the 1990s multidrug-resistant strains spread worldwide and have caused outbreaks in healthcare facilities. MDR-TB is TB that demonstrates resistance to at least isoniazid (INH) and rifampin, two first-line antituberculosis drugs. Several well-publicized hospital outbreaks of MDR-TB in the United States occurred among HIV-infected patients and healthcare workers in the early 1990s.[136,137,144,149] These outbreaks reflected the increased incidence of TB that occurred in many U.S. communities from 1988 through 1992. Factors that contributed to these outbreaks of MDR-TB included the following:[136]

- Delayed identification of patients with MDR-TB
- Delayed treatment of patients with MDR-TB
- Lack of proper isolation of patients with infectious MDR-TB
- Failure to keep patients in their isolation room
- Failure of patients to wear a mask when they were outside of their isolation room
- Inadequate respiratory protection for healthcare workers
- Inadequate environmental controls such as negative air pressure rooms

Between 2000 and 2006 extensively resistant strains of *M. tuberculosis* emerged worldwide.[173–175] XDR-TB is "TB showing resistance to at least rifampicin and isoniazid, which is the definition of MDR-TB, in addition to any fluoroquinolone, and to at least 1 of the 3 following injectable drugs used in anti-TB treatment: capreomycin, kanamycin, and amikacin."[176] XDR-TB presents a global health problem because it is difficult to treat and has a high mortality rate. The mode of transmission of MDR-TB and XDR-TB are the same as that of drug-sensitive strains of *M. tuberculosis*.

Mode of Transmission

M. tuberculosis is spread via the airborne route by droplet nuclei, particles that are produced when persons with pulmonary or laryngeal TB sneeze, cough, speak, or sing. Droplet nuclei are approximately 1–5 µm in size, have the ability to remain suspended in air for prolonged periods, and can be carried through a building on air currents.[157] Infection occurs when a susceptible person inhales these particles into the lungs.

Control Measures for Mycobacterium tuberculosis *in Healthcare Settings*

Guidelines for preventing the transmission of *M. tuberculosis* in healthcare settings have been published by the CDC,[157] the World Health Organization (WHO),[177,178] U.S. state health departments,[179] professional associations,[180] and public health agencies and coalitions worldwide.[181–184] The 2005 CDC *Guidelines for Preventing the Transmission of* Mycobacterium tuberculosis *in Health-Care Settings* provide a comprehensive discussion of TB in a variety of care settings, including inpatient, ambulatory and LTC, and includes forms and checklists for a TB prevention program (http://www.cdc.gov/mmwr/PDF/rr/rr5417.pdf. Accessed April 18, 2008).[157] These guidelines state that all healthcare settings need a "TB infection control program designed to ensure prompt detection, airborne precautions, and treatment of persons who have suspected or confirmed TB disease (or prompt referral of persons who have suspected TB disease for settings in which persons with TB disease are not expected to be encountered)."[157(p7)] They focus on measures that have been shown to prevent nosocomial transmission and present a three-level hierarchy of controls: administrative, environmental, and respiratory protection as shown in Exhibit 7–1.[157] SHEA published a position paper on prevention and control of TB in LTC facilities for older adults.[180] The SHEA position paper contains detailed information on the clinical presentation and management of TB in the elderly and provides recommendations for systematic screening of residents and personnel, diagnosis of active disease, and treatment of TB disease and latent TB infection in this population.

The first step in the development of a TB infection prevention and control program is an assessment of the risk of transmission of *M. tuberculosis* in each specific healthcare setting. A TB Risk Assessment Worksheet and the resulting TB Risk Classifications for Health-Care Settings can be found in the 2005 CDC guidelines.[157]

Because outbreaks of TB, especially those caused by MDR-TB, can result in significant morbidity and mortality, organizations should ensure that infection prevention and control measures that are appropriate for each healthcare setting are implemented. Regardless of the setting or the risk of transmission for *M. tuberculosis*, the most important measures for controlling the spread of TB are prompt identification and adequate treatment of persons with TB.[182]

Based on the results of the risk assessment for the likelihood of transmission of *M. tuberculosis* in a healthcare setting, the elements that should be considered for inclusion in a TB prevention and control program are discussed in the following sections.

Surveillance program and record-keeping system. All healthcare settings should have a surveillance program for the early identification of persons (patients, residents, personnel, and visitors) with signs and symptoms suggestive of pulmonary TB. Persons with signs and symptoms should receive prompt radiologic and bacteriologic evaluation. The surveillance program should include a mechanism for reporting all cases of TB to the health department. A record-keeping system should be developed to track and assess the facility's experience regarding TB infection and TB disease and should include TST results on patients, residents, and personnel and any follow-up performed. These records should be stored in a computerized retrievable database to allow ready access to obtain information for the periodic risk assessment or a contact investigation.

Isolation precautions. Persons with known or suspected TB should be promptly placed on airborne precautions in an airborne isolation room.[42] Personnel and patients must adhere to airborne isolation precautions: personnel must wear a respirator when entering, and patients must wear a mask when leaving the isolation room.[42] In the LTC setting, residents with suspected or confirmed infectious TB may remain in the setting if an airborne isolation room and a respiratory protection program for personnel are in place. If these are not available, then the resident must be transferred to another healthcare setting. In the outpatient setting, patients with known or suspected TB should be placed in a separate waiting area if no isolation room is available. They should be given a surgical mask and a box of tissues and should be instructed how to wear the mask and to use the tissues when coughing or sneezing. Because covering the mouth while coughing can reduce the number of tubercle bacilli expelled into the air, this simple intervention should not be overlooked.

Screening program for patients and residents of long-term care settings. There should be a screening program for patients and residents of LTC settings established according to evidenced-based guidelines.[157,183] As of this

Exhibit 7–1   Three-Level Hierarchy of Controls to Prevent Transmission
of *Mycobacterium tuberculosis* in Healthcare Settings

Administrative Controls	*Environmental Controls*
Assign responsibility for TB infection control in the setting	Primary environmental controls:
Conduct a TB risk assessment of the setting	Control the source of infection by using local exhaust ventilation (e.g., hoods, tents, or booths)
Develop and institute a written TB infection-control plan to ensure prompt detection, airborne precautions, and treatment of persons who have suspected or confirmed TB disease	Dilute and remove contaminated air by using general ventilation Secondary environmental controls:
Ensure the timely availability of recommended laboratory processing, testing, and reporting of results to the ordering physician and infection control team	Control the airflow to prevent contamination of air in areas adjacent to the source (airborne infection isolation rooms)
Implement effective work practices for the management of patients with suspected or confirmed TB disease	Clean the air by using high-efficiency particulate air filtration or ultraviolet germicidal irradiation.
Ensure proper cleaning and sterilization or disinfection of potentially contaminated equipment (usually endoscopes)	*Respiratory Protection Controls*
Train and educate healthcare workers regarding TB, with specific focus on prevention, transmission, and symptoms	Implement a respiratory protection program Train healthcare workers on respiratory protection
Screen and evaluate healthcare workers who are at risk for TB disease or who might be exposed to *M. tuberculosis* (i.e., TB screening program)	Train patients on respiratory hygiene and cough etiquette procedures
Apply epidemiologic-based prevention principles, including the use of setting-related infection-control data	
Use appropriate signage advising respiratory hygiene and cough etiquette	
Coordinate efforts with the local or state health department	

Source: Centers for Disease Control and Prevention. Guidelines for preventing the transmission of
Mycobacterium tuberculosis in health-care settings, 2005. *MMWR*. 2005;54(RR-17):1–141.

writing, the blood assay for *Mycobacterium tuberculosis* (BAMT) had not been recommended for use in the elderly.[185] The TST program should include administration and reading of the skin test at the time of admission and periodically thereafter, depending on the risk assessment and local jurisdiction rules and requirements. Residents that convert from TST-negative to TST-positive should have a chest radiograph and should be treated for LTBI if the radiograph is negative. If the radiograph is suggestive for TB, a medical evaluation, including sputum smear and culture for AFB, must be done.[183] Studies have shown that many LTC facilities lack an adequate surveillance program.[164,186] The mere existence of a TST program will not prevent TB outbreaks. In order for a skin-testing program to be effective, action must be taken based on the results of screening. This means that those who are found to be newly infected should be medically evaluated and given appropriate therapy, when indicated, to prevent the development of disease, and a search for the index case (i.e., the source of infection) should be conducted to prevent further transmission.

Screening program for patients and clients at risk for TB. In the inpatient and ambulatory care settings, there should be a screening program that includes use of a TST or BAMT for patients and clients at risk for TB (e.g., intravenous drug users and clients in drug treatment programs).[157,183–185]

Screening program for personnel. A screening program, including use of a TST or BAMT, should be implemented for personnel with occupational exposure to *M. tuberculosis*.[157,183–185] Personnel who are found to be TST-positive and have LTBI should be encouraged to accept and complete treatment. Failure to do so can result in progression to TB disease and exposure of patients, residents, co-workers, family, and others to *M. tuberculosis*.[156] Personnel that convert from TST-negative to TST-positive should have a chest radiograph and should be provided treatment for latent TB infection if the radiograph is negative. If the radiograph is suggestive for TB, a medical evaluation, including sputum smear and culture for AFB, must be done.[157,184]

Treatment of persons with TB disease. Prompt and effective treatment of persons who have clinical disease should be given in accordance with the latest public health service recommendations.[187,188] An infectious disease specialist should be consulted prior to administering antituberculosis therapy. Residents and patients who are given antituberculosis medications should be observed swallowing each dose to ensure that they are complying with therapy. (Note: There is no consensus on how long a patient who is sputum smear-positive for AFB should remain in isolation after treatment has begun. Several articles discuss the potential contagiousness of persons with active pulmonary TB;[189,190] however, relatively little is known about how long tubercle bacilli in the sputum remain infectious after effective therapy has been started. After reviewing the literature, Menzies concluded that "after initiation of therapy, patients who are still smear-positive should be considered still contagious."[189(p585)])

Contact investigation and management program for exposed persons. Whenever a person is diagnosed with infectious pulmonary TB (e.g., the person is coughing and has positive AFB sputum smears and an abnormal chest radiography compatible with TB), a contact investigation should be conducted. All close contacts, including those who care for, sleep, live, work, or share a common ventilation system for prolonged periods, should be screened for evidence of infection. Guidelines for investigating contacts have been published;[191] however, the local health department should be consulted for guidance. Contacts that have a documented skin test conversion, no clinical signs or symptoms of TB, and a negative chest radiograph should be diagnosed with LTBI and provided treatment for LTBI unless medically contraindicated.[191] Persons who refuse treatment for LTBI should be instructed to promptly seek medical evaluation if they develop signs or symptoms compatible with TB, such as a persistent cough, weight loss, fatigue, anorexia, or night sweats. Residents in LTC settings who are close contacts of an infectious person but who are not given prophylaxis should be carefully observed for the development of symptoms consistent with TB. Older patients, specially the frail elderly residents of nursing homes, have reduced reactivity to the TST and this must be kept in mind when conducting contact investigations. TB can cause significant morbidity and mortality in the LTC setting. Because healthcare workers and residents with exposure and documented TST conversion have developed clinical disease, it is important that preventive therapy be taken.[161,166] The author is personally aware of a nurse who converted from TST-negative to TST-positive following inadvertent occupational exposure to a patient with TB and who refused INH treatment. Six months later, the nurse developed infectious pulmonary TB and exposed family, friends, co-workers, and patients to *M. tuberculosis*.

Education. Regardless of the setting's risk for transmission of TB, training should be provided to healthcare providers about the signs and symptoms of TB and the control measures that should be implemented for suspected and known cases. The medical and nursing staffs should be instructed to remain alert for typical and atypical presentation of clinical disease, especially in the elderly, so that evaluation and treatment can be promptly initiated. Information on educational materials and training programs about TB can be found in the Resources section at the end of this chapter.

If TB is present in the community served, a screening program for personnel, patients, and residents is an integral part of an organization's overall infection control program and is essential for detecting unrecognized infection with *M. tuberculosis* and preventing the development of disease.

Clostridium difficile

Epidemiology

Clostridium difficile is a major healthcare-associated pathogen that can cause diarrhea, antibiotic-associated colitis, and pseudomembranous colitis in hospitalized patients and residents of LTC facilities. It is considered to be the most common cause of healthcare-associated infectious diarrhea.[42,192] The epidemiology of *C. difficile* is changing. Between 1996 and 2003 the incidence of *C. difficile*-associated disease (CDAD) increased in patients discharged from US hospitals.[193] In the early 2000s a new hypervirulent strain of *C. difficile* caused widespread hospital outbreaks in Canada that were associated with severe morbidity and increased mortality.[194] This more virulent strain is refractory to standard therapy, has emerged in several countries, and has caused healthcare-associated outbreaks in the United States, the United Kingdom, and Europe.[195–201]

A small percentage of healthy adults carry *C. difficile* in their gastrointestinal tract,[200] and neonates and infants are frequently asymptomatically colonized with *C. difficile*. Colonization rates in hospitalized adults and residents of LTC facilities vary widely.[202,203] Reported incidence rates of diarrhea caused by *C. difficile* in hospitals range from 1 to 30 cases per 1000 patient discharges and in nursing homes from 17 to 60 cases per 100,000 bed-days.[204–206] Nosocomial CDAD in adults is responsible for significant morbidity, increased length of stay, and rare fatalities in the acute and LTC settings.[196,207–210] Diarrhea can lead to volume depletion and wound infection and can significantly increase medical costs. Although the major risk factor for nosocomial CDAD is previous antibiotic therapy, other factors that have been found to increase the risk of disease include previous hospitalization, older age, hypoalbuminemia, leukemia and/or lymphoma, mechanical ventilation, surgery, and receipt of antimotility drugs, histamine-2 blockers, and proton pump inhibitors.[211] Traditionally considered to be associated with hospitals, CDAD has been increasingly recognized in persons who had no previous contact with the healthcare system.[212]

Once thought to arise solely from endogenous flora, it is now clear that nosocomial acquisition of *C. difficile* occurs, and outbreaks and clusters of CDAD have been reported in acute care hospitals,[199,202,204,210] skilled nursing facilities, geriatric units of hospitals, and rehabilitation hospitals.[213–219] When determining if a cluster or an outbreak exists in a healthcare setting, one of the first steps in the investigation is the development of a clear case definition. Clinical criteria for the diagnosis of CDAD are generally based on a combination of clinical and laboratory criteria. There is currently no nationally standardized clinical or surveillance definition for CDAD. In reviewing the literature it is clear that not all investigators use the same criteria for defining a case of CDAD. A following case definition is useful for surveillance and classification of hospital-acquired CDAD (published by the Canadian Nosocomial Infection Surveillance Program)[220]:

1. Diarrhea* or fever, abdominal pain, and/or ileus *and* laboratory confirmation of a positive toxin assay for *C. difficile*;

or

2. Diagnosis of pseudomembranes on sigmoidoscopy or colonoscopy, or histological/pathological diagnosis of CDAD.

*Diarrhea will be defined as one of the following: six watery stools in past 36 hours, three unformed stools in 24 hours for 2 days, or eight unformed stools over 48 hours.

The infection will be considered hospital-acquired if it meets the following criteria:

1. Patient's symptoms occur at least 72 hours after current admission.

or

2. Symptoms cause readmission in a patient who had been hospitalized within the previous 2 months of the current admission date, and who is not resident in a chronic care hospital or nursing home.

A variety of surveillance definitions for *C. difficile*, including healthcare facility-onset and community-onset, were published in 2007 by an ad hoc surveillance working group:[221]

A CDAD case is defined as a case of diarrhea (i.e., unformed stool that conforms to the shape of a specimen collection container) or toxic megacolon (i.e., abnormal dilation of the large intestine documented radiologically) without other known etiology that meets 1 or more of the following criteria: (1) the stool sample yields a positive result for a laboratory assay for C. difficile toxin A and/or B, or a toxin-producing C. difficile organism is detected in the stool sample by culture or other means; (2) pseudomembranous colitis is seen during endoscopic examination or surgery; and (3) pseudomembranous colitis is seen during histopathological examination.

A patient classified as having healthcare facility-onset, healthcare facility-associated CDAD is defined as a patient with CDAD symptom onset more than 48 hours after admission to an healthcare facility.

Clostridium difficile is a gram positive spore-forming bacillus. Its spores resist heat and drying, can persist in the environment for prolonged periods, and are resistant to commonly used disinfectants and antiseptics.[42,202] Environmental contamination of equipment, clothing, and the area surrounding *C. difficile*-infected patients and residents has long been recognized, and multiple strains may be isolated from the environment.[202–204,222,223] These factors, and the association of CDAD with antibiotic use, make outbreaks of *C. difficile* difficult to control.[42]

Mode of Transmission

Nosocomial acquisition and transmission via cross-infection has been demonstrated by molecular typing and fingerprinting.[203,202,210] The major reservoir for *C. difficile* is infected and colonized patients and residents, and newly admitted colonized patients have been responsible for introducing the organism into a hospital.[224] The mode of transmission is thought to be via the hands of personnel and contaminated equipment and devices.[42,202] *C. difficile* spores are readily found in the environment surrounding patients with CDAD. It is likely that environmental surface contamination and contaminated items, such as commodes and electronic thermometers, play a role in the transmission of *C. difficile* although that role is not clearly defined.[225–228]

Control Measures

Recommendations for preventing endemic and epidemic transmission of *C. difficile* in the acute and LTC settings have been published by SHEA,[229] Mc Farland et al.,[202] and the CDC HICPAC.[42,230] There are two major approaches for preventing healthcare-associated CDAD: (1) interrupting the transmission of *C. difficile* and thus preventing the patient or resident from acquiring the organism, and (2) promoting appropriate use of antibiotics to reduce an individual's risk of developing disease.

The global emergence of a fluroroquinolone-resistant, hypervirulent strain of *C. difficile* highlights the need to implement effective infection prevention and control programs to interrupt the transmission of this epidemiologically important organism. Control measures that have been effectively used to prevent nosocomial acquisition and to interrupt outbreaks include the following:

- Timely and accurate identification of patients and residents with CDAD
- Use of contact precautions that includes donning gown and gloves when entering the room of a person with CDAD. This helps to avoid transmission of *C. difficile* to hands and clothing from contact with the patient or the patient's contaminated environment, especially when handling feces and fecally contaminated items.[42,231]
- Either cohorting or providing a private room for persons with CDAD, especially for incontinent persons
- Hand washing with soap and water to mechanically remove *Clostridium* spores. Hand washing is the preferred method for hand hygiene when caring for persons with CDAD because alcohol hand rubs appear to have limited activity against spores.[42,46]
- Adherence to rigorous environmental cleaning and disinfection practices. *C. difficile* is resistant to many commonly used germicides.[232] Therefore, to control an outbreak most investigators recommend meticulous cleaning of the patient's room, especially fecally contaminated and high-touch surfaces, followed by disinfection with an agent that contains bleach or a 1:10 dilution of 5.25% sodium hypochlorite (household bleach) and water.[42,203,233]
- Use of disposable rectal thermometers. Several studies have shown that eliminating the use of electronic thermometers can reduce the incidence of CDAD.[234–236]

Because prior exposure to antibiotics is the major risk factor for disease, the most important control measure that can be used to reduce the risk of CDAD is the prudent use and restriction of antimicrobial agents.[237]

An active surveillance program must be in place in order to recognize clusters or outbreaks of CDAD.[42] Recommendations for surveillance programs for *C. difficile* have been published by Mylotte[238] and by a *C. difficile* Surveillance Working Group.[221] Mylotte described an easily conducted laboratory surveillance method that is based on the review of *C. difficile* stool toxin assays and is similar to the surveillance method that is used in many hospitals.[238]

Influenza Virus

Epidemiology

Influenza is characterized by abrupt onset of fever, chills, headache, severe malaise and myalgia, and by respiratory symptoms such as nonproductive cough, sore throat, and rhinitis.[239] It causes significant morbidity and mortality worldwide. In the United States and other countries with temperate climates, epidemics of influenza usually occur during the winter months, usually December through April. Outbreaks in the community can result in introduction of the virus into a healthcare setting by personnel, visitors, or newly admitted or transferred patients or residents.[240,241] Once introduced into a population, influenza can spread rapidly because it is highly contagious and has a fairly short incubation period, typically ranging from 1 to 4 days and averaging 2 days. Adults are considered infectious from the day prior to onset of symptoms through the fifth day after illness begins.[239] Persons over 65 years and those of any age with certain medical conditions, such as pulmonary and cardiovascular disorders, are at risk for complications and death from influenza.[239]

Although nosocomial transmission of influenza has been reported in both acute care[242-247] and LTC facilities,[248-256] outbreaks of influenza have been more commonly reported in the LTC setting. In the LTC setting, influenza has been shown to be spread from resident to resident,[248] from healthcare personnel to residents,[249,253] from residents to healthcare personnel, and among healthcare personnel.[257] Influenza outbreaks in LTC settings can result in considerable morbidity and mortality, with clinical attack rates as high as 70% and mortality rates averaging over 10%.[258] In one nursing home outbreak the attack rate among residents was 28% (11/39) with a 55% case-fatality rate.[249] Although most infected persons exhibit respiratory symptoms, asymptomatic infection can occur.

Mode of Transmission

Influenza is easily transmitted from person-to-person primarily through large-particle respiratory droplets, such as those produced when an infected person coughs or sneezes. Influenza transmission can also occur through contact with surfaces contaminated by respiratory secretions and via inhalation of small particles of evaporated droplets that can remain suspended in the air for an extended period of time.[239,259]

Control Measures

Recommendations and guidelines for preventing transmission of influenza in healthcare settings have been published by the CDCC,[42,50,239,260-262] the Association for Professionals in Infection Control and Epidemiology and SHEA,[263] Gravenstein et al.,[264] Gomolin et al.,[265] Kingston and Wright,[266] the WHO,[267] and many state health departments.[268,269] The most important measure for controlling transmission of influenza in the healthcare setting is annual immunization of all patients for whom the vaccine is recommended, all residents and patients of LTC settings, and healthcare workers.[260,262] It should be noted that, although studies have shown that immunization of residents in a LTC facility reduces the risk of transmission of influenza, outbreaks have been reported in nursing homes that had highly immunized populations.[251,253]

In addition to immunization, influenza-specific antiviral drugs (such as amantadine and rimantadine) are important components of an influenza prevention and control program.[260] Amantadine and rimantadine have been shown to be effective in preventing illness from influenza A when used as prophylaxis in healthy adults and children. In addition, these drugs can reduce the duration and severity of illness when they are used to treat persons with influenza A.[260] Emergence of amantadine/rimantadine-resistant strains of influenza virus have been reported when these drugs are used for therapy, so it is important to periodically perform susceptibility tests on influenza isolates to detect resistance.[270,271]

The following measures are recommended to reduce the risk of transmission of influenza in healthcare settings:

- Develop and implement an influenza prevention and control program based on published recommendations.[42,260–263]

- Conduct routine surveillance for respiratory illness, especially during flu season, to identify patients, residents, and personnel with influenza-like symptoms. Routine surveillance programs are essential to detect residents and personnel with influenza-like illness so control measures can be promptly instituted.[42,267]

- Institute a respiratory hygiene/cough etiquette program targeted to all persons who enter a healthcare setting, including healthcare personnel, patients, residents, and visitors. For instance, ask persons who are coughing to wear a surgical mask or cover their coughs with tissues.[42] (See Resources section at the end of this chapter.)

- Promptly institute droplet precautions for patients and residents suspected of having influenza. This includes restricting the resident or patient to his or her room during the period of greatest communicability (at least 3 days after onset of symptoms) or cohorting ill residents or patients, when possible, if private rooms are not available.[42,261]

- Implement an annual influenza immunization campaign aimed at increasing healthcare worker influenza vaccination acceptance and preventing an outbreak.[260,262,263]

- Annually vaccinate residents and patients in LTC settings. To avoid delay in providing vaccine to residents who may not be able to give consent, LTC facilities should obtain consent for vaccination from the resident or the healthcare decision maker at the time of admission to the facility. Ideally, all residents should be vaccinated annually at the same time, immediately preceding the influenza season. Residents who are admitted after completion of the annual vaccination program should be vaccinated at the time of their admission if they have not yet been immunized.[261,264]

- Document the influenza vaccination status of healthcare providers in all healthcare settings and residents and patients in LTC settings. This will allow rapid identification of unvaccinated individuals because these persons should be encouraged to receive the vaccine in the event of an outbreak. Store this information in a computer database so it can be easily accessed.

- Educate personnel on the signs and symptoms of influenza, the safety and efficacy of the influenza vaccine, and the importance of not coming to work if they have an influenza-like illness.[260,263]

In the event of an outbreak of influenza or influenza-like illness in a health-care setting, the following additional control measures are recommended:

- Report the outbreak to the health department. Some states require reporting of outbreaks of acute lower respiratory illness, including influenza, to the health department.

- Use a standardized case definition to identify persons with influenza-like illness. The Maryland Department of Health and Mental Hygiene guidelines for investigating influenza outbreaks in LTC facilities define an outbreak as one laboratory-proven case of influenza or three or more clinically-defined cases occurring in a facility within a 7-day period between October 1 and May 31.[269]

- Use rapid laboratory tests for influenza, such as the immunofluorescence assay or the enzyme immunoassay to confirm the diagnosis and establish the existence of an outbreak.[265]

- Offer influenza vaccine to any unvaccinated residents, patients, or health-care workers.[260]

- Administer antiviral agents such as amantadine or rimantadine to all well and ill residents and patients in an LTC setting. Follow the latest published public health recommendations.[260]

- Offer viral chemoprophylaxis (e.g., amantadine and rimantadine) to unvaccinated healthcare personnel for the duration of influenza activity or vaccinate unimmunized personnel and provide chemoprophylaxis for 2 weeks after vaccination (i.e., until immunity develops from the vaccination).[260]

- Develop a line listing of residents and healthcare workers with suspected influenza (see Appendix G. Appendix G is available for download at this text's Web site: http://www.jbpub.com/catalog/9780763757793/).

- Collect viral cultures on a representative number of cases to identify the strain of virus responsible for the outbreak.

- Consider closing the affected units to new admissions.

- Discourage visitors with influenza-like illness from visiting. Post signs at the entrances of the facility.

Additional Information on Seasonal Influenza

Much information on seasonal influenza is available on the Web sites of national and local public health departments. Excellent information on seasonal influenza, including guidelines for prevention and control of influenza and information for healthcare providers, can be obtained from the CDC influenza Web site at http://www.cdc.gov/flu.

Appendix G contains the Maryland Department of Health and Mental Hygiene "Guidelines for the Prevention and Control of Upper and Lower Acute Respiratory Illnesses (including Influenza and Pneumonia) in Long-Term Care Facilities" that contain information on preventing, detecting, investigating, and controlling an influenza outbreak and includes a form for documenting influenza vaccine administration, information on laboratory tests that can be used to confirm a clinical diagnosis of influenza, and respiratory illness questionnaires for residents and employees. Appendix G is available for download at this text's Website: http://www.jbpub.com/catalog/9980763757793.

Pandemic Influenza and Avian Influenza

A thorough discussion of pandemic influenza and avian influenza is beyond the scope of this text. However, it is important to note that widespread regional and pandemic outbreaks of influenza will affect all healthcare settings. At this time it is unlikely that enough vaccine, prophylactic medication, and personal protective equipment will be available for all who may be exposed during a pandemic. Therefore, it is imperative that those who are responsible for infection control programs in any healthcare setting ensure that their setting has a pandemic response and management plan. This plan should be updated as new information becomes available and should be integrated with local and regional healthcare institutions and public health services.

Much has published on pandemic and avian influenza, including guidelines and plans for response and emergency management. For more information, the reader is referred to national, international, state, and local public health agencies and their Web sites. Examples of Web sites with avian and pandemic influenza prevention and control information for healthcare settings include the following:

Centers for Disease Control and Prevention
> Avian Influenza (Bird Flu): http://www.cdc.gov/flu/avian/
>
> Prevention of Avian Influenza: http://www.cdc.gov/flu/avian/prevention.htm
>
> Emergency Preparedness and Response: http://www.bt.cdc.gov/preparedness/

U.S. Department of Health and Human Services
> PandemicFlu.gov: http://www.pandemicflu.gov
>
> Pandemic Flu Mitigation and Response: http://www.pandemicflu.gov/plan/community/mitigation.html

World Health Organization
> Influenza: http://www.who.int/csr/disease/influenza/en/
>
> Epidemic and Pandemic Alert and Response: http://www.who.int/csr/disease/influenza/en/
>
> WHO Global Influenza Preparedness Plan: http://www.who.int/csr/resources/publications/influenza/WHO_CDS_CSR_GIP_2005_5/en/index.html
>
> WHO Infection prevention and control in health care for preparedness and response to outbreaks: http://www.who.int/csr/bioriskreduction/infection_control/en/

All sites were accessed January 11, 2008.

Norovirus

Epidemiology

In the early 1990s, diagnostic assays using molecular techniques were developed to detect viral agents of gastroenteritis. The use of these tests has led to the recognition that noroviruses, formerly known as "Norwalk-like viruses," are the most common cause of acute nonbacterial gastroenteritis.[272] Noroviruses are highly contagious and are a frequent cause of outbreaks in healthcare settings worldwide, especially in hospitals and LTC facilities that care for the elderly.[273–288]

The incubation period for norovirus-associated gastroenteritis is short, 12 to 48 hours, with a median of approximately 33 hours.[282] Symptoms usually last from 12–60 hours and include acute-onset vomiting; watery, nonbloody diarrhea; abdominal cramps; nausea; myalgia; malaise; and headache.[282] Infected persons can remain infectious for several days after symptoms resolve.[289] The most common complication of illness is dehydration, and this may be severe enough to require intravenous replacement fluids.

Outbreaks in nursing homes and hospitals spread rapidly, can result in attack rates over 50%,[290,291] and can cause significant morbidity and mortality,[282] loss of revenue, staff shortages, and disruption of services.[275,277,279,281] Most reported outbreaks in healthcare settings affect patients, residents, and personnel,[275,277,279] and some have also involved visitors and family and friends of personnel.[279] Many outbreak are linked to ill food service workers.[274,292]

Because viral diagnostic and molecular tests are infrequently performed during many outbreaks in healthcare settings, the CDC has published the following criteria that can be used to identify if the likely cause of an outbreak is norovirus:

> An acute gastroenteritis outbreak is "considered consistent with norovirus if all of the following criteria are met: (1) vomiting in >50% of affected persons, (2) mean or median incubation period of 24–48 hours, (3) mean or median illness duration of 12–60 hours, and (4) no bacterial pathogens isolated from stool culture."[282(p846)]

Mode of Transmission

Noroviruses are transmitted primarily via the fecal-oral route and can be spread by direct person-to-person contact or via contaminated food, water, environmental surfaces, and fomites.[42,289] Droplet transmission also occurs via aerosolization of vomitus that can result in contamination of environmental surfaces and food.[42,279,280,282,293] Because noroviruses have a low infectious dose, less than 100 viral particles, they are easily transmitted from person to person and via contaminated food, items, and environmental surfaces.[289]

Noroviruses can cause extensive environmental contamination because they are relatively resistant to commonly used disinfectants and to freezing and heating and are able to survive for prolonged periods on environmental surfaces.[42,291] In the healthcare setting, transmission can occur by transferring the virus to the oral mucosa via hands that are contaminated after touching items and environmental surfaces contaminated with feces or vomitus. Wu et al. hypothesized that prolonged shedding of the virus in the feces, along with resident factors such as dementia, incontinence, and immobility, contributed to extensive environmental contamination in a prolonged norovirus outbreak that had a high attack rate in residents and personnel in a 240-bed veterans LTC facility.[291]

Control Measures

Noroviruses can spread rapidly from person to person, and outbreaks are difficult to control. Recommendations for controlling and preventing the transmission of noroviruses have been published by the CDC[42,289] and public health agencies[294,295] and in reports of outbreaks.[296] The following measures are recommended to prevent transmission of noroviruses in healthcare settings and to control an outbreak:

- Establish a surveillance system to allow early detection of a cluster or outbreak of gastrointestinal illness in patients, residents, and personnel.
- Enforce frequent and thorough hand hygiene by personnel, patients, residents, and visitors, especially when leaving an ill patient's room.
- Restrict ill personnel from work, especially from direct patient care and food handling, until 48 hours after vomiting and diarrhea resolve.
- Ensure that food handlers practice strict personal hygiene at all times and do not work if they have vomiting or diarrhea.
- Use contact precautions for persons with suspected norovirus infection including[42]:
  - Gloves and gowns when entering rooms with symptomatic patients
  - Mask if patient has uncontrolled diarrhea or vomiting and when cleaning up vomit and feces
  - Placement of infected patients and residents in a private room or cohort when an outbreak occurs
  - Restriction of ill residents in LTC facilities to their room and from participating in group activities until 48 hours after vomiting and diarrhea resolve
- Establish enhanced cleaning and disinfection protocols during an outbreak including:
  - Requirement to wear gloves, gowns, and surgical masks when cleaning
  - Prompt cleaning and disinfection of soiled environmental surfaces and equipment, especially toilet areas
  - Enhanced cleaning and disinfection of commonly touched surfaces such as bedrails, door knobs, and handrails
  - Use of chlorine bleach for environmental disinfection. Most authorities recommend that chlorine bleach be used to disinfect hard, non-porous, environmental surfaces at a minimum concentration of 1000 ppm (generally a dilution 1 part household bleach solution to 50 parts water). Healthcare personnel should use appropriate personal protection, such as gloves and goggles, when working with bleach.
  - As an alternative to bleach, use of a disinfectant registered by the US Environmental Protection Agency (EPA) as effective against norovirus.[297] Lists of EPA-approved disinfectants can be found on the EPA Web site at http://www.epa.gov/oppad001/chemregindex.htm. However, there is controversy as to whether or not nonchlorine disinfectants will inactivate norovirus.

- Limit sharing of equipment or ensure that equipment is cleaned and disinfected before use on another patient.

- Handle soiled linens and clothing as little as possible to avoid aerosolization of the virus.

Additional information on prevention and control measures for noroviruses can be found in the references noted at the beginning of this section,[42,289,293,294,295] in the Resources at the end of this chapter, and in Appendix H (Appendix H is available for download at this text's web site: http://www .jbpub.com/catalog/9780763757793/).

PARASITIC DISEASES

Introduction

Parasites that have the potential to cause healthcare-associated outbreaks fall into three broad categories: (1) enteric parasites, such as *Giardia lamblia*, *Entamoeba histolytica*, and *Cryptosporidium* species, (2) blood and tissue parasites, such as *Pneumocystis carinii*, and (3) ectoparasites, such as *Sarcoptes scabiei*. Although nosocomial transmission of parasitic and ectoparasitic diseases has been well documented, reports of outbreaks caused by healthcare-acquired parasites are rare, except for those caused by *Sarcoptes scabiei*, the scabies mite.[298–300] Outbreaks of scabies in healthcare settings, especially in LTC facilities, have long been recognized.[299,301–307] Despite the excessive fear that many healthcare workers have of catching head or body lice from an infested patient or resident, a search of the literature published from 1985 through early 2008 failed to detect any reports of outbreaks in the healthcare setting caused by lice.

In the past three decades, *Cryptosporidium parvum* and *Pneumocystis carinii* have emerged as important human pathogens, especially in persons with impaired natural host defense mechanisms, such as those with acquired immune deficiency syndrome or those undergoing immunosuppressive therapy. Only recently has nosocomial transmission and suspected outbreaks of these two organisms been reported.[298,299,308–320] Parasites that have been reported to cause outbreaks in the healthcare setting are listed in Table 7–1.[300–320]

Only those parasites that have been reported to cause outbreaks in healthcare settings will be discussed in this section. For further information on the nosocomial transmission of parasites, the reader is referred to the series of articles by Lettau, who reviewed published reports of transmission and outbreaks of parasitic diseases in hospitals, research laboratories, and institutions for the mentally ill.[298–300]

Sarcoptes scabiei (Scabies)

Scabies is caused by an itch mite, *Sarcoptes scabiei*, that is transmitted from person to person by direct skin-to-skin contact and can sometimes be spread via contact with underclothes and bedding that were recently contaminated.[300] The female mite burrows into the skin to lay her eggs, and this causes a reaction that is usually manifested as an intense pruritis but varies considerably, depending on the immune status of the host. The eggs hatch and mature into adults in 10 to 14 days.[324] The incubation period (time from infestation to observance of itching and rash) can be from several days to several weeks. Therefore, a person can transmit the mite to others before the symptoms are recognized. Most persons with scabies are said to harbor an average of 5 to 15 mites[324,325]; however, patients with compromised immune defenses can develop Norwegian, or crusted, scabies in which thousands of mites may be present. An adult mite can survive off the host and remain infective for only 24 to 36 hours at room temperature.[326] Fomites are not usually important modes of transmission; however, they have played a role in outbreaks when patients or residents had Norwegian scabies.[301,327] Mites have been found to survive in mineral oil for up to seven days;[324] therefore, oil-based ointments and creams could possibly serve as a reservoir. Because the appearance of the rash is so variable, a diagnosis of suspected scabies should routinely be confirmed by taking skin scrapings of the suspicious lesions and viewing them under a microscope.[301,302] The diagnosis can be confirmed if the adult mites, eggs, or scybala (feces) can be seen. Diagnosis should be relatively easy in a case of Norwegian scabies because of the large number of mites present; however, several scrapings may have to be done to confirm scabies infestation in a normal host because only a few mites may be present.

There are many published reports of scabies outbreaks in acute care[300,303,327–333] and LTC settings.[301,306,307,328,334–339] Most of these occurred after contact with a patient or resident with Norwegian scabies because this presentation is often unrecognized or misdiagnosed and is highly contagious due to the large number of mites on the body. Scabies is particularly problematic in the LTC setting where residents often have direct contact with each other and many require extensive hands-on care.

Outbreaks in both acute and LTC settings are difficult to control because continued spread frequently occurs due to (1) misdiagnoses and unrecognized cases among patients, residents, or personnel, and (2) ineffective or improperly applied treatment.[302,335,337] Continued exposure to unrecognized or inadequately treated cases can lead to prolongation of an outbreak. Treatment failures due to resistance to scabicides are well recognized.[331,336,338,339,340] Guidelines for managing outbreaks in acute and LTC settings have been published and include the following[50,301,339,341]:

- Education of personnel on recognizing signs and symptoms of typical and atypical scabies
- Education of personnel on measures used to prevent the transmission of scabies, especially the importance of thorough application of scabicides
- Development and implementation of a plan to evaluate and categorize patients, residents, personnel, and their contacts according to their probability of infestation[301]
- Identification of symptomatic patients, residents, and personnel
- Use of contact precautions for symptomatic patients and residents until 24 hours after treatment is applied
- Identification of symptomatic household contacts, significant others, and visitors of patients and residents

Table 7–1   Parasites That Have Caused Outbreaks in Healthcare Settings

Organism	Disease	Usual Mode of Transmission	Example of Healthcare-Associated Outbreak	Reference(s)
Cryptosporidium species	Diarrhea	Person to person via fecal-oral route; waterborne	Patient to patient in pediatric hospital in Mexico[313]	308–315
Dermanyssus gallinae; Ornithonyssus sylvarium (avian mites)	Mite infestation; dermatitis	Birds to man	Mites entered crevices in wall and infested patients in a surgical intensive care unit; source was pigeon roosts on roof	321
Entamoeba histolytica	Diarrhea	Person to person via fecal-oral route	Contaminated colonic irrigation equipment used in a chiropractic clinic	322
Giardia lamblia	Diarrhea	Person to person via fecal-oral route; waterborne	Food-borne and person-to-person outbreak in a nursing home	323
Pneumocystis carinii	Lower respiratory tract	Probably by inhalation of organism; possibly from person to person by droplet spread	Cluster of infections in pediatric hospital thought to be acquired by person-to-person spread[318]	316–320
Sarcoptes scabei	Dermatitis	Person to person by skin-to-skin contact	Multiple outbreaks in hospitals and long-term care facilities	300–307

- Identification of symptomatic household contacts and significant others of personnel
- Effective treatment of symptomatic persons (Note: It is important that the directions for scabicides are followed carefully and that treatment is applied to the entire body from the neck down including under the fingernails. For persons with Norwegian scabies, some scabicides should be

reapplied 7 days after the initial treatment. Instructions on the package insert for the medication used should be carefully followed.)

- Application of treatment to all identified persons within the same 24- to 48-hour period whenever possible
- Restriction of infested personnel from work until initial treatment is completed (after overnight application of scabicide)
- Reexamination of confirmed or suspected scabies cases at 14 and 28 days after initial treatment to evaluate treatment success
- Careful identification and surveillance of exposed patients and personnel who are asymptomatic
- For a continuing outbreak, prophylaxis for exposed patients and personnel who are asymptomatic (mass prophylaxis of asymptomatic contacts is generally not recommended.)
- Development of an ongoing surveillance program

The Maryland Department of Health and Mental Hygiene *Guidelines for Control of Scabies in Long-Term Care Facilities* are reprinted in Appendix I (Appendix I is available for download at this text's web site: http://www .jbpub.com/catalog/9780763757793/). These guidelines contain information on recognizing and diagnosing scabies, a procedure for performing skin scrapings, a protocol for the assessment and control of scabies outbreaks in LTC facilities, a line list for scabies cases, and a scabies fact sheet.[340]

Scabies outbreaks are extremely disruptive when they occur in healthcare facilities. They frequently result in adverse publicity and media coverage, overuse of prophylactic medication, and much fear and stress in personnel due to the stigma attached to having the disease and to the fact that their family members and significant others are frequently affected.[301,327,331,337,339] Once a scabies outbreak is confirmed (i.e., scabies has been diagnosed by skin scrapings), a carefully coordinated infection control plan must be implemented. This plan must be a multidisciplinary effort involving those responsible for infection control and employee health in the facility; the physicians caring for the residents or patients; all affected personnel; the household contacts of affected personnel, residents, or patients; the pharmacy; and the organization's administration and public relations departments. It is important that information on the extent of the outbreak and the control measures being taken be communicated consistently and frequently to personnel to avoid panic and misconceptions, especially if the outbreak is extensive or prolonged. To avoid providing conflicting information to personnel and the community, it is useful to appoint a single spokesperson for the organization.

The most important measure that can be taken to prevent a scabies epidemic in any healthcare setting is the prompt recognition and treatment of infested persons.

Cryptosporidium Species

Cryptosporidium parvum is an intestinal protozoan that causes diarrhea in humans and is spread directly from person to person via the fecal-oral route or indirectly via contaminated water or food.[298] Several highly publicized waterborne[342,343] and food-borne outbreaks[344,345] of *Cryptosporidium* have occurred in the United States, calling attention to the enteric parasites. In 1993, *Cryptosporidium* caused the largest waterborne disease outbreak ever documented in the United States when the municipal water in Milwaukee became contaminated with *Cryptosporidium* oocysts—an estimated 403,000 persons were infected.[342] *Cryptosporidium* has recently been recognized as a cause of nosocomial diarrhea in immunosuppressed patients and possibly in the elderly.[308–315] A few hospital outbreaks of cryptosporidiosis have been reported.[308,311,313,315] An outbreak of cryptosporidiosis has also been reported in a day care center associated with a hospital.[346] Outbreaks caused by this organism can be missed because many laboratories do not routinely test for *Cryptosporidium*.[347] Because infectious oocysts may be excreted in the stool of symptomatic and asymptomatic persons, control measures to prevent person-to-person transmission in the healthcare setting include standard precautions, hand hygiene, and careful handling of feces and fecally contaminated items. Contact precautions and use of a private room are recommended for persons who are diapered or incontinent.[42]

Giardia lamblia

Giardia lamblia is a common intestinal parasite in humans that can be transmitted via direct person-to-person contact or via contaminated water or food.[323] Although *G. lamblia* is a common cause of day care center epidemics[348] and waterborne outbreaks, a literature search revealed only one reported outbreak related to healthcare-associated acquisition and this occurred in residents and employees of an LTC facility and in children and staff of a day care center at the facility.[323] The outbreak investigation in this nursing home revealed that transmission probably occurred via two routes: (1) by direct transmission between the children in the day care center and from the children to the day care center staff and the nursing home residents who participated in an "adopted grandparents" program, and (2) by uncooked food prepared by infected food handlers, one of whom was the mother of an infected child in the day care center. Control measures used to terminate the outbreak included the following[323]:

- Education for employees regarding hand washing
- Instructions to the day care center staff to wash their hands after changing diapers and before preparing food
- Instructions to the nursing home staff to wash hands after caring for nursing home residents
- Treatment of symptomatic and asymptomatic persons who had *G. lamblia* in their stool
- Removal of infected food handlers until after they were treated and their symptoms resolved.

Pneumocystis carinii

Pneumocystis carinii is a protozoan parasite that genetically resembles a fungus. It is an opportunistic pathogen that causes lower respiratory tract infection in immunocompromised patients. Studies suggest that *P. carinii* can be transmitted from patient to patient in hospitals,[311,349] and there are several reports of healthcare-associated infection clusters.[316,318–320] All of these reports involved immunosuppressed patients. Although little is known about the epidemiology and mode of transmission of nosocomial pneumocystis, acquisition of *P. carinii* is believed to occur via inhalation.[299] The CDC guidelines for isolation precautions recommend that patients with *P. carinii* pneumonia not be placed in the same room with an immunocompromised patient.[42]

Ectoparasites Other Than Scabies

Several outbreaks of human infestation with avian mites have been reported in hospitals.[321,350] The source of these mites was pigeon roosts in close proximity to patient rooms. Since avian mites (*Ornithonyssus sylviarum* and *Dermanyssus gallinae*) can cause pruritic rashes in humans, healthcare personnel should be aware of the possible presence of these mites in the vicinity of areas used by nesting pigeons. These mites are larger than *Sarcoptes scabiei* and, unlike *S. scabiei*, they can be seen by the naked eye and do not burrow under the skin. It should be noted that *D. gallinae* is not affected by treatment with 1% gamma benzene hexachloride.[349]

DISEASE SYNDROMES—GASTROINTESTINAL ILLNESS

Epidemiology

Healthcare-associated diarrhea commonly occurs in hospitalized patients and residents of LTC facilities and may be caused by a variety of intrinsic and extrinsic factors: underlying diseases, gastric acidity, tube feedings, antacids, laxatives, antibiotics and other medications, and infectious agents. Gastrointestinal illnesses are caused by a variety of bacterial, viral, parasitic, fungal, and chemical agents; however, only a few of these agents have been involved in reported nosocomial outbreaks, and these are listed in Exhibit 7–2. A detailed discussion of each of these agents is beyond the scope of this chapter. For additional information on agents causing gastrointestinal illness in healthcare settings, the reader is referred to the references cited in this section and to the Suggested Reading and Resources section at the end of this chapter.

There are few data on the incidence of healthcare-associated gastroenteritis. Hospitals participating in the housewide surveillance component of the CDC NNIS system from 1985 to 1991 reported nosocomial gastroenteritis rates from 7.8 to 14.2 infections per 10,000 discharges, depending on the type and size of hospital.[351] Nicolle and Garibaldi reported the incidence of gastrointestinal infection in nursing homes to be from 0 to 2.5 infections per 1000 resident-days.[352] Noroviruses, *Salmonella*, and *Clostridium difficile* are the most commonly reported causes of outbreaks of nosocomial gastrointestinal infections in hospitals and LTC settings. Because the etiology for diarrhea is frequently not determined, it is likely that many outbreaks in healthcare facilities are not recognized—especially if they are caused by viral agents, because clinical microbiology laboratories do not routinely screen for viruses. Rotaviruses are among the most important causes of infectious diarrhea in infants, young children, and the elderly, and are responsible for causing both sporadic and epidemic gastroenteritis in acute and LTC facilities.

Mode of Transmission

Agents causing infectious gastroenteritis may be transmitted in the healthcare setting by contact with an infected individual [202,203,323,353–356] or a contaminated object[235,322,356,357] or by consuming contaminated food, water, or other beverages.[323,353,355,357–359] Examples of outbreaks of healthcare-associated gastrointestinal illness that have occurred in hospitals and LTC facilities, including the causative agent, the implicated source, and the probable mode of transmission, are shown in Table 7–2.[202,213,323,354,356,359–373] Once introduced into a healthcare setting, many of these agents can readily be spread from person to person, and outbreaks frequently involve both patients or residents and personnel[323,354,356,359,364,365,370,372,373] with occasional secondary spread to the household contacts of personnel.[363,364] Attack rates in the 50% range are frequently reported for the noroviruses (previously known as the small round structured viruses or SRSV).[354,364] In a Maryland nursing home outbreak, 62 of 121 residents (51%) and 64 of 136 staff (47%) developed vomiting and diarrhea that was subsequently determined to be caused by a SRSV.[354] The index case was a nurse who became ill at work and continued to work for 3 days, on three 12-hour shifts, although she was ill with explosive diarrhea. A nurse aide who worked with the nurse subsequently developed nausea, vomiting, and diarrhea and also continued to work. Both of these personnel were thought to be responsible for introducing the agent into the wards. The outbreak had an overall attack rate (staff and residents) of 50% and resulted in

Exhibit 7–2 Etiologic Agents Involved in Outbreaks of Gastrointestinal Illness in Healthcare Settings

Bacterial	Viral	Parasitic	Chemical
Aeromonas hydrophilia	Adenovirus	Cryptosporidium	Scombrotoxin
Campylobacter species	Astrovirus	Entamoeba histolytica	Niacin
Clostridium difficile	Coxsackievirus	Giardia lamblia	
Clostridium perfringens	Norovirus		
Escherichia coli O157:H7	Rotavirus		
Listeria monocytogenes			
Salmonella species			
Shigella species			
Staphylococcus aureus			
Yersinia enterocolitica			

three hospitalizations and two deaths among the 121 residents.[354] The investigators highlighted the importance of having a sick leave policy that encourages personnel to report gastrointestinal illnesses immediately and cease work until 48 hours after the resolution of vomiting and diarrhea.

Community outbreaks of rotavirus in temperate climates generally occur during the winter months and can result in nosocomial transmission via person-to-person spread.[373–376] Although the primary mode of transmission of the agents causing infectious gastroenteritis is fecal-oral, there is evidence that the noroviruses and rotavirus can be transmitted via aerosolization of feces or vomitus, such as may occur when a person handles contaminated laundry or has explosive vomiting or diarrhea.[357,377,378] Gastroenteritis caused by rotavirus can be characterized by severe diarrhea, vomiting, fever, and respiratory symptoms; however, there is little evidence that rotavirus is spread via respiratory secretions. Because rotavirus is fairly resistant to disinfectants and germicides and can survive on environmental surfaces for prolonged periods, fomites probably play a role in the transmission of this agent.[373]

Food-Borne Outbreaks

Food-borne and waterborne outbreaks may be caused by a variety of agents: bacteria, viruses, parasites, natural toxins, and chemicals.[353,357,379–389] A list of the incubation periods and clinical syndromes associated with food-borne agents that cause gastrointestinal disease can be found in the appendix of the 2006 CDC surveillance report on food-borne-disease outbreaks that is cited in the references.[389] Many recognized causes of community-acquired food-borne outbreaks are agents that have emerged or reemerged in the past three decades, such as *Campylobacter*, *Escherichia coli* O157:H7, *Helicobacter pylori*, *Listeria monocytogenes*, *Vibrio cholerae* and *vulnificus*, group A beta-hemolytic streptococcus, noroviruses, *Anisakis*, *Cryptosporidium*, *Giardia lamblia*, Microsporidia, *Toxoplasma gondii*, and *Cyclospora*. To date, those agents listed in Table 7–3 have been associated with nosocomial outbreaks.

Highly publicized outbreaks caused by widely distributed contaminated food products have occurred in the past 20 years. In 1993, a large multistate outbreak of *E. coli* O157:H57 in the Pacific Northwest was linked to hamburgers served by a fast-food chain.[385] Several outbreaks of cyclosporiasis have been associated with commercially distributed fresh raspberries, mesclun lettuce, and basil.[386] In 2002 a multistate outbreak of listeriosis caused by contaminated deli meat resulted in one of the largest food recalls in the United States.[387] These outbreaks call attention to the fact that contaminated water or commercially available products could affect healthcare workers through community exposure or could be served and consumed in a healthcare facility, thus infecting patients, residents, personnel, and visitors.

In 1995, the CDC, the US Department of Agriculture, the Food and Drug Administration, and the California, Connecticut, Georgia, Minnesota, and Oregon health departments initiated the Foodborne Disease Active Surveillance Network (FoodNet) to monitor the incidence of food-borne diseases in those states.[382] As of 2008, 10 states are members of FoodNet. The primary goals of the network are to characterize, understand, and respond to food-borne illnesses in

Table 7–2   Examples of Outbreaks of Healthcare-Associated Gastrointestinal Illness

Agent	Implicated Source	Probable Mode of Transmission	Healthcare Setting	Comments	Reference (year reported)
Aeromonas hydrophilia	Unknown	Unknown	LTC	Affected residents	369 (1990)
Bacillus cereus	Beef stew	Food-borne	LTC	Affected residents and personnel	368 (1988)
Campy-lobacter jejuni	Chicken liver	Food-borne	LTC	Affected residents and personnel	359 (1997)
Clostridium difficile	Infected residents	Person to person	LTC	Primary risk factor is prior antimicrobials	218 (1990)
	Infected patients	Person to person	Hospital	Primary risk factor is prior antimicrobials	202 (1989)
Clostridium perfringens	Meatloaf, split pea soup, roast beef, shepherd's pie, turkey	Food-borne	LTC	Multiple outbreaks	360 (1991)
	Canned tuna	Food-borne	Hospital	Affected personnel	366 (1994)
E. coli O157:H7	Sandwiches	Food-borne and person to person	LTC	Affected residents and personnel	370 (1987)
	Hamburger	Food-borne	LTC	Affected residents	371 (1986)
Giardia lamblia	Children and sandwiches	Person to person and food-borne	LTC and associated child day care center	Affected children, personnel, and residents	323 (1989)
Listeria mono-cytogenes	Raw vegetables	Food-borne	Hospital	Involved 20 patients in 8 hospitals	367 (1986)
Niacin intoxication	Cornmeal	Food-borne	LTC	Oversupple-mentation of cornmeal with vitamins and minerals	360 (1991)

Table 7–2 (*Continued*)

Agent	Implicated Source	Probable Mode of Transmission	Healthcare Setting	Comments	Reference (year reported)
Norovirus	Unknown	Person to person	LTC	Affected personnel and residents; was also transmitted to families of personnel	363 (1993)
	Ill nurse and nurse's aide	Person to person	LTC	Index case was ill nurse who worked while symptomatic; affected residents and personnel	354 (1996)
	Unknown	Person to person	LTC	Affected personnel and residents; was also transmitted to families of personnel	364 (1990)
	Ill nurse	Person to person	Hospital	Index case was hospitalized nurse; affected personnel and patients	365 (1998)
Rotavirus	Not identified	Person to person	LTC	Affected residents and personnel	372 (1980)
	Pediatric patients with community-acquired infection	Person to person	Hospital	Nosocomial transmission occurred in patients during community outbreak	373 (1990)
Salmonella species	Chicken liver	Food-borne	LTC	Affected residents and personnel	359 (1997)
	Eggs, chicken, turkey, pureed food	Food-borne	LTC	Multiple outbreaks reported	360 (1991)
	Soiled linen and asymptomatic cook	Food-borne, contact with laundry, person to person	LTC	Affected residents, laundry workers, and nurses	356 (1994)

Continues

Table 7–2   (*Continued*)

Agent	Implicated Source	Probable Mode of Transmission	Healthcare Setting	Comments	Reference (year reported)
	Unknown— probable chronic carrier	Food-borne, person to person	Hospital	Cases occurred over a 5-year period	361 (1985)
	Eggs	Food-borne	Hospital	Multiple out-breaks reported	362 (1998)
Staphylococcus aureus	Egg salad, chicken salad, potato salad, chicken, chopped beef livers	Food-borne	LTC	Multiple outbreaks reported	360 (1991)

LTC = Long-term care facility

the United States. FoodNet conducts active surveillance for nine organisms that cause food-borne illness (*Campylobacter*, *E. coli* O157:H7, *Listeria*, *Salmonella*, *Shigella*, *Vibrio*, *Yersinia*, *Cryptosporidium*, and *Cyclospora*) and for hemolytic uremic syndrome. Additional information is available on the Food-Net Web site at http://www.cdc.gov/foodnet.

Nosocomial outbreaks of food-borne pathogens have long been recognized.[360,362,379,380,382] Since 1973, the CDC has maintained a surveillance program for the collection and periodic reporting of data on the occurrence and causes of food-borne-disease outbreaks in the United States. The data are collected and submitted by state, local, and territorial health departments and periodically reported in the *MMWR Surveillance Summaries*.[387,388] Outbreaks in hospitals and nursing homes accounted for 3.3% of the food-borne outbreaks and 28.9% of the related deaths reported to the CDC from 1975 to 1992.[362] A confirmed causative agent was determined in 67 of 123 reported hospital outbreaks and 92 of 168 reported nursing home outbreaks. From 1975 to 1992 in hospitals, *Salmonella* was the most commonly reported agent (52%) followed by scombroid fish poisoning (12%), *Clostridium perfringens* (11%), and *Staphylococcus aureus* (8%) and in nursing homes, the most common agent was also *Salmonella* (66%) followed by *Staphylococcus aureus* (15%), *Clostridium perfringens* (9%), and *Campylobacter jejuni* (3%). In a CDC report of food-borne-disease outbreaks occurring in 1998 through 2002, the most common etiologic agent in hospital outbreaks was norovirus followed by *Salmonella*, *Clostridium perfringens*, and *Listeria monocytogenes*, and in nursing homes the most common etiologic agent was also norovirus, followed by *Salmonella*, *Listeria monocytogenes*, *Staphylococcus aureus*, and *E. coli*.[389] The

Table 7–3   Characteristics of Agents Causing Food-Borne Diseases

I. Diseases typified by vomiting (and little or no fever) after a short incubation period

Agent	Incubation Period Usual (Range)	Symptoms*	Characteristic Foods
Bacillus cereus	2–4 hours (1–6 hours)	N, V, D	Fried rice
Heavy metals (cadmium, copper, tin, zinc)	5–15 minutes (1–60 minutes)	N, V, C, D	Foods and beverages prepared, stored, or cooked in containers coated, lined, or contaminated with offending metal
Staphylococcus aureus	2–4 hours (0.5–8.0 hours)	N, C, V; D, F may be present	Sliced/chopped ham and meats, custards, cream fillings

II. Diseases typified by diarrhea (often with fever) after a moderate to long incubation period

Agent	Incubation Period Usual (Range)	Symptoms*	Characteristic Foods
Bacillus cereus	8–16 hours (6–24 hours)	C, D	Custards, cereals, puddings, sauces, meat loaf
Campylobacter jejuni	3–5 days (1–10 days)	C, D, B, F	Raw milk, poultry, water
Clostridium perfringens	10–12 hours (8–24 hours)	C, D (V, F rare)	Meat, poultry
Cyclospora species	1 week (1–14 days)	D, N, V, C	Berries, lettuce
Escherichia coli enterotoxigenic	24–72 hours (10–72 hours)	D, C	Uncooked vegetables, salads, water, cheese
Escherichia coli enteroinvasive	16–48 hours (10–48 hours)	C, D, F, H	Same
Escherichia coli enterohemorrhagic (E. coli O157:H7 and others)	72–96 hours (3–8 days)	B, C, D, H, F infrequent	Beef, raw milk, water

Continues

Table 7–3   *(Continued)*

II. Diseases typified by diarrhea (often with fever) after a moderate to long incubation period

Agent	Incubation Period Usual (Range)	Symptoms*	Characteristic Foods
Noroviruses	16–48 hours (range varies)	N, V, C, D	Shellfish, water
Rotavirus	24–72 hours	N, V, C, D	Food-borne transmission not well documented
Salmonella (nontyphoid)	12–36 hours (6–72 hours)	D, C, F, V, H septicemia or enteric fever	Poultry, eggs, milk, meat (cross-contamination important)
Shigella	24–48 hours (12–96 hours)	C, F, D, B, H, N, V	Foods contaminated by infected food handler; usually not food-borne
Vibrio cholerae non-01	16–72 hours	D, V	Shellfish
Vibrio cholerae O1	24–72 hours (3 hours to 5 days)	D, V	Shellfish, water, or foods contaminated by infected person or obtained from contaminated environmental source
Vibrio parahaemolyticus	12–24 hours (4–30 hours)	C, D N, V, F, H, B	Seafood
Yersinia enterocolitica	3 to 5 days usual (range unclear)	F, D, C, V, H	Pork products, foods contaminated by infected human or animal

III. Botulism

Agent	Incubation Period Usual (Range)	Symptoms*	Characteristic Foods
Clostridium botulinum	10–12 hours (6–24 hours)	V, D descending paralysis	Improperly canned or preserved foods that provide anaerobic conditions

Table 7–3   *(Continued)*

IV. Diseases most readily diagnosed from the history of eating a particular type of food

Agent	Incubation Period Usual (Range)	Symptoms*	Characteristic Foods
Ciguatera poisoning	1–6 hours	D, N, V, paresthesias, reversal of temperature sensation	Large ocean fish (i.e., barracuda, snapper)
Scombroid fish poisoning	5 minutes to 1 hour	N, C, D, H, flushing, urticaria	Mishandled fish (i.e., tuna)

*B = bloody stools; C = cramps; D = diarrhea; F = fever; H = headache; N = nausea; V = vomiting
Source: Adapted from Centers for Disease Control and Prevention. *Principles of Epidemiology. An Introduction to Applied Epidemiology and Biostatistics.* 2nd ed. US Department of Health and Human Services; 1992:493-497.

recognition of norovirus because the most common agent of food-borne disease in hospitals and nursing homes from 1998 through 2002 is likely due to the increased use of diagnostic testing for viral agents because these tests were not widely available until the early 1990s.

Hepatitis A virus (HAV) is an uncommon cause of nosocomial food-borne outbreaks but is an example of an enterically transmitted pathogen that can be spread in the healthcare setting via several routes: contaminated food, direct person-to-person transmission, and infusion of contaminated blood or blood products.[390] The primary risk factor in many nosocomial HAV outbreaks is poor hand hygiene. Outbreaks of HAV infection in healthcare personnel have been associated with poor hand hygiene and eating on the patient care unit.[391]

Additional information on food-borne pathogens and toxins and preventing food-borne outbreaks can be found in the Resources section at the end of this chapter.

Control Measures

Control measures for preventing the spread of agents that cause gastrointestinal infections depend on the mode of transmission and reservoir for the organism. It is important to remember that many of these agents have several modes of transmission and many can be spread by both the contact and food-borne routes. When an outbreak is first identified or suspected, neither the agent nor the mode of transmission may be known, so control measures should be implemented based on the most likely agent, reservoir, and mode(s) of transmission. This can be determined by evaluating the characteristic signs and symptoms of those affected and conducting an initial, quick epidemiologic study (i.e., identifying persons, place, time of onset, and incubation period). Guidelines for identifying the etiology of an outbreak of gastrointestinal disease can be found in Appendix H (Appendix H is available for download at this text's Web site: http://www.jbpub.com/catalog/9780763757793/). Foods that require handling and no subsequent cooking constitute the greatest risk of serving as vehicles for food-borne outbreaks. Many gastroenteritis outbreaks in healthcare settings are caused by the noroviruses, even though etiologic confirmation is frequently not made. Noroviruses generally cause a mild to moderate, self-limited disease characterized by nausea, vomiting, diarrhea, and abdominal pain with one or more of these symptoms lasting from 24 to 48 hours. The incubation period is usually from 12 to 48 hours with a median of 33 hours.[389]

Preventing Person-to-Person Transmission of Enteric Agents

The following control measures have been recommended to prevent the spread of enteric pathogens by direct person-to-person contact or indirect contact with contaminated items[42,46,50,354,357,392]:

- Instruct personnel, patients, residents, and visitors to practice careful hand hygiene; hand hygiene is the single most important measure for preventing the person-to-person transmission of enteric pathogens.
- Exclude ill personnel from patient care and food handling for at least 2 days after resolution of symptoms.
- Ensure that personnel adhere to standard and contact precautions, including the use of gloves when handling feces or fecally soiled articles or equipment.[42]
- Institute contact precautions for diapered or incontinent patients who have an acute diarrheal disease of suspected infectious etiology.[42]
- Instruct personnel to carefully handle feces and fecally contaminated items (especially bedpans and soiled laundry) to avoid aerosolization.[42]
- Use appropriate cleansers and disinfectants to clean and disinfect soiled environmental surfaces, articles, and equipment; some disinfectants are not active against rotavirus.[393] Guidelines for cleaning and disinfecting environmental surfaces and equipment can be found in Appendix F (Appendix F is available for download at this text's Web site: http://www.jbpub.com/catalog/9780763757793/).

During an outbreak, the following additional measures are recommended:

- To determine the likely causative agent, source, and mode of transmission so that appropriate measures can be identified and implemented, conduct an epidemiologic study by collecting information on the identity of affected persons, their characteristic symptoms, wards(s) affected, and date and time of onset; then determine the likely incubation period by drawing an epidemic curve. Outbreak investigation guidelines and data collection forms can be found in Appendix H (Appendix H is available for download at this text's Web site: http://www.jbpub.com/catalog/9780763757793/).

- Because the absence of routinely available laboratory tests for viral agents make it difficult to confirm the etiology of many outbreaks, consult with the laboratory regarding the collection of stool specimens.[357,394]

- Conduct active surveillance to identify new cases among patients, residents, personnel, and visitors.

- Isolate or cohort ill patients and residents.

- Ensure that ill personnel are reassigned to nonpatient care and nonfood handling duties or are restricted from work until at least 2 days after resolution of vomiting and/or diarrhea. (Note: Many states have specific regulations regarding work restrictions for food handlers and healthcare personnel and when they can return to work after salmonellosis or shigellosis is diagnosed.)

- Minimize contact between well and ill persons as much as possible (cohort personnel and patients/residents whenever possible).

- Alert visitors to wash their hands carefully or use an alcohol hand rub when visiting patients or residents.

- In LTC settings: (1) restrict ill residents from group activities, including meals, until 2 days after resolution of vomiting and/or diarrhea, and (2) depending on the organism involved and the extent of the outbreak, close the ward to new admissions.

- In pediatric settings: (1) close the playroom, (2) identify patients exposed to the index case and avoid placing them with unexposed patients for the duration of the incubation period, (3) depending on the organism involved and the extent of the outbreak, close the ward to new admissions, and (4) instruct parents and other household contacts in the use of proper hand hygiene and handling of feces and diapers.

- Emphasize careful handling of soiled linen, clothing, and diapers to avoid aerosolization of feces and contamination of the environment.

- If a norovirus is the likely cause of the outbreak, instruct personnel to wear masks when cleaning areas grossly soiled with feces or vomitus.

Many state public health agencies have guidelines for investigating and controlling gastroenteritis outbreaks in LTC facilities, and these should be followed when available. The Maryland Department of Health and Mental Hygiene Guidelines for the Epidemiological Investigation of Gastroenteritis Outbreaks in Long-Term Care Facilities can be found in Appendix H.[294] Appendix H is available for download at this text's Web site: http://www.jbpub.com/catalog/978076375779.

Preventing Food-Borne Transmission of Enteric Agents

The control measures for preventing the food-borne transmission of pathogens depend on the agent involved. For instance, because viral agents cannot multiply outside the host, the initial innoculum in the food source determines infectivity, and food storage is not as critical as if the contaminating agent were *Staphylococcus aureus,* which will readily multiply in food held at room temperature. Control measures for preventing and investigating food-borne outbreaks have been published by the CDC and state health departments and include[354,357,381]:

- Exclude ill personnel from handling food for at least 2 days after resolution of diarrhea and vomiting.
- Emphasize the importance of proper hand washing for all personnel who handle food.
- Train food handlers in food safety practices (i.e., the proper handling, storage, preparation, and cooking of food—especially the handling of eggs and the importance of maintaining proper temperatures for hot or cold foods and avoiding cross-contamination between cooked and uncooked foods).
- Follow state regulations, as appropriate, for food handlers with infectious gastroenteritis.

Control measures for interrupting and investigating a food-borne outbreak include the following:

- Exclude ill personnel from handling food for at least 2 days after resolution of diarrhea and vomiting.
- Consult with the laboratory regarding the collection of stool specimens.[357,394]
- Conduct active surveillance to identify new cases among patients, residents, personnel, and visitors.
- Isolate or cohort ill patients and residents.
- Ensure that ill personnel are reassigned to nonpatient care and nonfood handling duties or are restricted from work until at least 2 days after resolution of vomiting and/or diarrhea. (Note: Many states have specific regulations regarding work restrictions for food handlers and healthcare personnel and when they can return to work after salmonellosis or shigellosis is diagnosed.)

Pathogens introduced into a facility via food can be further transmitted from person to person by direct contact with an infected person or a contaminated item;[323,353,356,361,370] therefore, measures to prevent person-to-person transmission, as noted above, should also be implemented.

Although most cases of food-borne disease are caused by infectious agents, it is important to remember that pesticides and other chemicals have been responsible for outbreaks in healthcare settings resulting in gastrointestinal and neurologic illness.[388,395]

Outbreaks of gastrointestinal illness in healthcare settings can result in significant morbidity and mortality; affect patients, residents, and personnel; disrupt services; and cause economic loss.[396] To prevent these outbreaks, infection control professionals should implement infection surveillance, prevention, and control programs that reduce the risk of transmission of pathogens that are spread by the fecal-oral route.

REFERENCES

1. Smith L, Eberstadt I. *Selected Poems of Ogden Nash.* New York, NY: Little Brown & Company; 1975:59.

2. Jevons MP. "Celbenin"-resistant staphylococci. *BMJ* 1961;1:124–125.

3. Panlilo AL, Culver DH, Gaynes RP, et al. Methicillin-resistant *Staphylococcus aureus* in U.S. hospitals, 1975–1991. *Infect Control Hosp Epidemiol.* 1992;13:582–586.

4. Diekema DJ, Pfaller MA, Schmitz FJ, et al. Survey of infections due to *Staphylococcus* species: frequency of occurrence and antimicrobial susceptibility of isolates collected in the United States, Canada, Latin America, Europe, and the Western Pacific Region for the SENTRY Antimicrobial Surveillance Program, 1997–1999. *Clin Infect Dis.* 2001;32(Suppl 2): S114–S132.

5. The European Antimicrobial Resistance Surveillance System (EARSS). EARSS annual report 2006. http://www.rivm.nl/earss/news/index.jsp. Accessed November 25, 2007.

6. Andraševic AT, Tambic T, Kalenic S, Jankovic V and the Working Group of the Croatian Committee for Antibiotic Resistance Surveillance. Surveillance for antimicrobial resistance in Croatia. *Emerg Infect Dis.* 2002;8:14–8.

7. Nimmo GR, Pearson JC, Collignon PJ, et al and the Australian Group for Antimicrobial Resistance. Prevalence of MRSA among *Staphylococcus aureus* isolated from hospital inpatients, 2005: report of the Australian Group for Antimicrobial Resistance. *Commun Dis Intel.* 2007;31:288–296. http://www.antimicrobial-resistance.com/. Accessed November 25, 2007.

8. Centers for Disease Control and Prevention. National nosocomial infections surveillance (NNIS) system report, data summary from January 1992 through June 2004, issued October 2004. *Am J Infect Control.* 2004;32:470–485. http://www.cdc.gov/ncidod/dhqp/nnis_pubs.html. Accessed November 25, 2007.

9. Barrett FF, McGehee RP Jr, Finland M. Methicillin-resistant *Staphylococcus aureus* at Boston City Hospital. *N Engl J Med.* 1968;279:441–448.

10. Wenzel RP, Nettleman MD, Jones RN, Pfaller MA. Methicillin-resistant *Staphylococcus aureus*: implications for the 1990s and effective control measures. *Am J Med.* 1991;91: 3B-221S–3B-227S.

11. Harstein AI, LeMonte AM, Iwamoto PKL. DNA typing and control of methicillin-resistant *Staphylococcus aureus* at two affiliated hospitals. *Infect Control Hosp Epidemiol.* 1997;18: 42–48.

12. Lugeon C, Blanc DS, Wenger A, Francioli P. Molecular epidemiology of methicillin-resistant *Staphylococcus aureus* at a low-incidence hospital over a 4-year period. *Infect Control Hosp Epidemiol.* 1995;16:260–267.

13. Embil J, Ramotar K, Romance L, et al. Methicillin-resistant *Staphylococcus aureus* in tertiary care institutions on the Canadian prairies 1990–1992. *Infect Control Hosp Epidemiol.* 1994;15:646–651.

14. Layton MC, Hierholzer WJ, Patterson JE. The evolving epidemiology of methicillin-resistant *Staphylococcus aureus* at a university hospital. *Infect Control Hosp Epidemiol.* 1995;16:12–17.

15. Harstein AI, Denny MA, Morthland VH, LeMonte AM, Pfaller MA. Control of methicillin-resistant *Staphylococcus aureus* in a hospital and an intensive care unit. *Infect Control Hosp Epidemiol.* 1995;16:405–411.

16. Linnemann CC Jr, Moore P, Staneck JL, Pfaller MA. Reemergence of epidemic methicillin-resistant *Staphylococcus aureus* in a general hospital associated with changing staphylococcal strains. *Am J Med.* 1991;91:3B-238S–3B-244S.

17. Coombs GW, Van Gessel H, Pearson JC, Godsell MR, O'Brien FG, Christiansen KJ. Controlling a multicenter outbreak involving the New York/Japan methicillin-resistant *Staphylococcus aureus* clone. *Infect Control Hosp Epidemiol.* 2007;28(7):845–852.

18. Klein E, Smith DL, Laxminarayan R. Hospitalizations and deaths caused by methicillin-resistant *Staphylococcus aureus*, United States, 1999–2005. *Emerg Infect Dis.* 2007;13:1840–1846. http://www.cdc.gov/EID/content/13/12/1840.htm. Accessed December 10, 2007.

19. Troilett N, Carmeli Y, Samore MH, et al. Carriage of methicillin-resistant *Staphylococcus aureus* at hospital admission. *Infect Control Hosp Epidemiol.* 1998;19:181–185.

20. Klevens RM, Morrison MA, Nadle J, et al. for the Active Bacterial Core Surveillance (ABCs) MRSA Investigators. Invasive methicillin-resistant *Staphylococcus aureus* infections in the United States. *JAMA.* 2007;298(15):1763–1771.

21. Adcock PM, Pastor P, Medley F, Patterson JE, Murphy TV. Methicillin-resistant *Staphylococcus aureus* in two child care centers. *J Infect Dis.* 1998;178(2):577–580.

22. Centers for Disease Control and Prevention. Methicillin-resistant *Staphylococcus aureus* infections among competitive sports participants—Colorado, Indiana, Pennsylvania, and Los Angeles County, 2000–2003. *MMWR.* 2003;52(33):793–795.

23. Begier EM, Frenette K, Barrett NL, et al. A high-morbidity outbreak of methicillin-resistant *Staphylococcus aureus* among players on a college football team, facilitated by cosmetic body shaving and turf burns. *Clin Infect Dis.* 2004;39(10):1446–1453.

24. Centers for Disease Control and Prevention. Outbreaks of community-associated methicillin-resistant *Staphylococcus aureus* skin infections—Los Angeles County, California, 2002–2003. *MMWR.* 2003;52(5):88.

25. Centers for Disease Control and Prevention. Siegel JD, Rhinehart E, Jackson M, Chiarello L, and the Healthcare Infection Control Practices Advisory Committee. Management of multidrug-resistant organisms in healthcare settings, 2006. http://www.cdc.gov/ncidod/dhqp/index.html. Accessed November 25, 2007.

26. US Centers for Disease Control and Prevention. Methicillin resistant *Staphylococcus aureus* infections in correctional facilities—Georgia, California, and Texas, 2001–2003. *MMWR.* 2003; 52: 992–96.

27. Grundmann H, Aires-de-Sousa M, Boyce J, Tiemersma E. Emergence and resurgence of methicillin-resistant *Staphylococcus aureus* as a public-health threat. *Lancet.* 2006;368: 874–885.

28. O'Brien FG, Pearman JW, Gracey M, Riley TV, Grubb WB. Community strain of methicillin-resistant *Staphylococcus aureus* involved in a hospital outbreak. *J Clin Microbiol.* 1999;37: 2858–2862.

29. Saiman L, O'Keefe M, Graham PLIII, et al. Hospital transmission of community-acquired methicillin-resistant *Staphylococcus aureus* among postpartum women. *Clin Infect Dis.* 2003;37:1313–1319.

30. Bratu S, Eramo A, Kopec R, et al. Community-associated methicillin-resistant *Staphylococcus aureus* in hospital nursery and maternity units. *Emerg Infect Dis* 2005;11: 808–813.

31. Boyce JM. Methicillin-resistant *Staphylococcus aureus* in hospitals and long-term care facilities: microbiology, epidemiology, and preventive measures. *Infect Control Hosp Epidemiol.* 1992;13:725–737.

32. Meier PA, Carter CC, Wallace SE, Hollis RJ, Pfaller MA, Herwaldt LA. A prolonged outbreak of methicillin-resistant *Staphylococcus aureus* in the burn center of a tertiary medical center. *Infect Control Hosp Epidemiol.* 1996;17:798–802.

33. Thompson RL, Cabezudo I, Wenzel RP. Epidemiology of nosocomial infections caused by methicillin-resistant *Staphylococcus aureus*. *Ann Intern Med.* 1982;97:309–317.

34. Boyce JM, Landry M, Deetz TR, Dupont HL. Epidemiologic studies of an outbreak of methicillin-resistant *Staphylococcus aureus* infections. *Infect Control.* 1981;2:110–116.

35. Huang R, Mehta S, Weed D, Savor Price C. Methicillin-resistant *Staphylococcus aureus* survival on hospital fomites. *Infect Control Hosp Epidemiol.* 2006;27:1267–1269.

36. Sheretz RJ, Reagan DR, Hampton KD, et al. A cloud adult: the *Staphylococcus aureus* virus interaction revisited. *Ann Intern Med.* 1996;124:539–547.

37. Bertin ML, Vinski J, Schmidt S, et al. Outbreak of methicillin-resistant *Staphylococcus aureus* colonization and infection in a neonatal intensive care unit epidemiologically linked to a healthcare worker with chronic otitis. *Infect Control Hosp Epidemiol.* 2006;27:581–585.

38. Haley RW, Hightower AW, Khabbaz RF, et al. The emergence of methicillin-resistant *Staphylococcus aureus* in United States hospitals: the possible role of the house-staff patient transfer circuit. *Ann Intern Med.* 1982;97:297–308.

39. Reboli AC, John JF Jr, Platt CG, Cantey JR. Methicillin-resistant *Staphylococcus aureus* outbreak at a Veterans Affairs medical center: importance of carriage of the organism by hospital personnel. *Infect Control Hosp Epidemiol.* 1990;11:291–296.

40. Coombs GW, Van Gessel H, Pearson JC, et al. Controlling a multicenter outbreak involving the New York/Japan methicillin-resistant *Staphylococcus aureus* clone. *Infect Control Hosp Epidemiol.* 2007;28:845–852.

41. McDonald JR, Carriker CM, Pien BC, et al. Methicillin-resistant *Staphylococcus aureus* outbreak in an intensive care nursery: potential for interinstitutional spread. *Pediatr Infect Dis J.* 2007;26(8):678–683.

42. Centers for Disease Control and Prevention, Atlanta, Georgia. Siegel JD, Rhinehart E, Jackson M, Chiarello L, and the Healthcare Infection Control Practices Advisory Committee, 2007. Guideline for isolation precautions: preventing transmission of infectious agents in healthcare settings, June 2007. http://www.cdc.gov/ncidod/dhqp/gl_isolation.html. Accessed November 25, 2007.

43. Muto CA, Jernigan JA, Ostrowsky BE, et al. SHEA guideline for preventing nosocomial transmission of multidrug-resistant strains of *Staphylococcus aureus* and *Enterococcus*. *Infect Control Hosp Epidemiol.* 2003;24:362–386. http://www.shea-online.org/Assets/files/position_papers/SHEA_MRSA_VRE.pdf. Accessed December 13, 2007.

44. Coia JE, Duckworth GJ, Edwards DI, et al., for Joint Working Party of the British Society of Antimicrobial Chemotherapy, Hospital Infection Society, Infection Control Nurses Association. Guidelines for the control and prevention of methicillin-resistant *Staphylococcus aureus* (MRSA) in healthcare facilities. *J Hosp Infect.* 2006;63S:S1–S44.

45. Gerber SI, Jones RC, Scott MV, et al. Management of outbreaks of methicillin-resistant *Staphylococcus aureus* infection in the neonatal intensive care unit: a consensus statement. *Infect Control Hosp Epidemiol.* 2006;27:139–145.

46. Centers for Disease Control and Prevention. Guideline for hand hygiene in health-care settings-recommendations of the Healthcare Infection Control Practices Advisory Committee and the HICPAC/SHEA/APIC/IDSA Hand Hygiene Task Force. *MMWR.* 2003;51(RR-16):1–56.

47. Horan TC, Gaynes RP. Surveillance of nosocomial infections. In Mayhall CG, ed. *Hospital Epidemiology and Infection Control.* 3rd ed. Philadelphia:Lippincott Williams & Wilkins, 2004:1659–1702. http://www.cdc.gov/ncidod/dhqp/pdf/NNIS/NosInfDefinitions.pdf. Accessed April 16, 2008.

48. Centers for Disease Control and Prevention. The National Healthcare Safety Network (NHSN) Manual Patient Safety Component Protocol. CDC Division of Healthcare Quality Promotion. http://www.cdc.gov/ncidod/dhqp/nhsn_members.html. Accessed April 16, 2008.

49. Wenzel RP, Reagan DR, Bertino JS, Baron EJ, Arias K. Methicillin-resistant *Staphylococcus aureus* outbreak: a consensus panel's definition and management guidelines. *Am J Infect Control.* 1998;26:102–110.

50. Bolyard EA, Tablan OC, Williams WW, et al. Guideline for infection control in health care personnel, 1998. *Am J Infect Control.* 1998;26:289–354. http://www.cdc.gov/ncidod/dhqp/gl_hcpersonnel.html. Accessed April 19, 2008.

51. Strausbaugh L. Antimicrobial resistance: problems, laments, and hopes. *Am J Infect Control.* 1997;25:294–296.

52. Goetz AM, Muder RR. The problem of methicillin-resistant *Staphylococcus aureus*: a critical appraisal of the efficacy of infection control procedures with a suggested approach for infection control programs. *Am J Infect Control.* 1992;20:80–84.

53. Cooper BS, Stone SP, Kibbler CC, et al. Isolation measures in the hospital management of methicillin resistant *Staphylococcus aureus* (MRSA): systematic review of the literature. *BMJ.* 2004;329:533–540. http://www.bmj.com/cgi/content/full/329/7465/533. Accessed December 10, 2007.

54. Henderson DK. Managing methicillin-resistant staphylococci: a paradigm for preventing nosocomial transmission of resistant organisms. *Am J Infect Control.* 2006;34:S46–S54.

55. Jernigan JA, Titus M, Groschel DHM, Getchell-White SI, Farr BM. Effectiveness of contact isolation during a hospital outbreak of methicillin-resistant *Staphylococcus aureus*. *Am J Epidemiol.* 1996;143:496–504.

56. Nettleman MD, Trilla A, Fredrickson M, Pfaller M. Assigning responsibility: using feedback to achieve sustained control of methicillin-resistant *Staphylococcus aureus*. *Am J Med.* 1991;91:3B-228S–3B-232S.

57. Boyce JM. Preventing staphylococcal infections by eradicating nasal carriage of *Staphylococcus aureus*: proceeding with caution. *Infect Control Hosp Epidemiol.* 1996;17:775–779.

58. Gemmell CG, Edwards DI, Fraise AP, Gould FK, Ridgeway GL, Warren RE, for Joint Working Party of the British Society for Antimicrobial Chemotherapy, Hospital Infection Society, Infection Control Nurses Association. Guidelines for the prophylaxis and treatment of methicillin-resistant *Staphylococcus aureus* (MRSA) infections in the UK. *J Antimicrobial Chemother.* 2006;57(4):589-608. http://jac.oxfordjournals.org/cgi/content/full/57/4/589. Accessed December 10, 2007.

59. O'Toole RD, Drew WL, Dahlgren BJ, et al. An outbreak of methicillin-resistant *Staphylococcus aureus*. Observations in hospital and nursing home. *JAMA.* 1970;213:257–263.

60. Storch GA, Radcliff JL, Meyer PL, Hinrichs JH. Methicillin-resistant *Staphylococcus aureus* in a nursing home. *Infect Control.* 1987;8:24–29.

61. Strausbaugh LJ, Jacobson C, Sewell DL, Potter S, Ward TT. Methicillin-resistant *Staphylococcus aureus* in extended-care facilities: experiences in a Veterans' Affairs nursing home and a review of the literature. *Infect Control Hosp Epidemiol.* 1991;12:36–45.

62. Thomas JC, Bridge J, Waterman S, Vogt J, Kilman L, Hancock G. Transmission and control of methicillin-resistant *Staphylococcus aureus* in a skilled nursing facility. *Infect Control Hosp Epidemiol.* 1989;10:106–110.

63. Kauffman CA, Bradley SF, Terpenning MS. Methicillin-resistant *Staphylococcus aureus* in long-term care facilities. *Infect Control Hosp Epidemiol.* 1990;11:600–603.

64. Mylotte JM, Karuza J, Bentley DW. Methicillin-resistant *Staphylococcus aureus*: a questionnaire survey of 75 long-term care facilities in western New York. *Infect Control Hosp Epidemiol.* 1992;13:711.

65. Muder RR, Brennen C, Wagener MW, et al. Methicillin-resistant staphylococcal colonization and infection in a long-term care facility. *Ann Intern Med.* 1991;114:107–112.

66. Bradley SF, Terpenning MS, Ramsey MA, et al. Methicillin-resistant *Staphylococcus aureus*: colonization and infection in a long-term care facility. *Ann Intern Med.* 1991;115:417–422.

67. Bradley SF. Methicillin-resistant *Staphylococcus aureus*: long-term care concerns. *Am J Med.* 1999;106(5A):2S–10S.

68. Lee Y, Cesario T, Gupta G, et al. Surveillance of colonization and infection with *Staphylococcus aureus* susceptible or resistant to methicillin in a community skilled-nursing facility. *Am J Infect Control.* 1997;25:312–321.

69. Bradley SF. Methicillin-resistant *Staphylococcus aureus* in nursing homes. Epidemiology, prevention and management. *Drugs Aging.* 1997;10:185–198.

70. Mulhausen PL, Harrell LJ, Weinberger M, Kochersberger GG, Feussner JR. Contrasting methicillin-resistant *Staphylococcus aureus* colonization in Veterans Affairs and community nursing homes. *Am J Med.* 1996;100:24–31.

71. Gould CV, Rothenberg R, Steinberg JP. Antibiotic resistance in long-term acute care hospitals: the perfect storm. *Infect Control Hosp Epidemiol.* 2006;27:920–925.

72. Cretnik TZ, Vovko P, Retelj M, et al. Prevalence and nosocomial spread of methicillin-resistant *Staphylococcus aureus* in a long-term care facility in Slovenia. *Infect Control Hosp Epidemiol.* 2005;26:184–190.

73. Hsu CCS. Serial survey of methicillin-resistant *Staphylococcus aureus* nasal carriage among residents in a nursing home. *Infect Control Hosp Epidemiol.* 1991;12:416–421.

74. Lee YL, Gupta G, Cesario T, et al. Colonization by *Staphylococcus aureus* resistant to methicillin and ciprofloxacin during 20 months' surveillance in a private skilled nursing facility. *Infect Control Hosp Epidemiol.* 1996;649–653.

75. Pacio GA, Visintainer P, Maquire G, Wormser GP, Ratffalli J, Montecalvo MA. Natural history of colonization with vancomycin-resistant *Enterococcus*, methicillin-resistant *Staphylococcus aureus*, and resistant gram-negative bacilli among long-term care facility residents. *Infect Control Hosp Epidemiol.* 2003;24:246–250.

76. Mulligan ME, Murray-Leisure KA, Ribner BS, et al. Methicillin-resistant *Staphylococcus aureus*: a consensus review of the microbiology, pathogenesis, and epidemiology with implications for prevention and management. *Am J Med.* 1993;94:313–328.

77. McNeil SA, Mody L, Bradley SF. Methicillin-resistant *Staphylococcus aureus*. Management of asymptomatic colonization and outbreaks of infection in long-term care. *Geriatrics.* 2002;57(6):16–8, 21–4, 27.

78. Boyce JM, Jackson MM, Pugliese G, et al. Methicillin-resistant *Staphylococcus aureus* (MRSA): a briefing for acute care hospitals and nursing facilities. *Infect Control Hosp Epidemiol.* 1994;15:105–115.

79. McGeer A, Campbell B, Emori TG, et al. Definitions of infection for surveillance in long-term care facilities. *Am J Infect Control.* 1991;19:1–7.

80. Mylotte JM. Control of methicillin-resistant *Staphylococcus aureus*: the ambivalence persists. *Infect Control Hosp Epidemiol.* 1994;15:73–77.

81. Kauffman CA, Terpenning MS, Xiaogong H, et al. Attempts to eradicate methicillin-resistant *Staphylococcus aureus* from a long-term care facility with the use of mupirocin ointment. *Am J Med.* 1993;94:371–378.

82. Mody L, Kauffman CA, McNeil SA, Galecki AT, Bradley SF. Mupirocin-based decolonization of *Staphylococcus aureus* carriers in residents of 2 long-term care facilities: a randomized, double-blind, placebo-controlled trial. *Clin Infect Dis.* 2003;37(11):1467–1474.

83. Strausbaugh LJ, Jacobson C, Sewell DL, Potter S, Ward TT. Antimicrobial therapy for methicillin-resistant *Staphylococcus aureus* colonization in residents and staff of a Veterans Affairs nursing home care unit. *Infect Control Hosp Epidemiol.* 1993;13:151–159.

84. Willems RJL, Top J, van Santen M, et al. Global spread of vancomycin-resistant *Enterococcus faecium* from distinct nosocomial genetic complex. *Emerg Infect Dis.* 2005;11:821–828. http://www.cdc.gov/ncidod/EID/vol11no06/04-1204.htm. Accessed May 12, 2008.

85. Centikya Y, Falk P, Mayhall CG. Vancomycin-resistant enterococci. *Clin Microbiol Rev.* 2000; 13:686–707.

86. Centers for Disease Control and Prevention. Nosocomial enterococci resistant to vancomycin—United States, 1989–1993. *MMWR.* 1993;42:597–599.

87. Karanfil LV, Murphy M, Josephson A, et al. A cluster of vancomycin-resistant *Enterococcus faecium* in an intensive care unit. *Infect Control Hosp Epidemiol.* 1992;13:195–200.

88. Handwerger S, Raucher B, Altarac D, et al. Nosocomial outbreak due to *Enterococcus faecium* highly resistant to vancomycin, penicillin, and gentamicin. *Clin Infect Dis.* 1993;16:750–755.

89. Boyle JF, Soumakis SA, Rendo A, et al. Epidemiologic analysis and genotypic characterization of a nosocomial outbreak of vancomycin-resistant enterococci. *J Clin Microbiol.* 1993; 31:1280–1285.

90. Montecalvo MA, Horowitz H, Gedris C, et al. Outbreak of vancomycin, ampicillin, and aminoglycoside-resistant *Enterococcus faecium* bacteremia in an adult oncology unit. *Antimicrobiol Agents Chemother.* 1994;38:1363–1367.

91. Boyce JM, Opal SM, Chow JW, et al. Outbreak of multi-drug resistant *Enterococcus faecium* with transferable vanB class vancomycin resistance. *J Clin Microbiol.* 1994;32:1148–1153.

92. Quale J, Landman D, Atwood E, et al. Experience with a hospital-wide outbreak of vancomycin-resistant enterococci. *Am J Infect Control.* 1996;24:372–379.

93. Hanna H, Umphrey J, Tarrand J, Mendoza M, Raad I. Management of an outbreak of vancomycin-resistant enterococci in the medical intensive care unit of a cancer center. *Infect Control Hosp Epidemiol.* 2001;22:217–219.

94. Byers KE, Anglim AM, Anneski CJ, et al. A hospital epidemic of vancomycin-resistant *Enterococcus*: risk factors and control. *Infect Control Hosp Epidemiol.* 2001;22:140–147.

95. Pearman JW. 2004 Lowbury Lecture: the Western Australian experience with vancomycin-resistant enterococci—from disaster to ongoing control. *J Hosp Infect.* 2006;63:14–26.

96. Frieden TR, Munsiff SS, Low DE, et al. Emergence of vancomycin-resistant enterococci in New York City. *Lancet.* 1993;342:76–79.

97. Silverman J, Thal LA, Perri MB, Bostic G, Zervos MJ. Epidemiologic evaluation of antimicrobial resistance in community-acquired enterococci. *J Clin Micro.* 1998;36:830–832.

98. McDonald LC, Kuehneert MJ, Tenover FC, Jarvis WR. Vancomycin-resistant enterococci outside the health-care setting: prevalence, sources, and public health implications. *Emerg Infect Dis.* 1997;3:311–317.

99. Morris JT Jr, Shay DK, Hebden J, et al. Enterococci resistant to multiple antimicrobial agents, including vancomycin. Establishment of endemicity in a university medical center. *Ann Intern Med.* 1995;123:250–259.

100. Crossley K and Long-Term Care Committee of the Society for Healthcare Epidemiology of America. Vancomycin-resistant enterococci in long-term care facilities. *Infect Control Hosp Epidemiol.* 1998;19:521–525.

101. Edmond MB, Ober JF, Weinbaum DL, et al. Vancomycin-resistant *Enterococcus faecium* bacteremia; risk factors for infection. *Clin Infect Dis.* 1995;20:1126–1133.

102. Bonten MJM, Hayden MK, Nathan C, et al. Epidemiology of colonization of patients and environment with vancomycin-resistant enterococci. *Lancet.* 1996;348:1615–1619.

103. The Hospital Infection Control Practices Advisory Committee. Recommendations for preventing the spread of vancomycin resistance: recommendations of the Hospital Infection Control Practices Advisory Committee (HICPAC). *Am J Infect Control.* 1995;23:87–94.

104. Livornese LL, Dias S, Samel C, et al. Hospital-acquired infection with vancomycin-resistant *Enterococcus faecium* transmitted by electronic thermometer. *Ann Intern Med.* 1992;117: 112–114.

105. Martinez JA, Ruthazer R, Hansjosten K, Barefoot L, Snydman DR. Role of environmental contamination as a risk factor for acquisition of vancomycin-resistant enterococci in patients treated in a medical intensive care unit. *Arch Intern Med.* 2003;163(16):1905–1912.

106. Rhinehart E, Smith NE, Wennersten C. Rapid dissemination of beta-lactamase producing, aminoglycoside-resistant *Enterococcus faecalis* among patients and staff in an infant-toddler surgical ward. *N Engl J Med.* 323:1814–1818.

107. Eckstein BC, Adams DA, Ekstein EC, et al. Reduction of *Clostridium difficile* and vancomycin-resistant *Enterococcus* contamination of environmental surfaces after an intervention to improve cleaning methods. *BMC Infect Dis.* 2007;7:61–66. http://www.pubmedcentral.nih.gov/articlerender.fcgi?tool=pubmed&pubmedid=17584935. Accessed December 15, 2007.

108. Bhalla S, Pultz, NJ, Gries DM. Acquisition of nosocomial pathogens on hands after contact with environmental surfaces near hospitalized patients. *Infect Control Hosp Epidemiol.* 2004;2004;25:164–167.

109. Montecalvo MA, deLencastre H, Carraher M, et al. Natural history of colonization with vancomycin-resistant *Enterococcus faecium. Infect Control Hosp Epidemiol.* 1995;16:680–685.

110. Bonilla HF, Zervos MA, Lyons MJ, et al. Colonization with vancomycin-resistant *Enterococcus faecium*: comparison of a long-term care unit with an acute-care hospital. *Infect Control Hosp Epidemiol.* 1997;18:333–339.

111. Noskin GA, Stosor V, Cooper I, Peterson LR. Recovery of vancomycin-resistant enterococci on fingertips and environmental surfaces. *Infect Control Hosp Epidemiol.* 1995;16:577–581.

112. Bonilla HF, Zervos MJ, Kauffman CA. Long-term survival of vancomycin-resistant *Enterococcus faecium* on a contaminated surface [letter and comments]. *Infect Control Hosp Epidemiol.* 1996;17:770–772.

113. Boyce JM, Mermel LA, Zervos MJ, et al. Controlling vancomycin-resistant enterococci. *Infect Control Hosp Epidemiol.* 1995;16:634–637.

114. Wade JJ, Desai N, Casewell MW. Hygienic hand disinfection for the removal of epidemic vancomycin-resistant *Enterococcus faecium* and gentamicin-resistant *Enterobacter cloacae. J Hosp Infect.* 1991;18:211–218.

115. Brennen C, Wagener MM, Muder RR. Vancomycin-resistant *Enterococcus faecium* in a long-term care facility. *J Am Geriatr Soc.* 1998;46:157–160.

116. Padiglione AA, Grabsch E, Wolfe R, Gibson K, Grayson ML. The prevalence of fecal colonization with VRE among residents of long-term care—facilities in Melbourne, Australia. *Infect Control and Hosp Epidemiol.* 2001;22:576–578.

117. Terpenning MS, Bradley SF, Wan JY, Chenoweth CE, Jorgensen KA, Kauffman CA. Colonization and infection with antibiotic resistant bacteria in a long term care facility. *J Am Geriatr Soc.* 1994;42:1062–1069.

118. Trick WE, Weinstein RA, DeMarais PL, et al. Colonization of skilled-care facility residents with antimicrobial-resistant pathogens. *J Am Geriatr Soc.* 2001;49:270–276.

119. Safdar N, Maki DG. The commonality of risk factors for nosocomial colonization and infection with antimicrobial-resistant *Staphylococcus aureus, Enterococcus,* gram-negative bacilli, *Clostridium difficile,* and *Candida. Ann Intern Med.* 2002;136:834–844.

120. Donskey CJ, Ray AJ, Hoten CK, et al. Colonization and infection with multiple nosocomial pathogens among patients colonized with vancomycin-resistant *Enterococcus. Infect Control Hosp Epidemiol.* 2003;24:242–245.

121. Elizaga ML, Weinstein RA, Hayden MK. Patients in long-term care facilities: a reservoir for vancomycin-resistant enterococci. *Clin Infect Dis.* 2002;34:441–446.

122. Armstrong-Evans M, Litt M, McArthur MA, et al. Control of vancomycin-resistant *Enterococcus faecium* in a long-term care facility. *Infect Control Hosp Epidemiol.* 1999;20:312–317.

123. Trick WE, Kuehnert MJ, Quirk SB, et al. Regional dissemination of vancomycin-resistant enterococci resulting from interfacility transfer of colonized patients. *J Infect Dis.* 1999;180:391–396.

124. Boyce J. Environmental contamination makes an important contribution to hospital infection. *J Hsop Infect.* 2007;65:50–54.

125. Mody L, McNeil, Sun R, Bradley SF, Kauffman CA. Introduction of a waterless alcohol-based hand rub in a long-term care facility. *Infect Control Hosp Epidemiol.* 2003;24:165–171.

126. Hiramatsu K, Hanaki H, Ino T, Yabuta K, Oguri T, Tenover FC. Methicillin-resistant *Staphylococcus aureus* clinical strain with reduced vancomycin susceptibility. *J Antimicrobiol Chemother.* 1997;40:135–136.

127. Centers for Disease Control and Prevention. Update: *Staphylococcus aureus* with reduced susceptibility to vancomycin—United States, 1997. *MMWR.* 1997;46:813–815. http://www.cdc.gov/mmwr/preview/mmwrhtml/00053311.htm. Accessed April 17, 2008.

128. Ploy MC, Grelaud C, Martin C, de Lumley L, Denis F. First clinical isolate of vancomycin-intermediate *Staphylococcus aureus* in a French hospital. *Lancet.* 1998;351:1212.

129. Centers for Disease Control and Prevention. *Staphylococcus aureus* resistant to vancomycin—United States, 2002. *MMWR.* 2002;51(26);565–567. http://www.cdc.gov/mmwr/preview/mmwrhtml/mm5126a1.htm. Accessed April 17, 2008.

130. Hageman JC, Pegues DA, Jepson C, et al. Vancomycin-intermediate *Staphylococcus aureus* in a home health-care patient. *Emerg Infect Dis.* 2001;7:1023–1025. http://www.cdc.gov/ncidod/eid/vol7no6/hageman.htm. Accessed April 17, 2008.

131. Saha B, Singh B, Ghosh A, Bal M. Identification and characterization of a vancomycin-resistant *Staphylococcus aureus* isolated from Kolkata (South Asia). *Med Microbiol.* 2008;57(Pt 1):72–79.

132. Tenover FC, McDonald LC. Vancomycin-resistant staphylococci and enterococci: epidemiology and control. *Curr Opin Infect Dis.* 2005;18(4):300–305.

133. Howe RA, Monk A, Wootton M, Walsh TR, Enright MC. Vancomycin susceptibility within methicillin-resistant *Staphylococcus aureus* lineages. *Emerg Infect Dis.* 2004;10:855–857. http://www.cdc.gov/ncidod/EID/vol10no5/03-0556.htm. Accessed May 12, 2008.

134. Hageman JC, Patel JB, Carey RC, Tenover FC, McDonald LC. Investigation and control of vancomycin-intermediate and resistant *Staphylococcal aureus:* a guide for health departments and infection control personnel. Atlanta, GA. 2005. http://www.cdc.gov/ncidod/dhqp/pdf/ar/visa_vrsa_guide.pdf. Accessed April 17, 2008.

135. Edmond MB, Wenzel RP, Pasculle W. Vancomycin-resistant *Staphylococcus aureus:* perspectives on measures needed for control. *Ann Intern Med.* 1996;124:329–334.

136. Jarvis WR. Nosocomial transmission of multidrug-resistant *Mycobacterium tuberculosis. Am J Infect Control.* 1995;23:146–151.

137. Edlin BR, Tokars JI, Garieco MH, et al. An outbreak of multidrug-resistant tuberculosis among hospitalized patients with the acquired immunodeficiency syndrome. *N Engl J Med.* 1992;326:1514–1521.

138. Catanzaro A. Nosocomial tuberculosis. *Am Rev Respir Dis.* 1982;125:559–562.

139. Ehrenkranz NJ, Kicklighter JL. Tuberculosis outbreak in a general hospital: evidence of airborne spread of infection. *Ann Intern Med.* 1972;77:377–382.

140. Haley CE, McDonald RC, Rossi L, et al. Tuberculosis epidemic among hospital personnel. *Infect Control Hosp Epidemiol.* 1989;10:204–210.

141. Hutton MD, Stead WW, Cauthen GM, et al. Nosocomial transmission of tuberculosis associated with a draining tuberculous abscess. *J Infect Dis.* 1990;161:286–295.

142. Kantor HS, Poblete R, Pusateri SL. Nosocomial transmission of tuberculosis from unsuspected disease. *Am J Med.* 1988;84:833–838.

143. Lundgren R, Norman E, Asberg I. Tuberculous infection transmitted at autopsy. *Tubercle.* 1987;68:147–150.

144. Templeton GL, Illing LA, Young L, Cave MD, Stead WW, Bates JH. Comparing the risk for transmission of *Mycobacterium tuberculosis* at the bedside and during autopsy. *Ann Intern Med.* 1995;122:922–925.

145. CDC. *Mycobacterium tuberculosis* transmission in a health clinic—Florida, 1988. *MMWR.* 1989;38:256–258, 263–264.

146. Beck-Sague C, Dooley SW, Hutton MD, et al. Outbreak of multidrug-resistant *Mycobacterium tuberculosis* infections in a hospital: transmission to patients with HIV infection and staff. *JAMA.* 1992;268:1280–1286.

147. CDC. Nosocomial transmission of multidrug-resistant tuberculosis to health-care workers and HIV-infected patients in an urban hospital—Florida. *MMWR.* 1990;39:718–722.

148. CDC. Nosocomial transmission of multidrug-resistant tuberculosis among HIV-infected persons—Florida and New York, 1988–1991. *MMWR.* 1991;40:585–591.

149. Dooley SW, Jarvis WR, Martone WJ, Snider DE Jr. Multidrug-resistant tuberculosis [editorial]. *Ann Intern Med.* 1992;117:257–258.

150. Dooley SW, Villarino ME, Lawrence M, et al. Nosocomial transmission of tuberculosis in a hospital unit for HIV-infected patients. *JAMA.* 1992;267:2632–2634.

151. Centers for Disease Control. Transmission of multi-drug resistant tuberculosis from an HIV-positive client in a residential substance-abuse treatment facility—Michigan. *MMWR.* 1991:40:129–131.

152. Ikeda RM, Birkhead GS, DiFerdinando GT Jr, et al. Nosocomial tuberculosis: an outbreak of a strain resistant to seven drugs. *Infect Control Hosp Epidemiol.* 1995;16:152–159.

153. Huang WL, Jou R, Yeh PF, Huang A, and Outbreak Investigation Team. Laboratory investigation of a nosocomial transmission of tuberculosis at a district general hospital. *J Formos Med Assoc.* 2007;106:520–527.

154. Keijman J, Tjhie J, Olde Damink S, Alink M. Unusual nosocomial transmission of *Mycobacterium tuberculosis. Eur J Clin Microbiol Infect Dis.* 2001;20(11):808–809.

155. Centers for Disease Control and Prevention. Nosocomial transmission of *Mycobacterium tuberculosis* found through screening for severe acute respiratory syndrome—Taipei, Taiwan, 2003. *MMWR.* 2004;53(15);321–322. http://www.cdc.gov/mmwr/preview/mmwrhtml/mm5315a5.htm. Accessed December 14, 2007.

156. Centers for Disease Control and Prevention. *Mycobacterium tuberculosis* transmission in a newborn nursery and maternity ward—New York City, 2003. *MMWR.* 2005;54:1280–1283. http://www.cdc.gov/mmwR/preview/mmwrhtml/mm5450a2.htm. Accessed April 18, 2008.

157. Centers for Disease Control and Prevention. Guidelines for preventing the transmission of *Mycobacterium tuberculosis* in health-care settings, 2005. *MMWR.* 2005;54(RR-17):1–141. http://www.cdc.gov/mmwr/PDF/rr/rr5417.pdf. Accessed December 16, 2007.

158. CDC. Reported tuberculosis in the United States, 2006. Atlanta, GA: U.S. Department of Health and Human Services, CDC, September 2006. http://www.cdc.gov/tb/surv/default.htm. Accessed December 15, 2007.

159. Health Resources and Services Administration. Projected supply, demand, and shortage of registered nurses: 2000—2020. Rockville, MD: US Department of Health and Human Services, Health Resources and Services Administration; 2002. http://bhpr.hrsa.gov/healthworkforce. Accessed April 18, 2008.

160. Brennen C, Muder RR, Muraca PW. Occult endemic tuberculosis in a chronic care facility. *Infect Control Hosp Epidemiol.* 1988;9:548–552.

161. Stead WW. Tuberculosis among elderly persons: an outbreak in a nursing home. *Ann Intern Med.* 1981;94:606–610.

162. Stead WW. Special problems in tuberculosis. Tuberculosis in the elderly and in residents of nursing homes, correctional facilities, long-term care hospitals, mental hospitals, shelters for the homeless, and jails. *Clin Chest Med.* 1989;10:397–405.

163. Bentley DW. Tuberculosis in long-term care facilities. *Infect Control Hosp Epidemiol.* 1990;11:42–46.

164. Steimke EH, Tenholder MF, McCormick MI, Rissing JP. Tuberculosis surveillance: lessons from a cluster of skin test conversions. *Am J Infect Control.* 1994;22:236–241.

165. CDC. Tuberculosis—North Dakota. *MMWR.* 1979;27:523–525.

166. CDC. Tuberculosis in a nursing home—Oklahoma. *MMWR.* 1980;29:465–467.

167. CDC. Tuberculosis in a nursing care facility—Washington. *MMWR.* 1983;32:121–122, 128.

168. Stead WW, Lofgren JP, Warren E, Thomas C. Tuberculosis as an endemic and nosocomial infection among the elderly in nursing homes. *N Engl J Med.* 1985.312:1483–1487.

169. Malone JL, Ijaz K, Lamgert L, et al. Investigation of healthcare-associated transmission of *Mycobacterium tuberculosis* among patients with malignancies at three hospitals and at a residential facility. *Cancer.* 2004;101:2713–2721.

170. Lemaitre N, Sougakoff W, Coetmeur D, Vaucel J, Jarleir V, Grosset J. Nosocomial transmission of tuberculosis among mentally-handicapped patients in a long-term care facility. *Tuber Lung Dis.* 1996;77:531–536.

171. Centers for Disease Control. Prevention and control of tuberculosis in facilities providing long-term care to the elderly. Recommendations of the Advisory Committee for Elimination of Tuberculosis. *MMWR.* 1990;39(RR-10):7–20.

172. Ijaz K, Dillaha JA, Yang Z, Cave MD, Bates JH. Unrecognized tuberculosis in a nursing home causing death with spread of tuberculosis to the community. *J Am Geriatr Soc.* 2002; 50(7):1213–1218.

173. Emergence of *Mycobacterium tuberculosis* with extensive resistance to second-line drugs—worldwide, 2000–2004. *MMWR.* 2006;55,(11):301–305. http://www.cdc.gov/mmwr/preview/mmwrhtml/mm5511a2.htm. Accessed December 16, 2007.

174. Extensively drug-resistant tuberculosis—United States, 1993–2006. *MMWR.* 2007;56(11); 250–253. http://www.cdc.gov/mmwr/preview/mmwrhtml/mm5611a3.htm. Accessed December 16, 2007.

175. World Health Organization/International Union Against TB and Lung Disease Global Project on Anti-Tuberculosis Drug Resistance Surveillance. Anti-Tuberculosis Drug Resistance in the World: Fourth Global Report. Geneva; 2008. Report No. WHO/HTM?TB?2008.394. http://www.who.int/tb/publications/2008/drs_report4_26feb08.pdf. Accessed April 18, 2008.

176. WHO. Case definition for extensively drug-resistant tuberculosis. *Wkly Epidemiol Rec.* 2006;81(42):408. http://www.who.int/wer/2006/wer8142/en/index.ht. Accessed December 16, 2007.

177. World Health Organization. Guidelines for the prevention of tuberculosis in health care facilities in resource-limited settings. WHO/CDS/TB/99.269. http://www.who.int/tb/publications/who_tb_99_269/en/. Accessed April 18, 2008.

178. World Health Organization. Tuberculosis infection-control in the era of expanding HIV care and treatment. Addendum to WHO guidelines for the prevention of tuberculosis in health care facilities in resource-limited settings. http://www.who.int/tb/publications/who_tb_99_269/en/. Accessed April 18, 2008.

179. Maryland Department of Health and Mental Hygiene. Guidelines for prevention and treatment of tuberculosis, 2007. http://edcp.org/tb/guidelines.html. Accessed December 16, 2007.

180. Thrupp L, Bradley S, Smith P, et al and the SHEA Long-Term Care Committee. Tuberculosis prevention and control in long-term-care facilities for older adults. *Infect Control Hosp Epidemiol.* 2004;25:1097–1108.

181. Tuberculosis Infection Control: *A Practical Manual for Preventing TB.* http://www.nationaltbcenter.edu/products/product_details.cfm?productID=WPT-12. Accessed December 16, 2007.

182. Tuberculosis Coalition for Technical Assistance. International Standards for Tuberculosis Care (ISTC). The Hague: Tuberculosis Coalition for Technical Assistance, 2006. http://www.stoptb.org/resource_center/assets/documents/istc_report.pdf. Accessed December 18, 2007.

183. American Thoracic Society and CDC. Targeted tuberculin testing and treatment of latent tuberculosis infection. *MMWR.* 2000;49(RR-06):1–54 http://www.cdc.gov/mmwR/preview/mmwrhtml/rr4906a1.htm. Accessed April 18, 2008.

184. Centers for Disease Control and Prevention. Controlling tuberculosis in the United States: recommendations from the American Thoracic Society, CDC, and the Infectious Diseases Society of America. *MMWR.* 2005;54(No. RR-12):1–82. http://www.cdc.gov/mmwR /preview/mmwrhtml/rr5412a1.htm. Accessed April 18, 2008.

185. Centers for Disease Control and Prevention. Guidelines for using the QuantiFERON-TB Gold test for detecting *Mycobacterium tuberculosis* infection, United States. *MMWR Recomm Rep.* 2005;54(RR-15):49–55. [Erratum, *MMWR Morb Mortal Wkly Rep* 2005;54:1288.] http://www.cdc.gov/mmwR/PDF/rr/rr5415.pdf. Accessed April 18, 2008.

186. Naglie G, McArthur M, Simor A, et al. Tuberculosis surveillance practices in long-term care institutions. *Infect Control Hosp Epidemiol.* 1995;16:148–151.

187. American Thoracic Society, CDC, and Infectious Diseases Society of America. Treatment of tuberculosis. *MMWR.* 2003;52:(RR11):1–77. http://www.cdc.gov/mmwr/preview/mmwrhtml/rr5211a1.htm. Accessed December 18, 2007.

188. *Treatment of Tuberculosis: Guidelines for National Programmes*, 3rd ed. Geneva, World Health Organization, 2003 (WHO/CDS/TB/2003.313). http://www.who.int/tb/publications/cds_tb_2003_313/en/index.html. Accessed December 18, 2007.

189. Menzies D. Effect of treatment on contagiousness of patients with active pulmonary tuberculosis. *Infect Control Hosp Epidemiol.* 1997;18:582–586.

190. Sepkowitz K. How contagious is tuberculosis? *Clin Infect Dis.* 1996;23:954–962.

191. Centers for Disease Control and Prevention. Guidelines for the investigation of contacts of persons with infectious tuberculosis; recommendations from the National Tuberculosis Controllers Association and CDC. *MMWR Recomm Rep.* 2005;54(RR-15):1–48. http://www.cdc.gov/mmwR/PDF/rr/rr5415.pdf. Accessed April 18, 2008.

192. Johnson S, Gerding DN. *Clostridium difficile*-associated diarrhea. *Clin Infect Dis.* 1998; 26:1027–1034.

193. McDonald LC, Owings M, Jernigan DB. *Clostridium difficile* infection in patients discharged from US short-stay hospitals, 1996–2003. *Emerg Infect Dis.* 2006;12:409–415.

194. Pepin J, Valiquette L, Cossette B. Mortality attributable to nosocomial *Clostridium difficile*-associated disease during an epidemic caused by a hypervirulent strain in Quebec. *CMAJ.* 2005;173:1037–1042.

195. McFarland LV, Beneda HW, Clarridge JE, Raugi GJ. Implications of the changing face of *Clostridium difficile* disease for health care practitioners. *Am J Infect Control.* 2007;35:237–253.

196. CA Muto CA, Pokrywka M, Shutt K, et. al. A large outbreak of *Clostridium difficile*-associated disease with an unexpected proportion of deaths and colectomies at a teaching hospital following increased fluoroquinolone use. *Infect Control & Hosp Epidemiol.* 2005;26(3):273–280.

197. Bartlett JG. Narrative review: the new epidemic of *Clostridium difficile*-associated enteric disease. *Ann Intern Med.* 2006;145:758–764.

198. McDonald LC, Killgore GE, Thompson A, et al. An epidemic, toxin gene-variant strain of *Clostridium. N Engl J Med.* 2005;353:2433–2441.

199. McDonald LC. *Clostridium difficile*: responding to a new threat from an old enemy. *Infect Control Hosp Epidemiol.* 2005;26:672–675.

200. Warny M, Pepin J, Fang A, et al. Toxin production by an emerging strain of *Clostridium difficile* associated with outbreaks of severe disease in North America and Europe. *Lancet.* 2005;366:1079–1084.

201. Kuijper EJ, Coignard B, Tull P; ESCMID Study Group for *Clostridium difficile*; EU Member States; European Centre for Disease Prevention and Control. Emergence of *Clostridium difficile*-associated disease in North America and Europe. *Clin Microbiol Infect.* 2006;12 (Suppl 6):2–18.

202. McFarland LV, Mulligan ME, Kwok RYY, Stamm WE. Nosocomial acquisition of *Clostridium difficile* infection. *N Engl J Med.* 1989;320:204–210.

203. Gerding DN, Johnson S, Peterson LR, Mulligan ME, Silva J Jr. SHEA position paper. *Clostridium difficile*-associated diarrhea and colitis. *Infect Control Hosp Epidemiol.* 1995; 16:459–477.

204. Samore MH, Venkataraman L, DeGirolami PC, Arbeit RD, Karchmer AW. Clinical and molecular epidemiology of clustered cases of nosocomial *Clostridium difficile* diarrhea. *Am J Med.* 1996;110:32–40.

205. Thomas DR, Bennett RG, Laughon BE, Greenough WBIII, Bartlett JG. Postantibiotic colonization with *Clostridium difficile* in nursing home patients. *J Am Geriatr Soc.* 1990;38: 415–420.

206. Sohn S, Climo M, Diekema D, et al. Varying rates of *Clostridium difficile*-associated diarrhea at Prevention Epicenter Hospitals. *Infect Control Hosp Epidemiol.* 2005;26:676–679.

207. Simor AE, Yake SL, Tsimidis K. Infection due to *Clostridium difficile* among elderly residents of a long-term-care facility. *Clin Infect Dis.* 1993;17:672–678.

208. Sims RV, Hauser RJ, Adewale AO, et al. Acute gastroenteritis in three community-based nursing homes. *J Gerontol.* 1995;50A:M252–M256.

209. Olson MM, Stanholtzer CJ, Lee JT, Gerding DN. Ten years of prospective *Clostridium difficile*-associated disease surveillance and treatment at the Minneapolis VA Medical Center, 1982–1991. *Infect Control Hosp Epidemiol.* 1994;15:371–381.

210. Nath SK, Thornley JH, Kelly M, et al. A sustained outbreak of *Clostridium difficile* in a general hospital: persistence of a toxigenic clone in four units. *Infect Control Hosp Epidemiol.* 1994;15:382–389.

211. Dubberke ER, Reske KA, Yan Y, Olsen A, McDonald LC, Fraser VJ. *Clostridium difficile*-associated disease in a setting of endemicity: identification of novel risk factors. *Clin Infect Dis.* 2007;45:1543–1549.

212. Kyne L, Merry C, O'Connell B, Keane C, O'Neill D. Community acquired *Clostridium difficile* infection. *J Infect.* 1998;36:287–288.

213. Bentley DW. *Clostridium difficile*-associated disease in long-term care facilities. *Infect Control Hosp Epidemiol.* 1990;11:434–438.

214. Bennett GCJ, Allen E, Millard PH. *Clostridium difficile* diarrhoea: a highly infectious organism. *Age Ageing.* 1984;13:363–366.

215. Kerr RB, McLaughlin DI, Sonnenberg LW. Control of *Clostridium difficile* colitis outbreak by treating asymptomatic carriers with metronidazole. *Am J Infect Control.* 1990;18:332–335.

216. Cartmill TDI, Shrimpton SB, Panigrahi H, Khanna V, Brown R, Poxton IR. Nosocomial diarrhoea due to a single strain of *Clostridium difficile*: a prolonged outbreak in elderly patients. *Age Ageing.* 1992;21:245–249.

217. McNulty C, Logan M, Donald IP, et al. Successful control of *Clostridium difficile* infection in an elderly care unit through use of a restrictive antibiotic policy. *J Antimicrobiol Chemother.* 1997;40:707–711.

218. Gaynes R, Rimland D, Killum E, Lowery HK, Johnson TM, Killgore G. Outbreak of *Clostridium difficile* infection in a long-term care facility: association with gatifloxacin use. *Clin Infect Dis.* 2004;38:640–645.

219. Cherifi S, Delmee M, Van Broeck J, Beyer I, Byl B, Mascart G. Management of an outbreak of *Clostridium difficile*-associated disease among geriatric patients. *Infect Control Hosp Epidemiol.* 2006;11:1200–1205.

220. Canadian Nosocomial Infection Surveillance Program. Ongoing surveillance for *Clostridium difficile* associated diarrhea (CDAD) within acute-care institutions, February 2007. http://www.phac-aspc.gc.ca/nois-sinp/projects/pdf/cdad07_protocol_e.pdf. Accessed January 9, 2008.

221. McDonald LC, Coignard B, Dubberke E, et al.. Recommendations for surveillance of *Clostridium difficile*-associated disease. *Infect Control Hosp Epidemiol.* 2007;28:140–145. http://www.journals.uchicago.edu/doi/pdf/10.1086/511798. Accessed January 9, 2008.

222. Dubberke ER, Reske KA, Noble-Wang J, et al. Prevalence of *Clostridium difficile* environmental contamination and strain variability in multiple health care facilities. *Am J Infect Control.* 2007;35:315–318.

223. Perry C, Marshall R, Jones E. Bacterial contamination of uniforms. *J Hosp Infect.* 2001; 48(3):238–241.

224. Clabots CR, Johnson S, Olson MM, Peterson LR, Gerding DN. Acquisition of *Clostridium difficile* by hospitalized patients: evidence for colonized new admissions as a source of infection. *J Infect Dis.* 1992;166:561–567.

225. Zafar AB, Gaydos LA, Furlong WB, Nguyen MH, Mennonna PA. Effectiveness of infection control program in controlling nosocomial *Clostridium difficile*. *Am J Infect Control.* 1998;26:588–593.

226. Apisarnthanarak A, Zack JE, Mayfield JL, et al. Effectiveness of environmental and infection control programs to reduce transmission of *Clostridium difficile*. *Clin Infect Dis.* 2004;39: 601–602.

227. Beaulieu M, Thirion DJ, Williamson D, Pichette G. *Clostridium difficile* associated diarrhea outbreaks: the name of the game is isolation and cleaning. *Clin Infect Dis.* 2006;42:727–729.

228. Weiss K. Poor infection control, not fluoroquinolones, likely to be primary cause of *Clostridium difficile*-associated diarrhea outbreaks in Quebec. *Clin Infect Dis.* 2006;42:725–727.

229. Simor AE, Bradley SF, Strausbaugh LJ, Crossley K, Nicolle LE. SHEA position paper. *Clostridium difficile* in long-term-care facilities for the elderly. *Infect Control Hosp Epidemiol.* 2002;23:696–703.

230. Sehulster LM, Chinn RYW, Arduino MJ, et al. Guidelines for environmental infection control in health-care facilities. Recommendations from CDC and the Healthcare Infection Control Practices Advisory Committee (HICPAC). 2003. http://www.cdc.gov/ncidod/dhqp/gl_environinfection.html. Accessed January 10, 2008.

231. Kramer, et al. How long do nosocomial pathogens persist on inanimate surfaces? A systematic review. *BMC Infect Dis.* 2006;6:130.

232. Warren N, Fawley WN, Underwood S, et al. Efficacy of hospital cleaning agents and germicides against epidemic *Clostridium difficile* strains. *Infect Control Hosp Epidemiol.* 2007; 28:920–925.

233. Mayfield JL, Leet T, Miller J, Mundy LM. Environmental control to reduce transmission of *Clostridium difficile*. *Clin Infect Dis.* 2000;31(4):995–1000. http://www.journals.uchicago.edu/doi/pdf/10.1086/318149. Accessed January 9, 2008.

234. Brooks SE, Veal RO, Kramer M, Dore L, Schupf N, Adachi M. Reduction in the incidence of *Clostridium difficile*-associated diarrhea in an acute care hospital and a skilled nursing facility following replacement of electronic thermometers with single-use disposables. *Infect Control Hosp Epidemiol.* 1992;13:98–103.

235. Brooks SE, Khan A, Stoica D, et al. Reduction in vancomycin-resistant *Enterococcus* and *Clostridium difficile* infections following change to tympanic thermometers. *Infect Control Hosp Epidemiol.* 1998;19:333–336.

236. Jernigan JA, Siegman-Igra Y, Guerrant RC, Farr BM. A randomized crossover study of disposable thermometers for prevention of *Clostridium difficile* and other nosocomial infections. *Infect Control Hosp Epidemiol.* 1998;19:494–499.

237. Brown E, Talbot GM, Axelrod P, Provencher M, Hoegg C. Risk factors for *Clostridium difficile* toxin-associated diarrhea. *Infect Control Hosp Epidemiol.* 1990;11:283–290.

238. Mylotte JM. Laboratory surveillance method for nosocomial *Clostridium difficile* diarrhea. *Am J Infect Control.* 1998;26:16–23.

239. Centers for Disease Control and Prevention. Prevention and control of influenza: recommendations of the Advisory Committee on Immunization Practices (ACIP), 2007; *MMWR Early Release*. 2007;56:1–56.

240. Salgado CD, Farr BM, Hall KK, Hayden FG. Influenza in the acute hospital setting. *Lancet Infect Dis*. 2002;2(3):145–155.

241. Maltezou HC, Drancourt M. Nosocomial influenza in children. *J Hosp Infect*. 2003;55(2): 83–91.

242. Evans ME, Hall KL, Berry SE. Influenza control in acute care hospitals. *Am J Infect Control*. 1997;25:357–362.

243. Cunney RJ, Bialachowski A, Thornley D, Smaill FM, Pennie RA. An outbreak of influenza A in a neonatal intensive care unit. *Infect Control Hosp Epidemiol*. 2000;21:449–454.

244. Munoz FM, Campbell JR, Atmar RL, et al. Influenza A virus outbreak in a neonatal intensive care unit. *Pediatr Infect Dis J*. 1999;18(9):811–815.

245. Sagrera X, Ginovart G, Raspall E, et al. Outbreaks of influenza A virus infection in neonatal intensive care units. *Pediatr Infect Dis J*. 2002;21(3):196–200.

246. Singer R, Dennis P. Nosocomial influenza at a Canadian pediatric hospital from 1995 to 1999: opportunities for prevention. *Infect Control Hosp Epidemiol*. 2002;23:627–629.

247. Stott DJ, Kerr G, Carman WF. Nosocomial transmission of influenza. *Occ Med*. 2002;52: 249–253.

248. Morens DM, Rash VM. Lessons from a nursing home outbreak of influenza A. *Infect Control Hosp Epidemiol*. 1995;16:275–280.

249. Centers for Disease Control and Prevention. Update: influenza activity—United States, 1998–99 season. *MMWR*. 1999;48:177–181.

250. Libow LS, Neufeld RR, Olson E, Breuer B, Starer P. Sequential outbreak of influenza A and B in a nursing home: efficacy of vaccine and amantadine. *J Am Geriatr Soc*. 1996;44: 1153–1157.

251. Drinka PJ, Gravenstein S, Krause P, Schilling M, Miller BA, Shult P. Outbreak of influenza A and B in a highly immunized nursing home population. *J Fam Pract*. 1997;45:509–514.

252. Taylor JN, Dwyer DM, Coffman T, Groves C, Patel J, Israel E. Nursing home outbreak of influenza A (H3N2): evaluation of vaccine efficacy and influenza case definitions. *Infect Control Hosp Epidemiol*. 1992;13:93–97.

253. Coles FB, Balzano GJ, Morse DL. An outbreak of influenza A (H3N2) in a well immunized nursing home population. *J Am Geriatr Soc*. 1992;40:589–592.

254. Degelau J, Somani SK, Cooper SL, Guay DR, Crossley KB. Amantadine-resistant influenza A in a nursing facility. *Arch Intern Med*. 1992;152:390–392.

255. Patriarca PA, Weber JA, Parker RA, et al. Risk factors for outbreaks in nursing homes. A case-control study. *Am J Epidemiol*. 1986;124:114–119.

256. Staynor K, Foster G, McArthur M, McGeer A, Petric M, Simor AE. Influenza A outbreak in a nursing home: the value of early diagnosis and the use of amantadine hydrochloride. *Can J Infect Control*. 1994;9:109–111.

257. Gross PA, Rodstein M, LaMontagne JR, et al. Epidemiology of acute respiratory illness during an influenza outbreak in a nursing home. *Arch Intern Med*. 1988;148:559–561.

258. Smith PW, Rusnak PG. Infection prevention and control in the long-term care facility. *Am J Infect Control*. 1997;25:488–512.

259. Tellier R. Review of aerosol transmission of influenza A virus. *Emerg Infect Dis*. 2006;12:1657–1662. [serial on the Internet]. http://www.cdc.gov/ncidod/EID/vol12no11/ 06-0426.htm. Accessed April 19, 2008.

260. Centers for Disease Control and Prevention. Prevention and control of influenza: recommendations of the Advisory Committee on Immunization Practices (ACIP), 2007. *MMWR*. 2007;56(No RR-6):1–60. http://www.cdc.gov/mmwR/preview/mmwrhtml/rr5606a1.htm. Accessed April 19, 2008.

261. Centers for Disease Control and Prevention. Guidelines for preventing health-care-associated pneumonia, 2003. Recommendations of CDC and the Healthcare Infection Control Practices

Advisory Committee. http://www.cdc.gov/ncidod/dhqp/gl_hcpneumonia.html. Accessed April 19, 2008.

262. Centers for Disease Control and Prevention. Influenza vaccination of health-care personnel recommendations of the Healthcare Infection Control Practices Advisory Committee (HIC-PAC) and the Advisory Committee on Immunization Practices (ACIP). *MMWR.* 2006;55 (RR-2):1–20.

263. Association for Professionals in Infection Control and Epidemiology. 2004 APIC Immuniza-tion Practices Working Group. APIC position paper: improving health care worker influenza immunization rates. *Am J Infect Control.* 2004;32:123–125.

264. Gravenstein S, Miller BA, Drinka P. Prevention and control of influenza A outbreaks in long-term care facilities. *Infect Control Hosp Epidemiol.* 1992;13:49–54.

265. Gomolin IH, Leib HB, Arden NH, Sherman FT. Control of influenza outbreaks in the nursing home: guidelines for diagnosis and management. *J Am Geriatr Soc.* 1995;43:71–74.

266. Kingston BJ, Wright CW. Influenza in the nursing home. *Am Fam Physician.* 2002;65:75–78. http://www.aafp.org/afp/20020101/75.pdf. Accessed January 11, 2008.

267. World Health Organization. Infection prevention and control of epidemic and pandemic-prone acute respiratory diseases in health care. WHO interim guidelines, June 2007. http://www.who.int/csr/resources/publications/WHO_CD_EPR_2007_6/en/index.html. Accessed January 11, 2008.

268. California Department of Public Health, Division of Communicable Disease Control Infec-tious Diseases and Immunization Branches. Recommendations for the prevention, detection, and control of influenza in California long-term care facilities, 2007-2008. http://www.dhs .ca.gov/ps/dcdc/disb/disbindex.htm. Accessed April 20, 2008.

269. Maryland Department of Health and Mental Hygiene. Guideline for the prevention and con-trol of upper and lower acute respiratory illnesses (including influenza and pneumonia) in long term care facilities. http://www.cha.state.md.us/edcp/html/cd_guide.html. Accessed April 20, 2008.

270. Houck P, Hemphill M, LaCroix S, Hirsh D, Cox N. Amantadine-resistant influenza A in nurs-ing homes. Identification of a resistant virus prior to drug use. *Arch Intern Med.* 1995;155: 533–537.

271. Hota S, McGeer A. Antivirals and the control of influenza outbreaks. *Clin Infect Dis.* 2007;45(10):1362–1368.

272. Goodgame R. Norovirus gastroenteritis. *Curr Infect Dis Rep.* 2007;9(2):102–109.

273. Blanton LH, Adams SM, Beard RS, et al. Molecular and epidemiologic trends of caliciviruses associated with outbreaks of acute gastroenteritis in the United States, 2000–2004. *J Infect Dis.* 2006;193:413–421.

274. Widdowson MA, Sulka A, Bulens S, et al. Norovirus and foodborne disease, United States, 1991–2000. *Emerg Infect Dis.* 2005;11:95–102. http://www.cdc.gov/ncidod/EID/vol11no01/ pdfs/04-0426.pdf. Accessed April 15, 2008.

275. Grmek Kosnik I, Peternelj B, Pohar M, Kraigher A. Outbreak of norovirus infection in a nursing home in northern Slovenia, July 2007. *Eur Surveill.* 2007;12(10):E071011.3. http://www.eurosurveillance.org/ew/2007/071011.asp#3. Accessed April 15, 2008.

276. Ike AC, Broackman SO, Hartelt K, Marschang RE, Contzen A, Oehme RM. Molecular epi-demiology of norovirus in outbreaks of gastroenteritis in southwest Germany from 2001 to 2004. *J Clin Microbiol.* 2006;44:1262–1267.

277. Johnston CP, Qiu H, Ticehurst JR, et al. Outbreak management and implications of a nosoco-mial norovirus outbreak. *Clin Infect Dis.* 2007;45(5):534–540.

278. Vardy J, Love AJ, Dignon N. Outbreak of acute gastroenteritis among emergency department staff. *Emerg Med J.* 2007;24(10):699–702.

279. Marx A, Shay D, Noel J, et al. An outbreak of acute gastroenteritis in a geriatric long-term care facility: use of epidemiological and molecular diagnostic methods. *Infect Control Hosp Epidemiol.* 1999;20:306–311.

280. Lopman BA, Gallimore C, Gray JJ, et al. Linking healthcare associated norovirus outbreaks: a molecular epidemiologic method for investigating transmission. *BMC Infect Dis.* 2006;

6:108 doi:10.1186/1471-2334-6-108. http://www.biomedcentral.com/1471-2334/6/108. Accessed January 12, 2008.

281. Zingg W, Colombo C, Jucker T, et al. Impact of an outbreak of norovirus infection on hospital resources. *Infect Control Hosp Epidemiol.* 2005;26(3):263–267.

282. Centers for Disease Control and Prevention. Norovirus activity—United States, 2006–2007. *MMWR.* 2007;56(33);842–846. http://www.cdc.gov/mmwr/preview/mmwrhtml/mm5633a2 .htm. Accessed April 15, 2008.

283. Calderon-Margalit R, Sheffer R, Halperin T, Orr N, Cohen D, Shohat T. A large-scale gastroenteritis outbreak associated with norovirus in nursing homes. *Epidemiol Infect.* 2005; 133(1):35–40.

284. Costas L, Vilella A, Llupia A, Bosch J, Jimenez de Anta MT, Trilla A. Outbreak of norovirus gastroenteritis among staff at a hospital in Barcelona, Spain, September 2007. *Eurosurveillance Weekly Release.* 2007;12:(11). http://www.eurosurveillance.org/ew/2007/071122.asp#5. Accessed April 19, 2008.

285. Gellert GA, Waterman SH, Ewert D, et al. An outbreak of acute gastroenteritis caused by a small round structured virus in a geriatric convalescent facility. *Infect Control Hosp Epidemiol.* 1990;11(9):459–464.

286. Cooper E, Blamey S. A norovirus gastroenteritis epidemic in a long-term care facility. *Infect Control Hosp Epidemiol.* 2005;26(3):256.

287. Navarro G, Sala RM, Segura F, et al. An outbreak of norovirus infection in a long-term care. *Infect Control Hosp Epidemiol.* 2005;26(3):259.

288. Green KY, Belliot G, Taylor JL, et al. A predominant role for Norwalk-like viruses as agents of epidemic gastroenteritis in Maryland nursing homes for the elderly. *J Infect Dis.* 2002; 185(2):133–146.

289. CDC. Norwalk-like viruses. Public health consequences and outbreak management. *MMWR.* 2001;50(No. RR-9):1–17. http://www.cdc.gov/mmwr/preview/mmwrhtml/rr5009a1.htm. Accessed April 15, 2008.

290. Chadwick PR, Beards G, Brown D, et al. Management of hospital outbreaks of gastro-enteritis due to small round structured viruses. Report of the Public Health Laboratory Service, Viral Gastroenteritis Working Group. *J Hosp Infect.* 2000;45:1–10.

291. Wu HM, Fornek M, Schwab KJ, et al. A norovirus outbreak at a long-term care facility: the role of environmental surface contamination. *Infect Control Hosp Epidemiol.* 2005;26: 802–810.

292. Centers for Disease Control and Prevention. Norovirus outbreak associated with ill food-service workers—Michigan, January—February, 2006. *MMWR.* 2007;56(46);1212–1216. http://www.cdc.gov/mmwr/preview/mmwrhtml/mm5646a2.htm. Accessed April 15, 2008.

293. Marks PJ, Vipond IB, Regan FM, Wedgwood K, Fey RE, Caul EO. A school outbreak of Norwalk-like virus: evidence for airborne transmission. *Epidemiol Infect.* 2003;131:727–736.

294. Maryland Department of Health and Mental Hygiene. Guidelines for the epidemiological investigation of gastroenteritis outbreaks in long term care facilities. http://www.edcp .org/html/cd_guide.html. Accessed April 15, 2008.

295. Michigan Department of Community Health, Michigan Department of Agriculture. Viral gastroenteritis. Norovirus. Guidelines for environmental cleaning and disinfection of norovirus. http://www.michigan.gov/documents/Guidelines_for_Environmental_Cleaning_125846_7.pdf. Accessed April 15, 2008.

296. Lynn S, Toop J, Millar N. Norovirus outbreaks in a hospital setting: the role of infection control. *J N Z Med Assoc.* 2004;117(1189):771–779. http://www.nzma.org.nz/journal/117–1189/ 771/. Accessed April 15, 2008.

297. United States Environmental Protection Agency. List G: EPA's registered antimicrobial products effective against norovirus (Norwalk-like virus) January 7, 2008. http://www.epa .gov/oppad001/list_g_norovirus.pdf. Accessed April 15, 2008.

298. Lettau LA. Nosocomial transmission and infection control aspects of parasitic and ectoparasitic diseases: Part I. Introduction/enteric parasites. *Infect Control Hosp Epidemiol.* 1991; 12:59–65.

299. Lettau LA. Nosocomial transmission and infection control aspects of parasitic and ectoparasitic diseases: Part II. Blood and tissue Parasites. *Infect Control Hosp Epidemiol.* 1991; 12:111–121.

300. Lettau LA. Nosocomial transmission and infection control aspects of parasitic and ectoparasitic diseases: Part III. Ectoparasites/summary and conclusions. *Infect Control Hosp Epidemiol.* 1991;12:179–185.

301. Degelau J. Scabies in Long-term care facilities. *Infect Control Hosp Epidemiol.* 1992;13: 421–425.

302. Scheinfeld N. Controlling scabies in institutional settings: a review of medications, treatment models, and implementation. *Am J Clin Dermatol.* 2004;5(1):31–37.

303. Obasanjo OO, Wu P, Conlon M, et al. An outbreak of scabies in a teaching hospital: lessons learned. *Infect Control Hosp Epidemiol.* 2001;22(1):13–18.

304. Vorou R, Remoudaki HD, Maltezou HC. Nosocmial scabies. *J Hosp Infect.* 2007;65(1):9–14.

305. Achtari Jeanneret L, Erard P, Gueissaz F, Malinverni R. An outbreak of scabies: a forgotten parasitic disease still present in Switzerland. *Swiss Med Wkly.* 2007;137:695–699. http://www.smw.ch/docs/pdf200x/2007/49/smw-11904.pdf. Accessed October 6, 2000.

306. Wilson MM, Philpott CD, Breer WA. Atypical presentation of scabies among nursing home residents. *J Gerontol A Biol Sci Med Sci.* 2001;56(7):M424–M427.

307. Andersen BM, Haugen H, Rasch M, Heldal Haugen A, Tageson A. Outbreak of scabies in Norwegian nursing homes and home care patients: control and prevention. *J Hosp Infect.* 2000; 45(2):160–164.

308. Roncoroni AJ, Gomez MA, Mera J, Cagnoni P, Michel MD. Cryptosporidium infection in renal transplant patients. *J Infect Dis.* 1989;160:559.

309. Sarabia-Arce S, Salazar-Lindo E, Gilman RH, Naranjo J, Miranda E. Case-control study of *Cryptosporidium parvum* infection in Peruvian children hospitalized for diarrhea: possible association with malnutrition and nosocomial infection. *Pediatr Infect Dis J.* 1990;9:627–631.

310. Neill MA, Rice SK, Ahmad NV, Flanigan TP. Cryptosporidiosis: an unrecognized cause of diarrhea in elderly hospitalized patients. *Clin Infect Dis.* 1996;22:168–170.

311. Craven DE, Steger KA, Hirschorn LR. Nosocomial colonization and infection in persons infected with human immunodeficiency virus. *Infect Control Hosp Epidemiol.* 1996;17:304–318.

312. Gardner C. An outbreak of hospital-acquired cryptosporidiosis. *Br J Nurs.* 1994;3:152,154–158.

313. Navarrete S, Stetler HC, Avila C, Garcia Aranda JA, Santos-Preciado JI. An outbreak of *Cryptosporidium* diarrhea in a pediatric hospital. *Pediatr Infect Dis J.* 1991;10:248–250.

314. Weber DJ, Rutala WA. The emerging nosocomial pathogens *Cryptosporidium, Escherichia coli* O157:H7, *Helicobacter pylori*, and hepatitis C: epidemiology, environmental survival, efficacy of disinfection, and control measures. *Infect Control Hosp Epidemiol.* 2001;22(5): 306–315.

315. Ravn P, Lundgren JD, Kjaeldgaard P, et al. Nosocomial outbreak of cryptosporidiosis in AIDS patients. *BMJ.* 1991;302:277–280.

316. Perera DR, Western KA, Johnson HD, Johnson WW, Schultz MG, Akers PV. *Pneumocystis carinii* pneumonia in a hospital for children. Epidemiologic aspects. *JAMA.* 1970;214: 1074–1078.

317. Hennequin C, Page B, Roux P, Legendre C, Kreis H. Outbreak of *Pneumocystis carinii* pneumonia in a renal transplant unit. *Eur J Clin Microbiol Infect Dis.* 1995;14:122–126.

318. Fenelon LE, Keane CT, Bakir M, Temperley IJ. A cluster of *Pneumocystis carinii* infections in children. *BMJ.* 1985;291:1683.

319. Chaves JP, David S, Wauters JP, Van Melle G, Francioli P. Transmission of *Pneumocystis carinii* from AIDS patients to other immunosuppressed patients: a cluster of *Pneumocystis carinii* pneumonia in a renal transplant recipient. *AIDS.* 1991;5:927–932.

320. Schmoldt S, Schuhegger R, Wendler T, et al. Molecular evidence of nosocomial *Pneumocystis jirovecii* transmission among 16 patients after kidney transplantation. *J Clin Microbiol.* 2008;46(3):966–971.

321. Vargo JA, Ginsberg MM, Mizrahi M. Human infestations by the pigeon mite: a case report. *Am J Infect Control.* 1983;11:24–25.

322. Istre GR, Hreiss K, Hopkins RS, et al. An outbreak of amebiasis spread by colonic irrigation at a chiropractic clinic. *N Engl J Med.* 1982;307:339–342.

323. White KE, Hedberg CW, Edmonson LM, Jones DB, Osterholm MT, MacDonald KL. An outbreak of giardiasis in a nursing home with evidence for multiple modes of transmission. *J Infect Dis.* 1989;160:298–304.

324. Burkhart CG. Scabies: an epidemiologic reassessment. *Ann Intern Med.* 1983;98:498–503.

325. Green MS. Epidemiology of scabies. 1989;11:126–150.

326. Arlian LG, Runyan RA, Achar S, Estes SA. Survival and infectivity of *Sarcoptes scabiei* var. canis and var. hominis. *J Am Acad Dermatol.* 1984;11(2 Pt 1):210–215.

327. Paternak J, Richtman R, Ganme APP, et al. Scabies epidemic: price and prejudice. *Infect Control Hosp Epidemiol.* 1994;15:540–542.

328. Estes SA, Estes J. Therapy of scabies: nursing homes, hospitals, and the homeless. *Semin Dermatol.* 1993;12:26–33.

329. Sirera G, Rius F, Romeu J, et al. Hospital outbreak of scabies stemming from two AIDS patients with Norwegian scabies. *Lancet.* 1990;335:1227.

330. Purvis RS, Tyring SK. An outbreak of lindane-resistant scabies treated successfully with permethrin 5% cream. *J Am Acad Dermatol.* 1991;25(6 Pt 1):1015–1016.

331. Clark J, Friesen DL, Williams WA. Management of an outbreak of Norwegian scabies. *Am J Infect Control.* 1992;20:217–220.

332. Boix V, Sanchez-Paya J, Portilla J, Merino E. Nosocomial outbreak of scabies clinically resistant to lindane. *Infect Control Hosp Epidemiol.* 1997;18:677.

333. Bannatyne RM, Patterson TA, Wells BA, MacMillan SA, Cunninghan GA, Tellier R. Hospital outbreak traced to a case of Norwegian scabies. *Can J Infect Control.* 1992;7:111–113.

334. Holness DL, DeKoven JG, Nethercott JR. Scabies in chronic health care institutions. *Arch Dermatol.* 1992;128:1257–1260.

335. Yokonsky D, Ladi L, Gackenheimer L, Schultz MW. Scabies in nursing homes: an eradication program with permethrin 5% cream. *J Am Acad Dermatol.* 1990;23(6 Pt 1):1133–1136.

336. Haag ML, Brozena SJ, Fenske NA. Attack of the scabies: what to do when an outbreak occurs. *Geriatrics.* 1993;48:45–46, 51–53.

337. Jimenez-Lucho VE, Fallon F, Caputo C, Ramsey K. Role of prolonged surveillance in the eradication of nosocomial scabies in an extended care Veterans Affairs medical center. *Am J Infect Control.* 1995;23:44–49.

338. Paules SJ, Levisohn D, Heffron W. Persistent scabies in nursing home patients. *J Fam Pract.* 1993;37:82–86.

339. Centers for Disease Control and Prevention. Scabies in health-care facilities—Iowa. *MMWR.* 1988;37:178–179.

340. Strong M, Johnstone PW. Interventions for treating scabies. Cochrane Database of Systematic Reviews 2007; 3. doi: 10.1002/14651858.CD000320.pub2.

341. Maryland Department of Health and Mental Hygiene, Epidemiology and Disease Control Program. Guidelines for control of scabies in long-term care facilities. http://www.cha.state.md.us/edcp/html/cd_guide.html. Accessed April 16, 2008.

342. MacKenzie WR, Hoxie NJ, Proctor ME, et al. A massive outbreak in Milwaukee of cryptosporidium infection transmitted through the public water supply. *N Engl J Med.* 1994;331:161–167.

343. Centers for Disease Control and Prevention. Outbreak of gastroenteritis associated with an interactive water fountain at a beachside park—Florida, 1999. *MMWR.* 2000;49:565–568.

344. Centers for Disease Control and Prevention. Foodborne outbreak of cryptosporidiosis—Spokane, Washington, 1997. *MMWR.* 1998;47:565–567.

345. Millard PS, Gensheimer KF, Addiss DG, et al. An outbreak of cryptosporidiosis from fresh-pressed apple cider. *JAMA.* 1994;272:1592–1596.

346. Combee CL, Collinge ML, Britt EM. Cryptosporidiosis in a hospital-associated day care center. *Pediatr Infect Dis.* 1986;5:528–532.

347. Avgun G, Yilmaz M, Yasar H. Parasites in nosocomial diarrhoea: are they underestimated? *J Hosp Infect.* 2005;60(3):283–285.

348. Black RE, Dykes AC, Sinclair SP, Wells JG. Giardiasis in daycare centers: evidence of person-to-person transmission. *Pediatrics.* 1977;60:486-491.

349. Haron E, Bodey GP, Luna MA, Dekmezian R, Elting L. Has the incidence of *Pneumocystis carinii* pneumonia in cancer center patients increased with the AIDS epidemic? *Lancet.* 1988; 2:904–905.

350. Regan AM, Metersky ML, Craven DE. Nosocomial dermatitis and pruritis caused by pigeon mite infestation. *Arch Intern Med.* 1987;147:2185–2187.

351. Jarvis WR, Hughes JM. Nosocomial gastrointestinal infections. In: Wenzel RP, ed. *Prevention and Control of Nosocomial Infections.* 2nd ed. Baltimore, MD: Williams & Wilkins; 1992: 708–745.

352. Nicolle LE, Garibaldi RA. Infection control in long-term care facilities. *Infect Control Hosp Epidemiol.* 1995;16:348–353.

353. Steere AC, Craven PJ, Hall WJ, III, et al. Person-to-person spread of *Salmonella* after a hospital common-source outbreak. *Lancet.* 1975;1:319–322.

354. Rodriquez EM, Parrott C, Rolka H, Monroe SS, Dwyer DM. An outbreak of viral gastroenteritis in a nursing home: importance of excluding ill employees. *Infect Control Hosp Epidemiol.* 1996;17:587–592.

355. Schroeder SA, Askeroff, Brachman PS. Epidemic salmonellosis in hospitals and institutions: public health importance and outbreak management. *N Engl J Med.* 1968;279;674–678.

356. Standaert SM, Hutcheson RH, Schaffner W. Nosocomial transmission of *Salmonella gastroenteritis* to laundry workers in a nursing home. *Infect Control Hosp Epidemiol.* 1994; 15:22–26.

357. Centers for Disease Control. Viral agents of gastroenteritis. Public health importance and outbreak management. *MMWR.* 1990;39(RR-5):1–24.

358. Khuri-Bulos NA, Abu Khalaf M, Shehabi A, Shami K. Foodhandler-associated *Salmonella* outbreak in a university hospital despite routine surveillance cultures of kitchen employees. *Infect Control Hosp Epidemiol.* 1994;15:311–314.

359. Layton MC, Calliste SG, Gomez TM, Patton C, Brooks S. A mixed foodborne outbreak with *Salmonella heidelberg* and *Campylobacter jejuni* in a nursing home. *Infect Control Hosp Epidemiol.* 1997;18:115–121.

360. Levine WC, Smart JF, Archer DL, Bean NH, Tauxe RV. Foodborne disease outbreaks in nursing homes, 1975 through 1987. *JAMA.* 1991;266:2105–2109.

361. Linnemann CC Jr, Cannon CG, Stancek Jl, et al. Prolonged hospital epidemic of salmonellosis: use of trimethoprim-sulfamethoxazole for control. *Infect Control Hosp Epidemiol.* 1985; 6:221–225.

362. Slutsker L, Villarino ME, Jarvis WR, Goulding J. Foodborne disease prevention in healthcare facilities. In: Bennett JV, Brachman PS, eds. *Hospital Infections.* 4th ed. Philadelphia, PA: Lippincott-Raven; 1998;22:341.

363. Pegues DA, Woernle CH. An outbreak of acute nonbacterial gastroenteritis in a nursing home. *Infect Control Hosp Epidemiol.* 1993;14:87–94.

364. Gellert GA, Waterman SH, Ewert D, et al. An outbreak of acute gastroenteritis caused by a small round structured virus in a geriatric convalescent facility. *Infect Control Hosp Epidemiol.* 1990;11:459–464.

365. Caceres VM, Kim DK, Bresee JS, et al. A viral gastroenteritis outbreak associated with person-to-person spread among hospital staff. *Infect Control Hosp Epidemiol.* 1998;19:162–167.

366. Khatib R, Naber M, Shellum N, et al. A common source outbreak of gastroenteritis in a teaching hospital. *Infect Control Hosp Epidemiol.* 1994;15:534–535.

367. Ho JL, Shands, KN, Fredland G, et al. A outbreak of type 4b *Listeria monocytogenes* infection involving patients from eight Boston hospitals. *Arch Intern Med.* 1986;146:520–524.

368. DeBuono BA, Brondum J, Kramer JM, Gilbert RJ, Opal SM. Plasmid, serotype and entero-toxin analysis of *Bacillus cereus* in an outbreak setting. *J Clin Microbiol*. 1988;26:1571–1574.

369. Bloom HG, Bottone EJ. *Aeromonas hydrophilia* diarrhea in a long-term care setting. *J Am Geriatr Soc*. 1990;38:804–806.

370. Carter AO, Birczyk AA, Carlson JA, et al. A severe outbreak of *Escherichia coli* O157:H7—associated hemorrhagic colitis in a nursing home. *N Engl J Med*. 1987;317:1496–1500.

371. Ryan CA, Tauxe RV, Hosek GW, et al. *Escherichia coli* O157:H7 in a nursing home: clinical epidemiological, and pathological findings. *J Infect Dis*. 1986;154:631–638.

372. Halvorsrud J, Orstavik I. An epidemic of rotavirus-associated gastroenteritis in a nursing home for the elderly. *Scand J Infect Dis*. 1980;12:161–164.

373. Raad I, Sheretz RJ, Russell BA, Reuman PD. Uncontrolled nosocomial rotavirus transmission during a community outbreak. *Am J Infect Control*. 1990;18:24–28.

374. Smith MJ, Clark HF, Lawley D. The clinical and molecular epidemiology of community- and healthcare-acquired rotavirus gastroenteritis. *Pediatr Infect Dis J*. 2008;27(1):54–58.

375. Chandran A, Heizen RR, Santoshan M, Siberry G. Nosocomial rotavirus infections: a systematic review. *J Pediatri*. 2006;149(4):441–447.

376. Gleizes O, Desselberger U, Tatochenko V, et al. Nosocomial rotavirus infection in European countries: a review of the epidemiology, severity and economic burden of hospital-acquired rotavirus disease. *Pediatr Infect Dis J*. 2006;25(1 Suppl):S12–S21.

377. Emont SL, Cote TR, Dwyer DM, Horan JM. Gastroenteritis outbreak in a Maryland nursing home. *Md Med J*. 1993;42:1099–1103.

378. Sawyer LA, Murphy JJ, Kaplan JE, et al. 25 to 30-nm virus particle associated with a hospital outbreak of acute gastroenteritis with evidence for airborne transmission. *Am J Epidemiol*. 1988;127:1261–1271.

379. Wall PG, Ryan MJ, Ward LR, Rowe B. Outbreaks of salmonellosis in hospitals in England and Wales: 1992–1994. *J Hosp Infect*. 1996;33:181–190.

380. Collier PW, Sharp JC, MacLeod AF, et al. Food poisoning in hospitals in Scotland, 1978–1987. *Epidemiol Infect*. 1988;101:661–667.

381. Hedberg CW, Osterholm MT. Outbreaks of food-borne and waterborne viral gastroenteritis. *Clin Microbiol Rev*. 1993;6:199–210.

382. Centers for Disease Control and Prevention. Incidence of foodborne illnesses—FoodNet, 1997. *MMWR*. 1998;47:782–786.

383. Steiner TS, Theilman NM, Guerrant RL. Protozoal agents: what are the dangers for the public water supply? *Annu Rev Med*. 1997;48:329–340.

384. Center for Food Safety and Applied Nutrition. US Food and Drug Administration. *Foodborne Pathogenic Microorganisms and Natural Toxins Handbook*. College Park, MD: Center for Food Safety and Applied Nutrition; 1992.

385. Bell BP, Goldoft M, Griffin PM, et al. A multistate outbreak of *Escherichia coli* O157:H7-associated bloody diarrhea and hemolytic uremia syndrome from hamburgers: the Washington experience. *JAMA*. 1994;272:1349–1353.

386. Centers for Disease Control and Prevention. Outbreak of cyclosporiasis—Northern Virginia-Washington, DC-Baltimore, Maryland, Metropolitan Area, 1997. *MMWR*. 1997;46:689–691.

387. CDC. Outbreak of listeriosis—Northeastern United States, 2002. *MMWR*. 2002;51:950–951.

388. Bean NH, Gouldoft M, Griffin PM, et al. Surveillance for foodborne-disease outbreaks—United Sates, 1998–1992. In: CDC Surveillance Summaries, October 25, 1996. *MMWR*. 1996;45:1–67.

389. Centers for Disease Control and Prevention. Surveillance for foodborne-disease outbreaks United States, 1998–2002. Surveillance summaries. *MMWR*. 2006;55(No. SS-10):1–42. http://www.cdc.gov/mmwR/PDF/ss/ss5510.pdf. Accessed April 19, 2008.

390. Chodick G, Ashkenazi S, Lerman Y. The risk of hepatitis A infection among healthcare workers: a review of reported outbreaks and sero-epidemiologic studies. *J Hosp Infect*. 2006;62:414–420.

391. Doebbeling BN, Li N, Wenzel RP. An outbreak of hepatitis A among health care workers: risk factors for transmission. *Am J Public Health.* 1993;83:1679–1684.

392. Victorian Government Department of Human Services. Guidelines for the investigation of gastrointestinal illness, 1998. Victorian Government Department of Human Services. Melbourne, Victoria. http://www.health.vic.gov.au/ideas. Accessed April 19, 2008.

393. Sattar SA, Jacobsen H, Rahman H, Cusack TM, Rubino JR. Interruption of rotavirus spread through chemical disinfection. *Infect Control Hosp Epidemiol.* 1994;15:751–756.

394. Lew JF, LeBaron CW, Glass RI, et al. Recommendations for collection of laboratory specimens associated with outbreaks of gastroenteritis. *MMWR.* 1990;39(RR-14):1–13.

395. Centers for Disease Control and Prevention. Aldicarb as a cause of food poisoning—Louisiana, 1998. *MMWR.* 1999;48:269–271.

396. Lopman B, Reacher MH, Vipond IB, et al. Epidemiology and cost of nosocomial gastroenteritis, Avon, England, 2002–2003. *Emerg Infect Dis.* 2004;10(10):1827–1834. http://www.cdc.gov/ncidod/EID/vol10no10/pdfs/03-0941.pdf. Accessed April 16, 2008.

SUGGESTED READING AND RESOURCES

Resources

Foodborne and Gastrointestinal Diseases

CDC Outbreak Response and Surveillance Team (ORST): Foodborne disease surveillance and outbreak investigation toolkit. http://www.cdc.gov/foodborneoutbreaks/toolkit.htm. Accessed April 20, 2008.

Maryland Department of Health and Mental Hygiene. Guidelines for the epidemiological investigation of gastroenteritis outbreaks in long-term care facilities. http://www.edcp.org/html/cd_guide.html. Accessed April 15, 2008. These guidelines are reprinted in Appendix H (Appendix H is available for download at this text's Web site: http://www.jbpub.com/catalog/9780763757793/).

Ribes J, Thornton AC, Feola DJ, Murphy B. Diarrheal diseases. In: *APIC Text of Infection Control and Epidemiology.* Washington, DC: Association for Professionals in Infection Control and Epidemiology. 2005:100-1, 100-22.Legionnaires' Disease.

Norovirus

CDC. Norovirus in healthcare facilities fact sheet. Atlanta, GA: US Department of Health and Human Services, CDC; 2006. http://www.cdc.gov/ncidod/dhqp/id_norovirusFS.html#. Accessed April 20, 2008.

Michigan Department of Community Health, Michigan Department of Agriculture. Viral gastroenteritis. Norovirus. Guidelines for environmental cleaning and disinfection of norovirus. http://www.michigan.gov/documents/Guidelines_for_Environmental_Cleaning_125846_7.pdf. Accessed April 15, 2008.

Tuberculosis

World Health Organization TB publications: http://www.who.int/tb/ publications/2007/en/index.html.

American Association of Homes and Services for the Aging. Preventing TB in long term care: training modules for staff developers working in long term care, 2005. http://www2.aahsa.org/advocacy/nursing_homes/default.asp. Accessed December 20, 2007.

Guidelines for preventing the transmission of *Mycobacterium tuberculosis* in health-care settings, 2005. *MMWR.* 2005;54(No. RR-17):1–141. http://www.cdc.gov/mmwr/preview/mmwrhtml/rr5417a1.htm?s_cid=rr5417a1_e. Accessed May 12, 2008.

Tuberculosis (TB) risk assessment worksheet. Guidelines for preventing the transmission of *Mycobacterium tuberculosis* in health-care settings, 2005. *MMWR.* 2005;54(No. RR-

17):1–141. http://www.cdc.gov/tb/pubs/mmwr/Maj_guide/infectioncontrol.htm. Accessed December 16, 2007.

CDC guidelines relating to tuberculosis: http://www.cdc.gov/tb/pubs/mmwr/Maj_guide/default .htm. Accessed May 12, 2008.

CDC Division of Tuberculosis Elimination [homepage]. http://www.cdc.gov/tb/. Provides links to TB prevention and control guidelines, educational and training materials, *MMWR* articles relating to TB, and the CDC core curriculum course on TB.

Other

CDC vancomycin-intermediate/resistant (VISA/VRSA) *Staphylococcus aureus.* http://www.cdc .gov/ncidod/dhqp/ar_visavrsa.html. Accessed April 17, 2008.

CDC Division of Healthcare Quality Promotion: infection control in healthcare settings [homepage]. http://www.cdc.gov/ncidod/dhqp/index.html. Accessed April 17, 2008.

CDC respiratory hygiene/cough etiquette in healthcare settings. http://www.cdc.gov/flu/professionals/ infectioncontrol/resphygiene.htm. Accessed April 19, 2008.

Food and Drug Administration (FDA), United States: http://www.fda.gov. Information for consumers and health educators on food safety and medical devices.

Legionnaires' disease OSHA eTool. http://www.osha.gov/dts/osta/otm/legionnaires/index.html. Accessed December 20, 2007.

CHAPTER 8

Investigation, Prevention, and Control of Outbreaks in the Healthcare Setting

Kathleen Meehan Arias

> Sickness is catching.
> —William Shakespeare, *A Midsummer Night's Dream*

INTRODUCTION

Although outbreaks in healthcare settings account for only a small proportion of healthcare-associated infections (HAIs),[1-3] they can result in significant morbidity and mortality, disruption of services, and fear and anxiety among personnel, patients, residents, and the community. Chapters 3 through 7 describe outbreaks that have been reported in various healthcare settings and that have been associated with a variety of diseases, health-related conditions, organisms, products, procedures, devices, and technical errors. The investigations of these outbreaks have been instrumental in defining the sources, modes of transmission, and measures used to prevent and control the spread of healthcare-associated infections and in defining noninfectious risks associated with health care.

While most people associate the word *outbreak* with an infectious disease, it can also be used to describe an excess of noninfectious diseases, conditions, and health-related events. The epidemiologic methods used to identify and investigate outbreaks caused by infectious agents can also be applied to study outbreaks of noninfectious etiology.[4-9] Personnel who are responsible for the infection surveillance, prevention, and control programs in healthcare settings can gain a valuable perspective from studying the findings of outbreak investigations because this knowledge can help them identify potential risk factors and effective control measures if a similar outbreak occurs in their facility.[10,11] The purpose of this chapter is to discuss practical methods that can be used to recognize, investigate, prevent, and control outbreaks in the healthcare setting.

RECOGNIZING A POTENTIAL OUTBREAK

An outbreak is the occurrence of more cases of a disease or event than expected during a specified period of time in a given area or among a specific group of people. In a healthcare setting, an outbreak may be suspected when routine surveillance activities detect an unusual organism, a cluster of cases, or an apparent increase in the usual number or incidence of cases; when a clinician diagnoses an uncommon disease; or when an alert healthcare provider or laboratory worker notices a cluster of cases. A cluster is a group of cases of a disease or other health-related event that occurs closely related in time and place. In a cluster, the number of cases may or may not exceed the expected number—frequently, the expected number is not known.

Because the endemic rates for nosocomial diseases, injuries, and other adverse events are different for each healthcare setting, few definitive criteria exist for determining when to evaluate a potential problem or initiate an investigation. The following questions may be asked to help decide what action needs to be taken:

- Is there a documented increase in the number or incidence of observed cases? Is it unlikely that the increase is due to normal statistical variation? Is the increase significant? If the answers are yes, then an evaluation should be done to determine if an investigation should be initiated.

- Are there published criteria for evaluating the occurrence of the particular disease or event? There are published thresholds for evaluating the occurrence of several diseases: measles, staphylococcal infections in the nursery, tuberculosis in long-term care facilities (LTCF), and healthcare-associated infections caused by group A streptococci and *Legionella* species, as noted below and outlined in Table 8–1.[12–20] If these thresholds are reached or exceeded, enhanced surveillance and an investigation is recommended. In addition, some state and provincial health departments have threshold criteria for investigating specific diseases. For instance, the Maryland Department of Health and Mental Hygiene provides guidelines for investigating, preventing, and controlling acute respiratory illnesses, gastroenteritis, and scabies in LTCFs. These guidelines, which are printed in Appendices G, H, and I, provide criteria for defining an outbreak (Appendices G, H, and I are available for download at this text's Web site: http://www.jbpub.com /catalog/9780763757793/).

- Is the disease or organism of special interest for the healthcare setting? A healthcare organization can determine that an infectious agent or disease is "epidemiologically important" for a specific setting. The CDC has defined "epidemiologically important organisms" as having the following characteristics:[18(p21)]

  - A propensity for transmission within healthcare facilities based on published reports and the occurrence of temporal or geographic clusters of more than two patients, (e.g., *C. difficile*, norovirus, respiratory syncytial virus (RSV), influenza, rotavirus, *Enterobacter* spp., *Serratia* spp., group A streptococcus). A single case of healthcare-associated invasive disease caused by certain pathogens (e.g., group A streptococcus postoperatively,[12] in burn units,[13] or in a LTCF[14]; *Legionella* spp.[17]; *Aspergillus* spp.[21]) is generally considered a trigger for investigation and enhanced control measures because of the risk of additional cases and severity of illness associated with these infections.

  - Common and uncommon microorganisms with unusual patterns of resistance within a facility (e.g., the first isolate of *Burkholderia cepacia* complex or *Ralstonia* spp. in noncystic fibrosis patients or a quinolone-resistant strain of *Pseudomonas aeruginosa* in a facility)

Table 8–1   Suggested Thresholds for Investigating a Potential Outbreak

Disease or Condition	*Threshold*	*Recommended Action(s)*	*Reference Number(s)*
Group A streptococci (GAS)	One case of healthcare-associated infection caused by GAS	Initiate investigation; review medical and laboratory records to identify other cases; heighten surveillance to identify additional episodes; save isolates from infected patients	12–14
Measles	One case of suspected measles	Rapidly investigate all reports of suspected measles; identify contacts and promptly vaccinate susceptible persons; all persons who cannot provide proof of immunity should be vaccinated or excluded from the setting (e.g., health care facility school, day care center)	15
Staphylococcus aureus in a nursery	Two or more concurrent cases of staphylococcal disease related to a nursery	Investigate possibility of an outbreak; culture all lesions; examine healthcare personnel for draining lesions; save clinically important isolates for six months; institute isolation precautions for cases	16
Legionnaire's disease (LD)	Single case of lab-confirmed healthcare-associated LD or two or more lab-confirmed possible cases that occur within six months of each other	Conduct an epidemiologic investigation; begin intensive prospective surveillance for additional cases; conduct retrospective review of serologic, microbiologic, and postmortem data to identify previously unrecognized cases	17–19
Tuberculosis (TB)	One case of infectious TB in an LTCF	Report case to health department; do contact tracing; skin test (PPD) contacts; provide preventive therapy for contacts who have documented skin test conversion; provide treatment for those with TB disease	20

Source: Author.

- Difficult to treat because of innate or acquired resistance to multiple classes of antimicrobial agents (e.g., *Stenotrophomonas maltophilia*, *Acinetobacter* spp.)
- Association with serious clinical disease, increased morbidity, and mortality [e.g., methicillin-resistant *S. aureus* (MRSA) and methicillin-sensitive *S. aureus* (MSSA), group A streptococcus (GAS)]
- A newly discovered or reemerging pathogen

- Is the reported case an unusual disease or event? In addition to the characteristics and diseases noted above, certain adverse drug reactions and adverse events related to commercially available medical products and devices (for example, renal insufficiency[22] and endotoxin-like reactions[23]) should also prompt an investigation and, when appropriate, should be reported to the proper authorities (e.g., the local or state health department and the Food and Drug Administration's MedWatch Program by calling 1-800-FDA-1088 or reporting online at http://www.fda.gov/medwatch) and to the manufacturer. Adverse events such as clusters of excessive bleeding after surgery,[24] pyrogenic reactions after hemodialysis,[25] and unexplained deaths[7,9] should also be investigated.

INITIATING AN OUTBREAK INVESTIGATION

A full-scale outbreak investigation generally requires expert assistance (such as from the health department or the CDC) and consumes valuable time and resources. When investigating clusters and potential outbreaks in healthcare settings, an initial evaluation followed by a carefully conducted literature search and a basic investigation (i.e., a descriptive epidemiologic study that characterizes the cases by person, place, and time) will often be sufficient to verify the existence of an outbreak, identify the most likely risk factor(s), and identify control measures that have been shown to be effective in similar circumstances. Once these control measures are implemented, prospective (ongoing) surveillance will allow the investigator to determine if they are effective at preventing new cases. If these empirically applied measures are effective at interrupting the outbreak, then no further investigation may be needed. A basic investigation is all that may be needed if the only objective is to control the outbreak, and the investigators do not wish to publish their findings or identify the most likely causal factor by statistically demonstrating differences in exposures between the cases and a control population.

A full-scale investigation is warranted if a suspected outbreak is facility-wide, appears to be associated with a commercially available product or medical device, involves a disease or condition that causes considerable morbidity or mortality, or appears to be unique in that it has not been previously reported and there are no control measures that have previously been shown to be effective. A full-scale investigation consists of the steps conducted in a basic investigation plus a statistical (comparative) study of the suspected risk factors (i.e., formulation and testing of hypotheses to explain the observed disease pattern) as described in Chapter 10. Case-control or cohort studies are most commonly used to test associations between risk factors and disease in outbreak investigations in the healthcare setting.

It is important to keep in mind the objectives of an outbreak investigation:

- Describe the situation and occurrence of cases.
- Determine the most likely etiologic agent, source, and method of spread.
- Interrupt the outbreak.
- Prevent the recurrence of a similar episode.

STEPS IN CONDUCTING AN OUTBREAK INVESTIGATION

Many of the steps in an outbreak investigation occur simultaneously; however, whenever an outbreak or a cluster is suspected, the investigator must first conduct an initial evaluation of the reported cases to confirm that a potential outbreak exists, and then decide whether to initiate a basic or a full-scale investigation. Exhibit 8–1 is an outline for investigating an outbreak.

Exhibit 8–1   Outline for Investigating an Outbreak*

The initial evaluation

Verify the diagnosis of reported cases before initiating an outbreak investigation.
Evaluate the severity of the problem.
Conduct a retrospective review to identify other cases.
Develop a line listing of cases.
Review the existing data; determine if a potential problem exists.

The outbreak investigation

Identify and verify the diagnosis of new cases.
Develop a case definition.
Review clinical and laboratory findings.
Document and organize findings at each step in the investigation.
Confirm the existence of an epidemic.
Conduct a literature search.
Consult with the laboratory.
Notify those who need to know.
Assemble a team.
Appoint a spokesperson to assure that consistent information is disseminated; be prepared to answer questions and address the concerns of the community and personnel, patients or residents, and their families.
Record actions taken (keep records of communications such as memos, letters, and e-mails).
Decide if outside assistance is needed (consult with outside agencies and experts, as needed).
Communicate findings and recommendations frequently; distribute written reports.
Institute early control measures.
Seek additional cases; create a data collection form.
Orient the data as to person, place, and time.
Evaluate the problem; observe practices that are potentially related to the occurrence of the outbreak.

continues

Exhibit 8–1   *(Continued)*

The outbreak investigation (Continued)

Determine the need for additional cultures or other diagnostic testing.
Formulate a tentative hypothesis.
Institute control measures.
Evaluate efficiency of control measures.
Test the hypotheses; consult a statistician to assure that the appropriate study method and statistical tests are used.
Conduct further analysis and investigation.

Prepare and distribute a written report

* Many of these steps will occur simultaneously

Source: Author.

Initial Evaluation

The purpose of the initial evaluation is to provide a quick analysis of the likelihood that an important excess of cases has occurred and to determine if a potential problem exists.[26] The steps in the initial evaluation are as follows:

1. Verify the diagnosis of the reported cases. The diagnosis should be verified by reviewing laboratory reports and medical records. In addition, clinical findings can be discussed with the attending healthcare providers—especially when there appears to be a discrepancy between the clinical findings and the laboratory findings. If the clinical findings do not support the laboratory findings, then a pseudoinfection or a misdiagnosis should be suspected.

   Remember that rule number one in an outbreak investigation is to verify the diagnosis of the initial case(s) before any further steps are taken. Many investigators have started off on the proverbial wild goose chase only to discover later that the clinical or laboratory findings of the cases did not match the reported diagnoses. Much time and effort can be wasted investigating an outbreak that does not exist if the reported diagnoses are not verified before proceeding. For instance, several years ago *Pseudomonas* (now *Ralstonia*) *pickettii* was isolated from blood cultures of several infants in the neonatal intensive care unit (NICU) at a large university hospital. A review of the cases revealed that none of the infants had signs or symptoms consistent with *Pseudomonas* bacteremia, and the investigators suspected specimen or laboratory contamination. Serendipitously, one of the infection prevention and control professionals (ICPs) worked part-time in the microbiology laboratory of a nearby hospital and discovered that the other hospital had also experienced a recent cluster of *P. pickettii*-positive blood cultures. A little shoe leather epidemiology revealed that both hospitals used the same type of broth culture media and both had used the same lot number. The outbreak was actually a pseudo-outbreak that was attributable to intrinsically contaminated culture media.

2. Evaluate the severity of the problem. For example, is the disease or condition likely to affect many people or only a few? Is it associated with significant morbidity or mortality, or is it mild and inconsequential? If the condition is severe, a full-scale investigation may be needed. If it is mild or affects only a few people, then a basic investigation may be all that is needed.

3. Conduct a retrospective review of surveillance records, laboratory reports, and clinical records to identify other cases.

4. Develop a line listing of cases. A line listing may be created on a computer or by hand. Each row in a line listing represents one case, and each column represents an important characteristic that may aid in the investigation, such as name, record number, age, sex, unit(s) or ward(s), date of admission, date of onset, service, signs and symptoms, types of therapy, surgery, and dates and results of laboratory tests. When a line listing is created in a computer database or spreadsheet program, the cases can be sorted by specified characteristics—this makes it easier to detect common risk factors. Exhibit 8–2 is an example of a line listing developed to study a suspected increase in the incidence of surgical site infections following coronary artery bypass graft surgery.

5. Review the existing information and determine if a potential problem exists (i.e., does the number of cases or incidence rate appear to be greater than expected).

6. If a potential outbreak exists, decide whether to begin a basic or a full-scale outbreak investigation. Because the initial steps for both investigations are similar, no time will be lost if the investigator decides to begin a basic investigation and subsequently finds that a full-scale study is warranted.

Steps in Conducting an Outbreak Investigation

Identify and Verify the Diagnosis of Newly Reported Cases

Conduct prospective surveillance for new cases by monitoring laboratory results, clinical records, and reports from attending healthcare providers. Add any new cases to the line listing.

Develop a Case Definition

One of the first steps in an outbreak investigation is to develop a case definition that will be used to identify affected persons. A case definition uses epidemiologic, clinical, and laboratory criteria to define and classify cases and usually restricts cases to a specific time, place, and person. The definition may categorize cases as possible, probable, and definite. At the beginning of an investigation, the case definition should be broad to ensure that all those who have the disease or condition are included in the study. An example of a preliminary case definition for an outbreak of gastrointestinal illness in an LTCF may be "all residents and personnel in Nursing Home A with onset of vomiting or diarrhea

Exhibit 8–2   Sample Line-Listing Form

Surgical Site Infections Following Coronary Artery Bypass Graft (CABG)

Name	Record #	Date CABG	Surgeon	Date SSI onset	Chest SSI (note type)*	Leg SSI (note type)*	Date of Culture	Organism

NOTE: SSI = surgical site infection
* TYPE: S/I = superficial/incisional; DI = deep infection; O/S = organ/space infection

Source: Author.

(i.e., two or more loose stools per day or an unexplained increase in the number of bowel movements) during the month of April." The case definition can be refined and narrowed as the investigation progresses. Appendix B contains the CDC definitions for infectious conditions that are reportable to local and state health departments in the United States (Appendix B is available for download at this text's Web site: http://www.jbpub.com/catalog/9780763757793/). These may be useful for developing a case definition for an outbreak in a healthcare setting.

Review Clinical and Laboratory Findings

If the outbreak is of infectious etiology, clinical and laboratory findings should be reviewed early in the investigation to determine if the cases are infected or colonized or if they represent pseudoinfection (i.e., the cultures are false positives). It is important to recognize pseudoinfections promptly because they may lead to an incorrect diagnosis and unnecessary treatment and control measures.

Confirm the Existence of an Outbreak

Rule number two in an outbreak investigation is to confirm the existence of an epidemic. This is done by determining if the incidence rate or the number of cases is above the endemic, or expected, rate. This may be relatively easy if the disease or condition is unusual or serious, such as *Burkholderia cepacia* bacteremia or pyrogenic reactions after hemodialysis. If, however, cases occur at low levels over a prolonged period or if an outbreak is caused by a relatively common organism, such as *Escherichia coli*, then recognition will be more difficult. Frequently, the baseline or background rate of a disease or condition is not known, and it is difficult to determine if an outbreak truly exists. Many authors have described methods that can be used to identify significant increases.[1,12–20,27–38] Unfortunately, there is no standard method for determining statistically if an outbreak exists in a healthcare setting. In practice, many outbreaks are recognized when personnel detect an increase in the number of cases of a disease or health-related event—even without calculating rates.

Some questions should be answered before a decision is made to conduct a full-scale investigation:

- Is there a possibility that the perceived increase is due to surveillance artifact? It is important to recognize that a change in surveillance techniques, which may occur if there is a change in personnel that perform surveillance activities or a change in criteria used to define a particular disease, may produce artifactual changes that are perceived as increases or decreases in the incidence of a disease or event. It is also important to ensure that infections that were present at admission are not categorized as nosocomial. For instance, a cluster of methicillin-resistant *Staphylococcus aureus* (MRSA) in a healthcare setting may be due to the coincidental admission of several patients who had MRSA at the time of admission.

- If the suspected outbreak is of infectious etiology, have there been any changes in the way specimens are collected, transported, or processed? It is important to determine if (1) there has been any change in the way specimens are collected, or (2) there has been any change in the laboratory procedures used to process specimens or to identify the suspect agent. Changes in the way specimens are collected or processed may produce a change in the incidence of an organism and have been responsible for many reported pseudo-outbreaks as discussed in Chapter 6. For instance, a pseudo-outbreak of *Pseudomonas aeruginosa* in neutropenic patients in a hematology unit occurred when several personnel collected stool cultures by sampling feces from the toilet. The toilet water contaminated the specimens.[39] Once the personnel were instructed how to properly collect the stool cultures, the outbreak subsided.

Conduct a Literature Search

A literature search should be conducted early in the investigation, as discussed in Chapter 9, to determine if other healthcare facilities have had a similar experience and have identified risk factors, sources, reservoirs, modes of transmission, and effective control measures. When conducting a literature search for outbreaks caused by a specific organism, the investigator should keep in mind that the nomenclature of microorganisms may change, as shown in Table 8–2, and older articles may use a previous name.

Consult with the Laboratory

If the outbreak is of infectious etiology, laboratory personnel should be notified as soon as possible about the likelihood of an outbreak, and they should be instructed to save sera and all isolates of the suspected agent, as appropriate, for possible future study (e.g., molecular typing of bacterial isolates to determine strain relatedness). Chapter 11 provides a discussion of the laboratory's role in outbreak investigation.

Table 8–2 Changing Nomenclature of Selected Organisms Associated with Outbreaks in the Healthcare Setting

Bacteria

Current Name	Other Names
Acinetobacter baumanii	Acinetobacter anitratus
Burkholderia cepacia	Pseudomonas cepacia
Citrobacter koseri	Citrobacter diversus
Enterococcus faecalis	Streptococcus faecalis (group D enterococcus)
Enterococcus faecium	Streptococcus faecium (group D enterococcus)
Ralstonia pickettii	Pseudomonas pickettii, Burkholderia pickettii
Stenotrophomonas maltophilia	Pseudomonas maltophilia, Xanthomonas maltophilia
Streptococcus agalactiae	Group B streptococcus
Streptococcus pyogenes	Group A streptococcus
Xanthomonas maltophilia	Pseudomonas maltophilia

Fungi

Current Name	Other Names
Candida albicans	Candida stellatoidea, Monilia albicans
Candida glabrata	Torulopsis glabrata
Malassezia furfur	Cladosporium mansonii, Pityrosporum orbiculare, Pityrosporum ovale
Malassezia pachydermatis	Pityrosporum pachydermatis

Viruses

Current Name	Other Names
Norovirus	Norwalk and Norwalk-like viruses, small round structured viruses, Calicivirus
Rhinovirus	Common cold virus

Source: Author.

Notify Essential Personnel

The organization's administrative staff should be notified as soon as possible of the likelihood of an outbreak—especially if the epidemic involves considerable morbidity or mortality. If the suspected outbreak involves a disease that is likely to attract media attention, such as Legionnaires' disease, scabies, salmonellosis, or meningitis, then the public relations department should also be notified. It would be unfortunate if either of these were to first learn about an outbreak in their facility through a reporter calling to request information.

Personnel in affected departments should be alerted as soon as the existence of an outbreak is confirmed. If likely prevention and control measures, such as hand hygiene or contact isolation, can be identified, then personnel should be instructed to use those precautions. The local health department should be notified if a reportable disease is involved or if local regulations require that outbreaks in healthcare facilities be reported. Risk management personnel should also be notified because outbreaks frequently result in lawsuits being filed against a healthcare organization.

Assemble a Team

An investigative team should be assembled and a member of the team should be appointed to be the primary contact person who will answer questions and communicate findings and recommendations. The team may be composed of personnel from infection prevention and control, infectious disease, quality management, risk management, laboratory, pharmacy, employee health, nursing, patient/resident care services, and administration, as needed. If the outbreak is covered by the media, it is helpful to have a spokesperson for the organization that is not actively involved in the investigation so that a person is not pulled away from the investigation to do interviews.

Outbreaks usually generate much fear and anxiety in personnel, patients or residents, and their families, and the team should anticipate overreaction, and possibly panic, and should be prepared to answer many questions and allay fears. For instance, in the early 1980s, a community hospital in Pennsylvania experienced an outbreak of *Citrobacter diversus* (now *koseri*) meningitis in neonates in the normal newborn nursery. The local health department and the CDC participated in the outbreak investigation, which attracted extensive media coverage. An employee who did not work in patient care and did not work in the nursery asked "to be tested for meningitis" because she was "afraid of bringing meningitis home" to her family. In addition, one of the investigators was pregnant and experienced pressure from her family to "let someone else" work on the investigation so she would not "catch something."

Determine the Need for Outside Assistance

The investigative team should decide if outside assistance is needed. When conducting an extensive investigation that involves a case control or cohort study, the investigators should seek the assistance of a trained statistician. Local and state health departments can arrange for assistance in conducting an outbreak investigation, and in many localities disease outbreaks of known or unknown etiology are reportable to the health department. In the United States, a health department will frequently call the CDC if an outbreak involves an unusual condition, a disease with high morbidity or mortality, or a common source outbreak believed to be linked to a commercially available product such as food or medication. The CDC personnel provide epidemiologic, laboratory, statistical, and technical assistance.

In addition, if a full-scale investigation is conducted, it will be necessary to arrange secretarial, clerical, technical, and laboratory support for the investigative team.

Institute Early Control Measures

Because the major objective of an outbreak investigation is to interrupt the outbreak, control measures should be identified and instituted as soon as possible. These should be based on the magnitude and nature of the problem and relevant findings from the literature search.

Seek Additional Cases

A thorough retrospective and concurrent search should be conducted to detect additional cases. This can be done by reviewing laboratory reports, surveillance records, medical records, and health department reports; calling area healthcare facilities to determine if they have detected cases; and encouraging personnel and physicians to report new cases. If the disease or condition has a long incubation period and it is likely that patients may be discharged before symptoms develop, then active surveillance for new cases can be conducted by calling physicians' offices to uncover additional cases. If the illness can be asymptomatic, it may be necessary to test for infection in order to detect cases (e.g., if a resident in an LCTF is diagnosed with infectious tuberculosis, then tuberculin skin testing must be done to detect M. tuberculosis infection in the resident's contacts).

Create a Data Collection Form

The investigators should create a data collection form to collect information on each case. The data elements to be included on the form will depend on the disease, condition, or event being studied. This form must be designed carefully to (1) include the information needed to determine if a case fits the case definition, (2) avoid wasting time collecting too much information, and (3) avoid missing data that are later found to be needed.

If data will be entered into a computer database, it is helpful to design the form so that the data elements are in the same order as they are entered into the computer. As noted, the information that should be collected depends on the disease being studied. Data elements may include the following:

- Identification information, such as name, record number, unit or ward, address, phone, and admission date
- Demographic information such as age, sex, and race
- Clinical information such as date of onset, signs and symptoms, underlying diseases, dates of collection and types of specimens, laboratory results, radiology results, and outcome
- Name and service of attending physician or surgeon
- Risk factors that are relevant to the disease or condition being studied (e.g., food and date/time eaten, medications and date/time given, therapeutic and diagnostic procedures and dates done, exposures to personnel,

types of intravascular devices used and dates/time inserted and removed, and presence of urinary catheters and dates used). Information collected during the literature search should be used to identify potential risk factors.

Investigators should take care to avoid collecting data that will not be used because this is a waste of time and resources. For example, a patient's address and phone number would not be needed unless the patient will likely be contacted for follow-up or the outbreak involves a reportable disease and this information is needed to complete a communicable disease report form.

Selected information is then abstracted from each data collection form and recorded on the line listing. Examples of a line-listing form and its corresponding data collection tool are shown in Chapter 12. Additional examples of line listing and data collection forms can be found in Appendices G and H (Appendices G and H are available for download at this text's Web site: http://www.jbpub .com /catalog/9780763757793/).

Describe the Epidemic: Person, Place, and Time

Once data are collected, the investigators can conduct the descriptive phase of the investigation by characterizing the outbreak with respect to person, place, and time. For instance, did the cases occur in one area of a facility or during a short period of time?

Person. Cases should be identified and entered on the line listing so that risk factors common to the affected persons can be identified. The population at risk should then be determined and, when possible, attack rates should be calculated. It is not always possible to calculate an attack rate because the denominator (the population at risk) cannot always be quantified. The use and calculation of attack rates are discussed in Chapter 10.

Place. The location of the cases, such as hospital unit, ward in an LTCF, or an ambulatory care center should be identified. It may be helpful to construct a spot map to illustrate the location of cases in a facility. By showing the distribution of cases, it may be possible to formulate a hypothesis on the mode of transmission or a potential source. Figure 12–11 in Chapter 12 is an example of a spot map. It illustrates the occurrence of mumps cases in the trading pits of stock exchange A in Chicago, Illinois, from August 18, 1987, to December 25, 1987.

Time. The date of onset should be recorded for each case. Both date and time of onset should be determined for acute diseases such as gastroenteritis that have an abrupt onset and a short incubation period (i.e., the period between when exposure occurs and symptoms develop). Both date and time of occurrence should be recorded for adverse events such as falls and other injuries, because if adverse events are found to occur on a particular shift, then attention can be focused on identifying risk factors that exist on that shift but not on another. Several investigations have implicated personnel as the cause of an outbreak because data on the shifts on which the events occurred were recorded and analyzed. For example, an investigation of cardiac arrests in an intensive care unit revealed that the patients of a particular nurse on the evening shift were 47.5 times more likely to experience a cardiac arrest than were the other nurses' patients.[7] Many of the implicated nurse's patients were found to have unexplained hyperkalemia and unexpected cardiac arrests. The outbreak ended when the nurse stopped working in the ICU.

For some infectious diseases, once the causative agent is identified and the incubation period is determined, the probable period of exposure can be postulated. The incubation periods of selected food-borne gastrointestinal diseases are listed in Table 7–3 in Chapter 7.

Outbreaks may involve cases that are not temporally related (i.e., do not occur closely spaced in time). There are several reported nursery outbreaks of *C. koseri* (formerly *C. diversus*) meningitis in which the cases were separated by many months.[40,41] In an unpublished outbreak that occurred at one hospital, the cases occurred in May, September, and the following February.

Draw an Epidemic Curve

An epidemic curve is a graph (a histogram) that is constructed by plotting the number of cases on the *y*-axis and the date of onset on the *x*-axis as discussed in Chapter 12. A properly constructed epidemic curve can often be used to distinguish between a common source and a propagated outbreak.

In a common source outbreak, the cases are exposed to a common noxious influence. If this exposure is brief and essentially simultaneous, then disease develops within one incubation period, and the outbreak is called a point source outbreak. Examples of a point source outbreak would be food poisoning caused by consumption of contaminated food at a single meal, gastrointestinal illness associated with a recreational water activity,[42] and the 1976 Legionnaires' disease (LD) outbreak among the attendees of the American Legion convention in Philadelphia. Figure 8–1 shows the epidemic curve for a point source outbreak of cryptosporidiosis associated with a water sprinkler fountain.[42] A common source outbreak may occur over a wide geographic area (e.g., multistate outbreaks have occurred when a widely distributed food or medical product from a single source is contaminated) or may extend over a prolonged period, as may occur if LD occurs sporadically in persons exposed to a contaminated air conditioning unit, but the cases are not readily detected and the outbreak is not recognized for many months.

Some outbreaks will originate from a common source and then spread further via person-to-person contact. This often occurs in outbreaks of diseases that have several modes of transmission, such as salmonellosis or hepatitis A, as these can be introduced into a population through contaminated food and then spread to others by direct person-to-person contact and by contact with feces.[43]

In a propagated or progressive outbreak, the disease is transmitted from person to person such as during an outbreak of chickenpox, measles, or influenza. Figure 8–2 shows the epidemic curve for a propagated outbreak of measles.[44] The case shown on August 10 was the index (or first) case, a visitor from another country, who introduced the disease into the population.

Evaluate the Problem

Existing data should be reviewed to determine the nature of the disease or event. If the outbreak is of infectious etiology, the identity and characteristics of the infecting organism will often indicate where to look further. For instance, *S. aureus* outbreaks are spread by person-to-person contact, and the reservoir is an infected or colonized person. If an *S. aureus* outbreak occurs

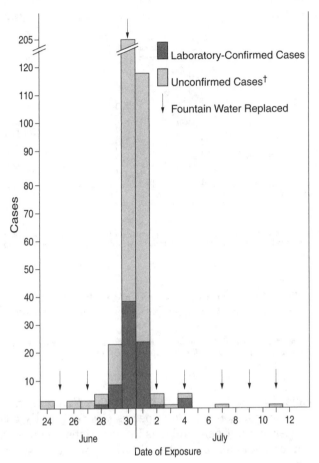

* $n = 369$.

† Defined as vomiting or three or more loose stools within a 24-hour period, with onset 3–15 days after fountain exposure of at least 3 days.

Figure 8–1 Epidemic Curve for a Point Source Outbreak: Reported Cases of Cryptosporidiosis Associated with a Water Sprinkler Fountain, by Date of Exposure— Minnesota, 1997 ($n = 369$)

Source: Centers for Disease Control and Prevention. Outbreak of cryptosporidiosis associated with a water sprinkler fountain—Minnesota, 1997. *MMWR*. 1998;47:856–860.

among postoperative patients or is clustered on a single unit and occurs abruptly, a potential source would be an infected or colonized healthcare worker, and therefore personnel should be evaluated for signs and symptoms of infection, such as a lesion.[45] If the outbreak spreads slowly, it may be the result of a breakdown in proper infection control practices, such as inadequate hand hygiene or aseptic technique.[46]

Group A streptococci outbreaks in healthcare settings are invariably associated with a healthcare worker who is infected or is an asymptomatic carrier.[47–49] Environmental reservoirs have not been implicated in group A streptococcal outbreaks; however, there have been food-borne outbreaks of group A streptococcal pharyngitis in which the source was an infected food handler who contaminated the food while preparing it.[50]

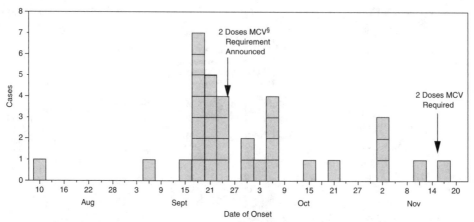

Figure 8–2. Epidemic Curve for a Propagated Outbreak: Number of Confirmed* Measles Cases, by Date of Rash Onset, by Three-Day Interval—Anchorage, Alaska, August 10–November 23, 1998 (n = 33)

Source: Centers for Disease Control and Prevention. Transmission of measles among a highly vaccinated school population—Anchorage, Alaska, 1998. *MMWR*. 1999;47:1109–1111.

Outbreaks caused by certain organisms, such as *Pseudomonas, Burkholderia*, or nontuberculous *Mycobacterium* species, are frequently associated with contaminated water or solutions, and this information can guide the investigators to look for aqueous reservoirs by evaluating common risk factors such as medications and solutions diluted with water or procedures involving fluid.[51]

If the outbreak involves postoperative infections, the investigator needs to determine if a personnel carrier or an environmental source is most likely by reviewing the characteristics of the infecting organism. This information can usually be found by conducting a careful literature search. For example, outbreaks of postoperative infections caused by group A streptococcus are generally associated with a human carrier,[49] and those caused by gram negative rods are frequently associated with an environmental reservoir.[52]

Data should be reviewed for evidence of person-to-person spread or a common source reservoir. For instance, if all of the infected and colonized patients had the same procedure (such as bronchoscopy) or therapy (such as mechanical ventilation),[51] or all of the ill persons ate the same meal, then the investigator could hypothesize that the disease occurred as a result of this common exposure.

The investigator should observe practices that may possibly contribute to the occurrence of the outbreak. Depending on the circumstances of the outbreak, these practices could involve patient or resident care, preparation of food, or cleaning, disinfection, and sterilization of equipment and medical devices.

Note that rule number three in outbreak investigation is to observe the practices being reviewed. Although policies and procedures may reflect appropriate infection prevention and control practices, personnel frequently do not adhere to written protocols. Personnel will often state the proper method that should be used; however, one should not assume that personnel are actually practicing what they say. Careful observation, done in a nonthreatening manner, will sometimes discover unrecognized breaks in proper technique. If an outbreak involves postoperative infections, it is particularly important to observe operating room and instrument and equipment processing practices.

Two cases illustrate the importance of observing practices. The first case involved an investigation of an outbreak of *Burkholderia cepacia* lower respiratory tract infection and colonization that occurred in the ICUs of a large tertiary care hospital.[51] Since 38 of the 44 case patients were on mechanical ventilators, respiratory therapy was thought to play a role in the outbreak. A literature search revealed a report of an outbreak of *B. cepacia* respiratory tract infections that was associated with nebulized albuterol. A review of the cases in the tertiary care hospital found that all 44 patients had received albuterol bronchodilator therapy.[51] Albuterol solutions were then tested and *B. cepacia* was isolated from an opened in-use multidose vial of albuterol, and polymerase chain reaction ribotyping showed that the albuterol isolate and 12 patient isolates had identical banding patterns. Observation of the practices of the respiratory therapists revealed that the albuterol was dispensed from a multidose vial via a plastic eyedropper. The personnel would frequently touch the tip of the eyedropper to the side of the nebulizer reservoir and then insert the eyedropper back into the vial, which they placed in their pockets for use on the next patient. After aseptic technique and proper use of multidose vials were reviewed with the respiratory therapy staff, no new cases occurred. The most likely source of the *B. cepacia* was determined to be extrinsically contaminated albuterol.

The second case involved an outbreak of gram-negative bacteremia in open-heart surgery patients that was traced to probable contamination of pressure-monitoring equipment.[52] The equipment (disposable transducers, intravenous extension tubing, heparinized saline, and stopcocks) was frequently set up at the end of the day for possible emergency use during the evening or night shifts. If it was not used overnight, it was used for the first case of the day. The equipment was not covered. When housekeeping practices were observed, it was discovered that the housekeeping staff used a hose to spray a water-disinfectant mixture into the operating room when they were cleaning the room. This mixture was sprayed very close to the pressure-monitoring equipment. Contamination of the equipment by the spray was thought to be responsible for the bacteremias because the outbreak was terminated when cleaning practices were changed and pressure-monitoring equipment was set up immediately before each open-heart procedure.[52]

Investigators should consider using the opportunity of an outbreak investigation to identify other practices that may contribute to a future outbreak. These practices can than be reviewed, analyzed, and corrected after the outbreak investigation is completed.

Determine the Need for Additional Cultures or Other Diagnostic Tests

The investigative team must determine the need for collecting microbiologic cultures or conducting other diagnostic tests, such as serologic studies or skin tests. Additional testing will depend on the circumstances of the outbreak.

Microbiologic cultures. If microbiologic culturing of personnel, patients, residents, or the environment is to be done, arrangements should be made with the laboratory, with personnel in areas where testing will occur, and with the organization's administrator, who must determine how to cover the expenses involved. The required specimens and culture methods should then be identified, and the specimens should be collected and processed. The appropriate typing methods for the organism being studied must also be identified and arrangements must be made to have these tests done on any isolates of epidemiologic importance.

The decision whether or not to culture personnel, equipment, devices, or environmental surfaces should be based on evidence that a person or an environmental reservoir is epidemiologically linked to the outbreak.[2] It is important to remember that a person, item, or surface is not necessarily the source of the outbreak just because it is culture positive; any of these may have become contaminated by the true source or by an infected or colonized person. Extensive microbiologic culturing of personnel or the environment is generally not warranted and should not be done unless a full-scale epidemiologic study is conducted, the study implicates a personnel carrier or an environmental source, and the significant isolates are typed for evidence of strain relatedness.

If culturing is done, the isolates should be typed to determine strain relatedness. There are many methods for typing microbial isolates.[53] Phenotypic techniques, which detect characteristics that are expressed by an organism, include biotyping, serotyping, antimicrobial susceptibility, bacteriophage and bacteriocin typing, polyacrylamide gel electrophoresis (PAGE), multilocus enzyme electrophoresis (MLEE), and immuno-blotting. Genotypic (or molecular) techniques, which examine an organism's genetic content, include plasmid analysis, restriction endonuclease analysis (REA), ribotyping, pulsed-field gel electrophoresis (PFGE), and polymerize chain reaction (PCR).[53] Typing systems have been shown to be a powerful tool for investigating outbreaks of healthcare-associated infection when they are used as an adjunct to an epidemiologic investigation.[54] They must be used and interpreted with caution, however, to avoid erroneous conclusions. For instance, the finding that there is only one strain circulating in a healthcare setting does not necessarily mean that all of the infections are related—there may be only a single strain circulating in the community even though there may be many reservoirs or sources. Conversely, if multiple strains are found, there may still be an outbreak, as multiple strains have been found to cause an outbreak (based on epidemiologic evidence). The use, advantages, and disadvantages of the various typing methods are discussed in Chapter 11.

If culturing of personnel is done, specimens should be labeled with a code, rather than with a healthcare worker's name, to protect the identity of anyone who is culture positive for the organism being studied. Only one person should hold the key connecting the codes and names. Culturing creates substantial anxiety among personnel because they will be concerned that they may be involved in causing the outbreak. Therefore, the decision to culture personnel must be made carefully, based on epidemiologic evidence, and personnel need to be assured that the results of testing will remain confidential—to allay concerns that they will be blamed for the outbreak if they are culture positive.

If an infectious agent has a carrier state or can cause colonization, it may sometimes be desirable to culture patients or residents to determine the extent of the spread in the population at risk. Culture surveys should not be done unless the significant organisms that are isolated are typed or otherwise characterized to determine if they are related strains.

Other diagnostic tests. For those diseases in which infection may occur without signs or symptoms, other tests may be needed to determine if persons were infected as a result of exposure during the outbreak. For instance, tuberculin skin testing would be needed to identify persons who become infected following exposure to *M. tuberculosis* because most infections with this organism are asymptomatic. Those who are identified as newly infected could then be given prophylaxis to prevent the development of disease. When investigating an outbreak of measles, serologic testing is frequently done to identify susceptible persons so they can be immunized to prevent infection and further transmission of the disease.

Formulate a Tentative Hypothesis

One of the objectives of an outbreak investigation is to determine why certain individuals in a population develop disease. This is done by collecting information on possible risk factors (exposures) and generating hypotheses. Based upon an evaluation of the information collected up to this point, a tentative hypothesis should be formulated regarding the likely causative factors of the outbreak (e.g., reservoir, source, and mode of transmission of the agent if the outbreak is of infectious etiology).

For example, a multidrug-resistant *Pseudomonas aeruginosa* has been isolated from the respiratory tract of three patients in the ICU during a three-week period. The ICU, laboratory, and previously established ICP personnel recognize that this represents more cases of this organism than expected. An initial review of the cases shows that one patient has pneumonia and two are colonized. All three patients are on ventilators. Since mechanical ventilation has been shown to be a risk factor for infection and colonization with *P. aeruginosa*, a tentative hypothesis could be that exposure to mechanical ventilation is associated with the nosocomial acquisition of a multidrug-resistant strain of *P. aeruginosa*.

Implement Control Measures

Control measures should be implemented as soon as possible during the investigative process. For an infectious disease outbreak of known etiology, preventive interventions should be based on the characteristics of the causative agent, including possible reservoirs and sources and the most likely mode of transmission. Measures that have been shown to be effective in interrupting the transmission of a variety of organisms have been discussed in Chapters 3 through 7. The identified control measures could be as simple as emphasizing good hand hygiene and adherence to contact precautions to help control an outbreak or cluster of MRSA. To interrupt outbreaks of noninfectious etiology, control measures should be based on the nature of the disease or event. For example, in one published report, an excess number of needlestick injuries in hospital personnel was traced to needles piercing the walls of infectious waste containers.[6] The outbreak was terminated when a different type of container was used.

Evaluate the Efficacy of Control Measures

Surveillance activities should be continued to determine if any new cases are occurring. If new cases continue to occur, control measures must be reevaluated, and a more extensive epidemiologic investigation may be needed.

Evaluate and Test the Hypothesis

In a full-scale investigation, statistical tests are done to test the hypotheses that explain the likely risk factors contributing to the outbreak. Many investigations do not reach this stage. The investigation may end prior to this point if the control measures are working and if the situation does not require further study. The following outbreak situations should be pursued further: those associated with considerable morbidity or mortality, those that continue to occur despite the implementation of control measures, those that are suspected to be facility-wide, and those adverse events that are associated with a medical device or a commercial product.

This phase poses one of the greatest challenges when conducting an outbreak investigation. The investigators must carefully review the clinical, laboratory, and epidemiologic findings and hypothesize which risk factors or exposures could plausibly lead to disease. The hypotheses are then tested by comparing the population with the disease (cases) with a population without the disease (controls) in regards to exposures to postulated risk factors. These comparisons are usually done by conducting a case-control or cohort study, as discussed in Chapter 10. To ensure that the appropriate study design and statistical tests are used, those who are investigating an outbreak should consult a trained statistician before beginning a case-control or cohort study. For a discussion of the use of case-control studies in outbreak investigations, the reader is referred to a review article by Dwyer et al.[55]

When testing a hypothesis, investigators need to keep in mind the criteria that should be used to judge if an association is causal: strength of association, dose–response relationship, consistency of association, chronological relationship, specificity of association, and biological plausibility, as discussed in Chapter 1. Data should also be evaluated to determine if (1) there are any persons who were not exposed to a particular risk factor who are affected, or (2) if there are persons who were exposed to a particular risk factor who are not affected.

For example, over a 9-day period, 5 personnel and 15 residents in an LTCF develop a febrile illness with diarrhea or vomiting. *Salmonella enteritidis* is isolated from several cases and is determined to be the etiologic agent of the outbreak. Because an investigation shows that no other cases have recently been reported in the community, the investigators hypothesize that exposure to the source of the organism occurred in the LTCF. Because *S. enteritidis* outbreaks are most frequently associated with a food-borne source, a further hypothesis could be that consumption of some food or beverage in the facility was the exposure necessary to develop disease. Therefore, the likely period of exposure, based on the usual incubation period of the disease (6 to 48 hours), would be identified and the cases would be interviewed to determine what they had to eat or drink at the facility during that period. To determine if exposure to certain foods eaten by the ill persons (cases) was associated with disease, these exposures would be compared with exposures of persons who were not ill (controls) by conducting statistical tests of association and significance, as explained in Chapter 10.

To increase efficiency and promote accuracy, computers and appropriate software programs should be used as much as possible to collect and organize data and to calculate statistical tests. Epi Info, a software program developed by the CDC to manage and analyze data collected during an epidemiologic investigation, can be downloaded from the CDC's Web site at http://www .cdc.gov/epiinfo. Epi Info can be used to calculate statistical measures such as odds ratios, relative risk, 95% confidence intervals (CIs), chi-squares, and P values.

Continue Surveillance, Analysis, and Investigation

Investigators should continue to seek additional cases by searching both retrospectively and concurrently. Concurrent (ongoing) surveillance should be used to assess the effectiveness of the implemented control measures. The investigative team should meet to review findings up to this point and to formulate and evaluate additional hypotheses, as needed.

If other testing is warranted, such as microbiologic culturing or serologic tests for hepatitis A or measles, these tests should be completed. The results of all laboratory tests should be carefully recorded and analyzed by the investigative team.

Prepare and Distribute Written Reports

Investigators should carefully document their actions and organize their findings at each step in the investigation. Interim reports should be prepared and distributed, as needed, to the organization's administrative staff, to those who are affected by the outbreak, to the infection prevention and control committee, and to relevant government or public health agencies. When the investigation is completed, a final report should be prepared and submitted to the departments, areas, or units involved in the outbreak, to the organization's administrative staff, to the infection prevention and control committee, and to the health department and other authorities, as appropriate.

The final report should follow the usual scientific format: introduction and background, methods, results, discussion, and summary and recommendations. The report should include the names and titles of those who prepared it and those to whom it was provided. Guidelines for preparing a report of an outbreak investigation are shown in Table 8–3. A good example of a detailed report of an outbreak is the article by White et al. who describe an epidemic of giardiasis in an NH.[56]

Table 8–3   Guideline for Preparing a Report of an Outbreak Investigation

Section	Describes or explains, when appropriate
1. Introduction/Background	Similar outbreaks that were previously reported; how the outbreak was detected; who conducted the investigation; the type of facility and area(s) where the outbreak occurred
2. Methods	
a. Laboratory methods	Types of culture media used; method for collecting specimens; identification and typing systems used for microorganisms isolated; serologic or other tests used
b. Epidemiologic methods	Type of study used (e.g., case-control or cohort); case definition (possible, probable, definite; asymptomatic vs. symptomatic); how the cases and controls were selected; sources of the data collected (e.g., patient or resident medical records, infection control surveillance data, quality management data, laboratory records, reports from healthcare workers, health department records, phone or written surveys, interviews with patients, personnel, or visitors)
c. Statistical methods	Statistical tests used
3. Results	Findings of the study (facts only, with no discussion); may also include tables of cases and risk factors, an epidemic curve, and spot maps, as appropriate
4. Discussion	The interpretation and discussion of the results
5. Summary/Recommendations	The summary of the findings and recommendations
6. Distribution of report	Notes the names and titles of those to whom the report was given
7. Author(s)	Notes the names and titles of those who prepared the report

Source: Author.

PUBLISHING AN ARTICLE ABOUT AN OUTBREAK INVESTIGATION

A literature search is one of the crucial steps in conducting an outbreak investigation because it helps the investigator identify potential risk factors associated with a disease and control measures that have been shown to be effective in preventing that disease in similar situations. Preparing a written report of an outbreak investigation using the outline provided in Table 8–3, provides the investigator the basis for writing an article and submitting it for publication. Personnel who conduct outbreak investigations in healthcare settings should consider publishing their findings—especially if the outbreak involves an unusual organism or a previously unrecognized risk factor, source, reservoir, or mode of transmission of an infectious agent. Since outbreak investigations frequently advance knowledge of the epidemiology of infections and other adverse outcomes in healthcare institutions, healthcare professionals who investigate clusters and outbreaks of healthcare-related events should publish their findings to assist others who are investigating similar conditions.[10,11,57]

RISK MANAGEMENT ISSUES

Outbreaks can result in claims and lawsuits being filed against a healthcare organization. In rare cases, members of the ICP department have been named in these suits. Healthcare personnel, including the infection control staff, may be subpoenaed to give a deposition or testify in court. In addition, during the discovery process of a lawsuit, the defendant(s) will be required to produce documents relating to the case. During an outbreak investigation, the investigators should be careful to record facts, and not speculations or personal comments, because documents produced during the investigation may be subpoenaed. The organization's risk management and legal departments should be consulted to answer questions about risk and legal issues surrounding an outbreak investigation.

OUTBREAK INVESTIGATION SKILLS

According to Goodman et al., "The concepts and techniques used in field investigations derive from clinical medicine, epidemiology, laboratory science, decision analysis, skilled communications, and common sense."[58(p10)] To successfully apply epidemiologic methods to recognizing, investigating, and controlling an outbreak, the investigator must be skilled in a unique set of tasks:[59]

- Surveillance—the ongoing, systematic collection of data
- Investigation—careful observation and gathering of data for a detailed descriptive study
- Analysis—observation followed by comparison of groups
- Evaluation—the assessment of the effectiveness of the actions and control measures taken to resolve a problem

In addition, the investigator should possess skills in communication, management, consultation, presenting epidemiologic findings, and human relations.[59]

OUTBREAK PREVENTION

Outbreaks can result in significant morbidity and mortality; fear and anxiety among personnel, patients, residents and the community; disruption of services; lost revenue; and temporary closure of medical departments, patient/resident care units, or even an entire facility.[60,61] Many outbreaks that have occurred in healthcare settings could have been prevented if healthcare workers had routinely used appropriate infection prevention practices. To prevent healthcare-associated infections and recognize potential outbreaks, each healthcare organization should have an infection surveillance, prevention, and control program that is appropriate for the setting. The program should incorporate evidence-based infection prevention practices, comply with applicable regulations and requirements, and have a surveillance system that is capable of detecting clusters and increases in the numbers and rates of infections and epidemiologically significant organisms. A mechanism should be in place to address clusters, increases in infections, and the occurrence of epidemiologically significant organisms as soon as possible so that measures can be implemented to interrupt an outbreak or prevent one from occurring.

PUBLIC HEALTH ISSUES

Recognizing and Reporting Clusters and Suspected Outbreaks

Healthcare providers are well suited to assisting health departments in the recognition and follow-up of community outbreaks of disease because persons who are ill frequently present to a hospital emergency department or to a healthcare provider for treatment. Community outbreaks of infectious diseases such as salmonellosis and staphylococcal food poisoning have been first recognized by hospital personnel, especially those in emergency departments, when several patients presented during a short time period with gastrointestinal illnesses.[62,63] In 1994 the staff of a community hospital reported a cluster of community-acquired cases of LD, and this led to the detection of an outbreak of LD among passengers of a cruise ship.[64]

Phares et al. described an investigation prompted by the discovery of two cases of LD in residents of an LTCF.[65] The investigation led to the detection of seven confirmed cases of legionellosis: two residents of the LTCF, one visitor to the LTCF, one inpatient in the hospital attached to the LTCF, one visitor to the hospital, one patient seen in a nearby outpatient medical office building, and one resident of the nearby community. No Legionella was isolated from multiple samples of water and biofilm collected throughout the LTCF. However, Legionella pneumophila was isolated from an industrial cooling tower located 0.4 km from the LTCF and was the same strain as that isolated from the cases. The investigators concluded that the most likely source of infection for the LTCF residents was the community cooling tower, and the occurrence of LD in the LTCF residents was a sentinel event that led to the detection of a community outbreak.

Healthcare organizations should have a mechanism for reporting suspected community outbreaks of infectious and noninfectious conditions to the local health department as soon as possible. All 50 states in the United States have reportable disease requirements, and healthcare providers have the responsibility for reporting cases of communicable diseases and other conditions to the health department. Even though one case may not seem important, that one individual may be involved in a larger outbreak that may not be recognized unless several cases are reported.

Community Outbreaks Can Affect Healthcare Facilities

Widespread community outbreaks of infectious diseases such as salmonellosis and influenza may cause community-acquired infections in healthcare personnel and their families and may result in increased admissions of persons with communicable diseases and in nosocomial spread to other patients, residents, or personnel.[66] In addition, healthcare organizations may be asked to assist health departments provide prophylaxis, immunization, or other follow-up for persons potentially exposed to a communicable disease. Many hospital ICPs have assisted local and state health departments in providing prophylaxis for family members of patients with meningococcal meningitis and immunization for contacts of a patient with measles. If outbreaks affect many persons, it may be necessary to set up special clinics and telephone hotlines.[67] Guidelines for developing a written plan to address infectious disease emergencies have been published by many organizations and health departments, and these can be used to develop a facility-specific plan.

When widespread outbreaks are associated with commercial products, such as food or medication, healthcare personnel must determine if their organization has received that product and has used it. Food-borne outbreaks associated with intrinsically contaminated commercial products put patients, residents, personnel, visitors, and guests at risk—especially if the organization is involved in catering meetings attended by members of the community.[68]

Emerging Infectious Diseases, Biological Weapons, and Terrorist Attacks

ICPs, healthcare epidemiologists, healthcare providers, and clinical laboratory personnel play a critical role in detecting, reporting, and responding to diseases and events of public health significance, such as emerging infectious diseases and infections that could potentially be related to a bioterrorist attack. A widespread outbreak or pandemic will affect many healthcare settings, and each setting should have a system for detecting and reporting emerging infectious diseases so that prevention and control measures can be quickly implemented.[69]

The use of biological agents during a war or for a terrorist attack could cause widespread outbreaks and paralyze the healthcare system. A religious cult intentionally contaminated salad bars at 10 restaurants in Oregon, and this resulted in at least 751 cases of *Salmonella typhimurium* in a county that typically reports fewer than five cases per year.[70] The bioterrorism-related release of *Bacillus anthracis* spores in several states and Washington, DC, in late 2001 resulted in 22 cases of anthrax, hundreds of persons receiving antimicrobial prophylaxis, the closure of several buildings for decontamination, and considerable disruption of services at local hospitals.[71] Healthcare personnel should be familiar with the biological agents most likely to be used in a bioterrorist attack—especially with their disease manifestations and modes of transmission and with the measures that can be used to control their spread.[72]

ICPs, healthcare administrators, and healthcare providers also play an important role in ensuring that their organizations have emergency plans in place to address a surge of infectious patients and reduce the adverse impacts these events have on healthcare settings.[69] These plans should be developed by a multidisciplinary task force composed of personnel from the healthcare organization that is developing its plan and personnel from surrounding healthcare organizations, public health agencies, emergency responders, and other stakeholders.

A discussion of emergency preparedness is beyond the scope of this text; however, much information can be found on the websites of national, state, and provincial government and public health agencies worldwide. Resources for information on emerging infections and emergency planning include the CDC's Emergency Preparedness and Response website (http://www.bt.cdc.gov /planning/), the online journal *Emerging Infectious Diseases* (http://www.cdc .gov/nciod/EID), the World Health Organization (http://www.who.int/en/), and the Agency for Healthcare Research and Quality's Public Health Emergency Preparedness website (http://www.ahrq.gov/prep/).

USING TECHNOLOGY TO AID IN OUTBREAK DETECTION AND INVESTIGATION

Computers have greatly aided in the management and analysis of data collected during routine surveillance activities and during outbreak investigations. Information technology is regularly used in the detection and investigation of outbreaks worldwide. For instance, following a report that several attendees of a conference developed salmonellosis, the CDC initiated an epidemiologic investigation by sending a questionnaire to conference attendees via the e-mail system of the organization that sponsored the conference.[73] The attendees were instructed to complete the survey and return it to the CDC via fax. Since the attendees had come from all 50 states, this electronic communication facilitated the search for cases and aided in the identification and investigation of a food-borne outbreak in a widely dispersed population. Using information supplied by the attendees, the source of the organism was eventually traced to an infected food handler at a restaurant near the convention site.

Many healthcare professionals subscribe to electronic notification systems and e-mail lists that allow instant communication locally, nationally, and internationally. These systems can be used to inquire about the experiences of others during an outbreak and to alert healthcare institutions about outbreaks associated with medical procedures or with commercial products and devices. Technologies such as e-mail and e-mail lists play an integral role in detecting and responding to outbreaks. The use of information technology for outbreak detection and investigation is discussed in Chapter 9.

SUMMARY

Although outbreaks in healthcare settings account for only a small proportion of healthcare-associated infections, they can result in significant morbidity and mortality, disruption of services, and fear and anxiety among personnel, patients, residents, and the community. Healthcare organizations should have an infection surveillance, prevention, and control program that is based on the needs and characteristics of the healthcare setting for which it is designed. The personnel responsible for the program should have the ability to (1) recognize clusters and potential outbreaks, (2) act promptly to evaluate and investigate the situation, (3) follow the standard outbreak investigation steps outlined in this chapter, and (4) implement appropriate prevention and control measures to interrupt the outbreak and prevent it from recurring.

ICPs, healthcare providers, and administrators play a critical role in recognizing, reporting, and responding to public health emergencies that may result when a natural or man-made outbreak or pandemic occurs.

REFERENCES

1. Haley RW, Tenney JH, Lindsey JO, Garnet JS, Bennett JV. How frequent are outbreaks of nosocomial infection in community hospitals? *Infect Control*. 1985;6:233–236.

2. Beck-Sague C, Jarvis WR, Martone WJ. Outbreak investigations. *Infect Control Hosp Epidemiol*. 1997;18:138–145.

3. Smith PW, Rusnak PG. Infection prevention and control in the long-term care facility. *Am J Infect Control*. 1997;25:488–512.

4. Martone WJ, Williams WW, Mortensen ML, et al. Illness with fatalities in premature infants: association with intravenous vitamin E preparation, E-Ferol. *Pediatr*. 1986;78:591–600.

5. Shay DK, Fann LM, Jarvis WR. Respiratory distress and sudden death associated with receipt of a peripheral parenteral nutrition admixture. *Infect Control Hosp Epidemiol*. 1997;18:814–817.

6. Anglim AM, Collmer JE, Loving J, et al. An outbreak of needlestick injuries in hospital employees due to needles piercing infectious waste containers. *Infect Control Hosp Epidemiol*. 1995;16:570–576.

7. Sacks JJ, Stroup DF, Will ML, Harris EL, Israel E. A nurse-associated epidemic of cardiac arrests in an intensive care unit. *JAMA*. 1988;295:689–695.

8. Franks A, Sacks JJ, Smith JD, Sikes RK. A cluster of unexplained cardiac arrests in a surgical intensive care unit. *Crit Care Med*. 1987;15:1075–1076.

9. Kafrissen ME, Grimes DA, Hogue CJ, Sacks JJ. Cluster of abortion deaths at a single facility. *Obstet Gynecol*. 1986;68:387–389.

10. Gastmeier P, Stamm-Balderjahn S, Hansen S, et al. How outbreaks can contribute to prevention of nosocomial infection: analysis of 1022 outbreaks. *Infect Control Hosp Epidemiol*. 2005;26:357–361.

11. Gastmeier P, Stamm-Balderjahn S, Hansen S, et al. Where should one search when confronted with outbreaks of nosocomial infection? *Am J Infect Control*. 2006;34(9):603–605.

12. CDC. Prevention of invasive group A streptococcal disease among household contacts of case patients and among postpartum and postsurgical patients: recommendations from the Centers for Disease Control and Prevention. *Clin Infect Dis*. 2002;35(8):950–959.

13. Gruteke P, van Belkum A, Schouls LM, et al. Outbreak of group A streptococci in a burn center: use of pheno and genotypic procedures for strain tracking. *J Clin Microbiol*. 1996;34(1):114–118.

14. Greene CM, Van Beneden CA, Javadi M, et al. Cluster of deaths from group A streptococcus in a long-term care facility—Georgia, 2001. *Am J Infect Control*. 2005;33(2):108–113.

15. Centers for Disease Prevention and Control. Measles. *Vaccine Preventable Diseases Surveillance Manual*. 3rd ed. Atlanta, GA: CDC; 2002. http://www.cdc.gov/vaccines/pubs/surv-manual/downloads/chpt06_measles.pdf. Accessed March 21, 2008.

16. Heyman DL. *Control of Communicable Diseases Manual*. 18th ed. Washington, DC: American Public Health Association; 2005.

17. Tablan OC, Anderson LJ, Besser R, Bridges C, Hajjeh R. Guidelines for preventing healthcare associated pneumonia, 2003. Recommendations of CDC and the Healthcare Infection Control Practices Advisory Committee. http://www.cdc.gov/ncidod/dhqp/index.html. Accessed March 21, 2008.

18. Siegel JD, Rhinehart E, Jackson M, Chiarello L, and the Healthcare Infection Control Practices Advisory Committee, 2007. Guideline for isolation precautions: preventing transmission of infectious agents in healthcare settings, June 2007. http://www.cdc.gov/ncidod/dhqp/pdf/isolation2007.pdf. Accessed March 21, 2008.

19. Sabria M, Campins M. Legionnaires' disease: update on epidemiology and management options. *Am J Respir Med*. 2003;2(3):235–243.

20. Centers for Disease Control and Prevention. Prevention and control of tuberculosis in facilities providing long-term care to the elderly. Recommendations of the Advisory Committee for Elimination of Tuberculosis. *MMWR.* 1990;39(10):7–20.

21. Bille J, Marchetti O, Calandra T. Changing face of health-care associated fungal infections. *Curr Opin Infect Dis.* 2005;18(4):314–319.

22. Centers for Disease Control and Prevention. Renal insufficiency and failure associated with immune globulin intravenous therapy—United States, 1985–1998. *MMWR.* 1999;48:518–521.

23. Centers for Disease Control and Prevention. Endotoxin-like reactions associated with intravenous gentamicin—California, 1998. *MMWR.* 1998;47:877–880.

24. Geiss HK, Schmitt J, Frank SC. Bleeding after cardiovascular surgery caused by detergent residues in laparotomy sponges. *Infect Control Hosp Epidemiol.* 1997;18:579–581.

25. Beck-Sague CM, Jarvis WR, Bland LA, Arduino MJ, Aguero SM, Verosic G. Outbreak of gram-negative bacteremia and pyrogenic reactions in a hemodialysis center. *Am J Nephrol.* 1990; 10:397–403.

26. Centers for Disease Control. Guidelines for investigating clusters of health events. *MMWR.* 1990;39(11):1.

27. Birnbaum D. Analysis of hospital infection surveillance data. *Infect Control.* 1984;5:332–338.

28. McGuckin MB, Abrutyn E. A surveillance method for early detection of nosocomial outbreaks. *Am J Infect Control.* 1979;7:18–21.

29. Childress JA, Childress JD. Statistical test for possible infection outbreaks. *Infect Control.* 1981;2:247–249.

30. Mylotte JM. The hospital epidemiologist in long-term care: practical considerations. *Infect Control Hosp Epidemiol.* 1991;12:439–442.

31. Birnbaum D. Nosocomial infection surveillance programs. *Infect Control.* 1987;8:474–479.

32. Jacquez GM, Waller LA, Grimson R, Wartenberg D. The analysis of disease clusters, part I: state of the art. *Infect Control Hosp Epidemiol.* 1996;17:319–327.

33. Jacquez GM, Waller LA, Grimson R, Wartenberg D. The analysis of disease clusters, part II: introduction to techniques. *Infect Control Hosp Epidemiol.* 1996;17:385–397.

34. Selleck JA. Statistical process control charts in hospital epidemiology. *Infect Control Hosp Epidemiol.* 1993;14:649–656.

35. Brewer JH, Gasser CS. The affinity between continuous quality improvement and epidemic surveillance. *Infect Control Hosp Epidemiol.* 1993;14:95–98.

36. Benneyan JC. Statistical quality control methods in infection control and hospital epidemiology, part I: introduction and basic theory. *Infect Control Hosp Epidemiol.* 1998;19:194–214.

37. Benneyan JC. Statistical quality control methods in infection control and hospital epidemiology, part II: chart use, statistical properties, and research issues. *Infect Control Hosp Epidemiol.* 1998;19:265–283.

38. Birnbaum D. CQI tools: sentinel events, warning, and action limits. *Infect Control Hosp Epidemiol.* 1993;14:537–539.

39. Verweij PE, Bilj D, Melchers W, et al. Pseudo-outbreak of multiresistant *Pseudomonas aeruginosa* in a hematology unit. *Infect Control Hosp Epidemiol.* 1997;18:128–131.

40. Kline MW. *Citrobacter meningitis* and brain abscess in infancy: epidemiology, pathogenesis, and treatment. *J Pediatr.* 1988;113:430–434.

41. Graham DR, Anderson RL, Ariel FE, et al. Epidemic nosocomial meningitis due to *Citrobacter diversus* in neonates. *J Infect Dis.* 1981;144:203–209.

42. Centers for Disease Control and Prevention. Outbreak of cryptosporidiosis associated with a water sprinkler fountain—Minnesota, 1997. *MMWR.* 1998;47:856–860.

43. Standaert SM, Hutcheson RH, Schaffner W. Nosocomial transmission of *Salmonella* gastroenteritis to laundry workers in a nursing home. *Infect Control Hosp Epidemiol.* 1994;15:22–26.

44. Centers for Disease Control and Prevention. Transmission of measles among a highly vaccinated school population—Anchorage, Alaska, 1998. *MMWR.* 1999;47:1109–1111.

45. Sheretz RJ, Bassetti S, Bassetti-Wyss B. "Cloud" health-care workers. *Emerg Infect Dis.* 2001;7:241–244.

46. Boyce JM. Methicillin-resistant *Staphylococcus aureus* in hospitals and long-term care facilities: microbiology, epidemiology, and preventive measures. *Infect Control Hosp Epidemiol.* 1992;13:725–737.

47. Ridgeway EJ, Allen KD. Clustering of group A streptococcal infections on a burns unit: important lessons in outbreak management. *J Hosp Infect.* 1993;25:173–182.

48. Viglionese A, Nottebart V, Bodman HA, Platt R. Recurrent group A streptococcal carriage in a health care worker associated with widely separated nosocomial outbreaks. *Am J Med.* 1991;91(Suppl 3B):329S–333S.

49. Paul SM, Genese C, Spitalny K. Postoperative group A beta-hemolytic *Streptococcus* outbreak with the pathogen traced to a member of a health care worker's household. *Infect Control Hosp Epidemiol.* 1990;11:643–646.

50. Decker MD, Lavely GB, Hutcheson RHU, Schaffner W. Food-borne streptococcal pharyngitis in a hospital pediatrics clinic. *JAMA.* 1986;353:679–681.

51. Reboli AC, Koshinski R, Arias K, Marks-Austin K, Stieritz D, Stull TL. An outbreak of *Burkholderia cepacia* lower respiratory tract infection associated with contaminated albuterol nebulization solution. *Infect Control Hosp Epidemiol.* 1996;17:741–743.

52. Redneck JR, Beck-Sague CM, Anderson RL, Schable B, Miller JM, Jarvis WR. Gram-negative bacteremia in open-heart-surgery patients traced to probable tap-water contamination of pressure-monitoring equipment. *Infect Control Hosp Epidemiol.* 1996;17:281–285.

53. Singh A, Goering RV, Simjee S, Foley SL, Zervos MJ. Application of molecular techniques to the study of hospital infection. *Clin Micro Rev.* 2006;19:512–530.

54. Jarvis WR. Usefulness of molecular epidemiology for outbreak investigations. *Infect Control Hosp Epidemiol.* 1994;15:500–503.

55. Dwyer DM, Strickler H, Goodman RA, Armenian HK. Use of case-control studies in outbreak investigations. *Epidemiol Rev.* 1994;16:109–123.

56. White KE, Hedberg CW, Edmonson LM, Jones DBW, Osterholm MT, MacDonald KL. An outbreak of giardiasis in a nursing home with evidence for multiple modes of transmission. *J Infect Dis.* 1989;160:298–304.

57. Gastmeier P, Loui A, Stamm-Balderjahn S, et al. Outbreaks in neonatal intensive care units - they are not like others. *Am J Infect Control.* 2007;35:172–176.

58. Goodman RA, Buehler JW, Kaplan JP. The epidemiologic field investigation: science and judgment in public health practice. *Am J Epidemiol.* 1990;132:9–16.

59. Last JM, Tyler CW. Epidemiology. In: Last JM, Wallace RB, eds. *Maxcy-Rosenau-Last Public Health and Preventive Medicine.* 13th ed. Norwalk, CT: Appleton & Lange; 1992:11–39.

60. Baggett HC, Duchin JS, Shelton W, Zerr DM, Heath J, Ortega-Sanchez IR, Tiwari T. Two nosocomial pertussis outbreaks and their associated costs—King County, Washington, 2004. *Infect Control Hosp Epidemiol.* 2007;28(5):537–543.

61. Hansen S, Stamm-Balderjahn S, Zuschneid I, et al. Closure of medical departments during nosocomial outbreaks: data from a systematic analysis of the literature. *J Hosp Infect.* 2007;65(4):348–353.

62. Goodman LJ, Lisowski JM, Harris AA, et al. Evaluation of an outbreak of foodborne illness initiated in the emergency department. *Ann Emerg Med.* 1993;22:62–65.

63. Centers for Disease Control and Prevention. Outbreak of staphylococcal food poisoning associated with precooked ham—Florida, 1997. *MMWR.* 1997;46:1189–1191.

64. Guerrero IC, Filippone C. A cluster of Legionnaires' disease in a community hospital—a clue to a larger epidemic. *Infect Control Hosp Epidemiol.* 1996;17:177–178.

65. Phares CR, Russell E, Thigpen MC, et al. Legionnaires' disease among residents of a long-term care facility: The sentinel event in a community outbreak. *Am J Infect Control.* 2007;35:319–323.

66. Jarosch MJ, Sinwell G, Galviz CJ, et al. Activities of infection control practitioners during an outbreak of *Salmonella typhimurium. Am J Infect Control.* 1989;17:159–161.

67. Frace RM, Jahre JA. Policy for managing a community infectious disease outbreak. *Infect Control Hosp Epidemiol.* 1991;12:364–367.

68. Gellert GA, Tormay M, Rodriguez G, Brougher G, Dessey D, Pate C. Food-borne disease in hospitals: prevention in a changing food environment. *Am J Infect Control.* 1989;17:136–140.

69. Petrosillo N, Puro V, DiCarlo A, Ippolito G. The initial hospital response to an epidemic. *Arch Med Res.* 2005;36(6):706–712.

70. McDade JE, Franz D. Bioterrorism as a public health threat. *Emerg Infect Dis.* 1998;4:493–494.

71. Centers for Disease Control and Prevention. Update: investigation of bioterrorism-related anthrax, 2001. *MMWR.* 2001;50(45):1008–1010.

72. Centers for Disease Control and Prevention. Medical examiners, coroners, and biologic terrorism: a guidebook for surveillance and case management. *MMWR.* 2004;53(8):1–36.

73. Mahon BE, Rohn DD, Pack SR, Tauxe RV. Electronic communication facilitates investigation of a highly dispersed foodborne outbreak: *Salmonella* on the superhighway. *Emerg Infect Dis.* 1995;1:94–95.

SUGGESTED READING AND RESOURCES

Additional Information

For additional information on investigating outbreaks in the healthcare setting, refer to the Web sites of national, state, and provincial public health agencies and to the chapter on outbreak investigation in one of the infection prevention and control texts (Bennett and Brachman, Mayhall, Association for Professionals in Infection Control and Epidemiology, and Wenzel) in the Suggested Reading list.

Suggested Reading

APIC Text of Infection Control and Epidemiology. 2nd ed. Washington, DC: Association for Professionals in Infection Control and Epidemiology; 2005.

Beck-Sague C, Jarvis WR, Martone WJ. Outbreak investigations. *Infect Control Hosp Epidemiol.* 1997;18:138–145.

Heyman DL. *Control of Communicable Diseases Manual.* 18th ed. Washington, DC: American Public Health Association; 2005.

Jarvis WR, ed. *Bennett and Brachman's Hospital Infections.* 5th ed. Philadelphia, PA: Lippincott Williams & Wilkins; 2007.

Centers for Disease Control and Prevention. *Principles of Epidemiology in Public Health Practice: An Introduction to Applied Epidemiology and Biostatistics.* 3rd ed. Atlanta, GA: Centers for Disease Control and Prevention, Office of Workforce and Career Development; 2005. p. 1–46. http://www2a.cdc.gov/TCEOnline/registration/detailpage.asp?res_id=1394. Accessed May 12, 2008.

Dwyer DM, Strickler H, Goodman RA, Armenian HK. Use of case-control studies in outbreak investigations. *Epidemiol Rev.* 1994;16:109–123.

Mayhall CG. *Hospital Epidemiology and Infection Control.* 3rd ed. Baltimore, MD: Lipincott, Williams & Wilkins; 2004.

Pickering LK, ed. *Red Book: 2008 Report of the Committee on Infectious Diseases*, 27th ed. Elk Grove Village, IL: American Academy of Pediatrics; 2008.

Reingold AL. Outbreak investigations—a perspective. *Emerg Infect Dis.* 1998;4:21–27.

Roueche B. The Medical Detectives. New York, NY: Washington Square Press; 1986.

Roueche B. The Medical Detectives, Vol. II. New York, NY: Washington Square Press; 1986.

Roueche B. The Medical Detectives. Reprint edition. New York, NY: Plume; 1991.

Smolinski MS, Hamburg MA, Lederberg J. eds. Committee on emerging microbial threats to health in the 21st century. Microbial threats to health: emergence, detection, and response. Washington, DC: National Academies Press; 2003. http://www.nap.edu/catalog.php?record_id=10636. Accessed March 26, 2008.

Wallace RB. *Public Health and Preventive Medicine* (Maxcy-Rosenau-Last Public Health and Preventive Medicine), 15th ed. Columbus: McGraw-Hill; 2007.

Wenzel RP, ed. *Prevention and Control of Nosocomial Infections.* 4th ed. Baltimore, MD: Lippincott Williams & Wilkins; 2002.

Resources

The Centers for Disease Control and Prevention's Web site (http://www.cdc.gov) can be used to access the *Morbidity and Mortality Weekly Report*, the online journal *Emerging Infectious Diseases*, the Division of Healthcare Quality and Promotion, and other information on outbreaks, infection prevention and control, and infectious diseases.

Centers for Disease Control and Prevention. Epi Info. http://www.cdc.gov/epiinfo. Accessed March 13, 2008. Epi Info is free downloadable software that the user can use to develop a questionnaire or form, customize the data entry process, enter and analyze data, and produce epidemiologic statistics, tables, graphs, and maps.

CHAPTER 9

Information Technology and Outbreak Investigation

Kathleen Meehan Arias

> *Information technology is the use of modern technology to create, store, exchange, and manipulate information and use this as a basis for reasoning, discussion, or calculation.*
>   —L. Goss. *APIC Text of Infection Control and Epidemiology*[1]

INTRODUCTION

In 2003 news of an outbreak of a mysterious atypical pneumonia that was causing much morbidity and mortality in the People's Republic of China was reported on the Program for Monitoring Emerging Diseases (ProMED)-mail.[2] Details of the outbreak, which was affecting hundreds of people, including nurses, doctors, and other healthcare workers, were rapidly transmitted worldwide via the Internet. Within a few months, the illness, now known as severe acute respiratory syndrome (SARS), had spread to over 20 countries in Asia, North America, Europe, and South America.[3] The information posted on ProMED-mail provided the opportunity for information exchange among numerous entities (public health agencies, professional organizations, and the healthcare community) and allowed these groups to prospectively follow the progression of the outbreak and rapidly contribute to the development of infection control strategies to prevent further transmission of the disease.

The term *information technology* (IT), as used in this chapter, is the use of computer systems (hardware, software, and Internet based) that are used to collect, store, manipulate, analyze, report, and transmit data and information. IT plays an increasingly essential role in infection surveillance, prevention, and control programs. Events of the past decade, such as the emergence of SARS and the intentional release of *Bacillus anthracis* spores in the United States, have highlighted the critical need for accurate surveillance data and rapid transfer of information when responding to outbreaks and other public health emergencies.

This chapter focuses on the use of IT for detecting, investigating, preventing, and controlling outbreaks in the healthcare setting. It provides an overview of the role of IT in infection surveillance, prevention, and control programs in healthcare settings; supplies information on public domain software programs for outbreak investigation; gives examples of public health surveillance systems, e-mail lists, and electronic notification and reporting systems; discusses the use of electronic methods for conducting literature and information searches; and provides a list of resources relating to outbreak investigation and infection prevention and control. The information is presented here under the assumption that the reader knows how to use a personal computer, an e-mail program, a search engine, and how to enter an address (i.e., a uniform resource locator or URL) into a Web browser.

USING INFORMATION TECHNOLOGY FOR SURVEILLANCE IN HEALTHCARE SETTINGS

The use of information technology for healthcare epidemiology and surveillance has rapidly grown as a broad range of patient data has become accessible electronically. As healthcare organizations expand their use of computerized data management systems and electronic patient records, infection prevention and control professionals (ICPs) gain the ability to access this data for use in the surveillance of infections and other adverse events.

The traditional method of conducting surveillance solely by manual chart review is labor intensive and time consuming. Because efficiency and accuracy can be improved by computerizing the data collection, management, and reporting processes, many manual surveillance steps have been effectively replaced by information systems and computer programs.[4-7] The time needed to collect and analyze data is decreased, and more time is gained to guide infection prevention activities. ICPs should routinely use computers to collect, manage, store, review, analyze, and report data used for both routine surveillance and outbreak investigation.

Data Collection, Management, and Storage

Because manual chart review is labor intensive, data collection should be automated as much as possible. ICPs should work with the information services personnel in their organization to identify how they can extract and download data from a variety of sources, such as patient records, the laboratory, pharmacy, radiology, operating room, and admissions departments. For instance, microbiology laboratory results and patient demographic data should be provided electronically to the infection prevention and control department. Ideally, these data should be downloaded directly into a retrievable database so they can be easily accessed for review and analysis.

Data collection is frequently done using paper forms; however, the data collected on paper should be transferred into a computerized system. Storage on paper forms should be avoided as much as possible because the data is not readily retrievable for analysis if a cluster or outbreak is suspected. When data are stored in a database program such as Microsoft Access it can be queried and retrieved quickly when needed. Data stored in a spreadsheet program, such as Microsoft Excel, can be manipulated and sorted using pivot tables.

Some ICPs enter data collected during chart review directly into a personal notebook computer or a handheld device such as a personal digital assistant (PDA).[8]

Data Review, Analysis, and Reporting

Routine surveillance data should be reviewed and analyzed with the aid of computer programs that can sort and group the data for analysis and calculate incidence rates and other statistics used in healthcare epidemiology, as discussed in Chapter 10. The information derived from data analysis should be reported using computer-generated tables, graphs, and charts, as appropriate, as discussed in Chapter 12.

Computerized systems for screening patients for potential nosocomial or healthcare-associated infections (HAIs) and for automating infection surveillance have been developed and effectively used by many hospitals.[4,5,9–13] However, developing and maintaining these systems is beyond the ability of many hospital information services departments, and in-house programs are not widely used.[14] Commercial programs for automated surveillance and data mining are used by many healthcare organizations. At the time of press, these include Premier SafetySurveillor (http://www.premierinc.com/quality-safety/index.jsp), Vecna Technologies QC Pathfinder (http://www.vecna.com/), TheraDoc Infection Control Assistant (http://www.theradoc.com/), and Cardinal Health's MedMined (http://www.cardinalhealth.com/medmined/). These programs can provide real-time data access and reporting capabilities and will alert the user if significant events, such as a cluster or potential outbreak, are detected.[15]

In addition to automated and data mining systems, there are commercial software programs for infection surveillance data management and reporting, such as the ICPA AICE! programs (http://www.icpa.net), EpiQuest Healthcare Epidemiology and Statistics programs (http://www.epiquest.com), and ICNet software (http://www.icnet.org.uk).

The CDC National Healthcare Safety Network (NHSN) developed an Internet-based data management and reporting system that is used by healthcare organizations that submit data to the NHSN (http://www.cdc.gov/ncidod/dhqp/nhsn_members.html).

The use of computerized data management and automated surveillance and data mining systems in healthcare settings is expected to grow as regulators, government agencies, and healthcare payers worldwide expand mandatory reporting requirements for HAI-related data.

PUBLIC DOMAIN SOFTWARE FOR OUTBREAK INVESTIGATION

Two data management programs that are useful for investigating an outbreak are Epi Info and EpiData. Epi Info can store data and perform statistical analyses. Although it was developed for use in outbreak investigation, it is used by some ICPs for routine surveillance activities.

Epi Info was developed by the CDC in the 1970s to allow public health personnel to efficiently manage data collected on-site during an outbreak investigation. Epi Info can be used to create data collection forms; store and analyze data; perform a variety of statistical calculations; and produce tables, graphs, and maps. Although Epi Info is a CDC trademark, the programs, documentation, and teaching materials are in the public domain and may be freely copied, distributed, and translated. The various programs that are part of Epi Info are available in Microsoft Windows and DOS formats. Information, tutorials, and the Microsoft Windows version are available at http://www.cdc.gov/epiinfo/. A DOS version, including user manual, frequently asked questions, and tutorials, is still available at http://www.cdc.gov/epiinfo/Epi6/ei6.htm.

EpiData software is based on Epi Info. An initiative to create the EpiData software was established by Jens M. Lauritsen, MD, PhD, in 1999 in Denmark. The goal was to produce a Windows-based version of Epi Info that uses simple text files (ASCII) instead of the Microsoft Access database used by the Windows version of Epi Info. The first version of EpiData software was released in 2000. The EpiData Entry and EpiData Analysis software programs, including supporting documents and a field guide (users manual), are available free of charge through the EpiData Association at http://www.epidata.dk/index.htm.

USING INFORMATION TECHNOLOGY FOR PUBLIC HEALTH SURVEILLANCE SYSTEMS

Public health surveillance systems are used worldwide to collect and monitor data on disease trends and to detect outbreaks. These systems may be local, state, regional, or national. Many of the programs also have a mechanism for disseminating information on outbreaks to public health agencies, healthcare organizations, and healthcare providers.

One example is the CDC's National Electronic Disease Surveillance System (NEDSS). It is designed to detect outbreaks rapidly, facilitate the electronic transfer of information from clinical information systems in the healthcare system to public health departments, enhance both the timeliness and quality of information provided, and advance the development of efficient and integrated surveillance systems at federal, state, and local levels. NEDSS is a major component of the CDC's Public Health Information Network (PHIN) (http://www.cdc.gov/phin/about.html).

Another example is the European Centre for Disease Prevention and Control's Enter-Net. Enter-Net is an international surveillance network for human gastrointestinal infections and involves 15 countries of the European Union (EU), plus Australia, Canada, Japan, South Africa, Switzerland, and Norway (http://ecdc.europa.eu/Activities/surveillance/ENTER_NET/index.html).

There are many state, local, and regional public health agency surveillance programs. Each state in the United States has a public health agency that is responsible for collecting data on notifiable diseases and providing guidelines for infection prevention and control. Contact information and a link to state and territory public health agency Web sites can be obtained at StatePublicHealth.org (http://www.statepublichealth.org/index.php). Links to state health departments can also be found on the CDC Web site (http://www.cdc.gov/mmwR/international/relres.html).

Another surveillance system is the World Health Organization Global Outbreak Alert and Response Network (GOARN). GOARN is a network of public health agencies and technical and operational resources from scientific institutions in member states, laboratories, United Nations organizations, the Red Cross, and international humanitarian nongovernmental organizations that pool human and technical resources for the rapid identification, confirmation, and response to outbreaks of international importance (http://www.who .int/csr/outbreaknetwork/en/).

In addition to surveillance for specific diseases, syndromic surveillance is used in many countries to monitor disease trends at the local, state, regional, and national levels by collecting data on disease syndromes.[16–26] Syndrome surveillance systems collect information such as patient signs, symptoms, and laboratory results before final diagnoses are made. Although data is frequently collected from health information systems already in place in emergency departments, some programs monitor over-the-counter medications purchased at pharmacies and stores.[27] The purpose of syndrome surveillance is to provide an early detection system for naturally occurring or terrorism-related events and outbreaks. There is much variation in existing syndrome surveillance programs and their ability to detect outbreaks and other events of public health significance; many of these systems are still evolving.[28,29]

ELECTRONIC NOTIFICATION, REPORTING SYSTEMS, AND E-MAIL LISTS

Many government agencies and infection prevention and control organizations have electronic systems that send or receive information on outbreaks. Some are set up only to send alerts to users, and some are capable of two-way communication. Several systems that are useful for ICPs and epidemiologists in healthcare settings are listed here.

Notification systems may use e-mail alerts and/or RSS (rich site summary or really simple syndication) feeds to send notification to users about outbreaks and other public health issues. It is easy to subscribe to these services by going to the Web site of the organization, clicking on the box or link to the specific system and following the instructions.

To receive RSS feeds on a computer, one must first install a program called a news reader or feed reader that will allow the RSS feed from the sender to be received and displayed. There are many different news readers available for free download or purchase on the Internet. The sender's Web site will provide instructions for those who wish to subscribe to the RSS feed and install the reader needed for its system. A feed reader allows the user to subscribe to news, blogs, and other frequently updated content and view the new information separate from an e-mail inbox. RSS feeds can also be read on PDAs and cell phones.

E-mail lists are programs that allow subscribers to send an e-mail to one address from which that message is broadcast to all of the other subscribers to the list.

Examples of notification systems and e-mail lists are:

- Agency for Healthcare Research and Quality (AHRQ) Public Health Preparedness Update—The AHRQ provides e-mail alerts to subscribers when it updates its Public Health Emergency Preparedness Web site

(http://www.ahrq.gov/prep/). Subscribe at https://subscriptions.ahrq
.gov/service/user.html?code=USAHRQ.

- APICList—The APICList is a moderated e-mail list provided by the Association for Professionals in Infection Control and Epidemiology that is open to those interested in infection prevention and control. Subscribe at http://www.apic.org/AM/Template.cfm?Section=Networking_and_Communities&Template=/CM/HTMLDisplay.cfm&ContentID=9479.

- CDC Clinician Communication Updates—This free communication network was developed by the CDC to provide clinicians with real-time information to help prepare for (and possibly respond to) public health emergencies. Subscribers receive regular e-mail updates on terrorism and other emergency issues. Subscribe at http://www.bt.cdc.gov/clinregistry.

- CDC Rapid Notification System for Healthcare Professionals—The CDC Division of Healthcare Quality Promotion (formerly Hospital Infections Program) provides occasional time-sensitive e-mail messages about important healthcare events (e.g., outbreaks, product recalls) and publications (e.g., new health care guidelines) to persons interested in the prevention of healthcare-acquired infections and antimicrobial resistance. Subscribe either at http://www2.cdc.gov/ncidod/hip/rns/hip_rns_subscribe.html or address an e-mail to LISTSERV@CDC.GOV. Leave the subject line blank and in the message box type: subscribe HIP-RNS. The RNS is not an interactive system; however, in September 2007 the CDC used this e-mail list to solicit reports of infections or clusters of infections that occurred in total joint recipients and were caused by *Enterococcus galinarum* or *E. faecium*. The CDC was collecting information for an investigation that it was conducting on a cluster of deep surgical site infections caused by these organisms.

- FDA MedWatch—MedWatch, the US Food and Drug Administration's Safety Information and Adverse Event Reporting Program, has two functions:

  1. To provide information about safety issues involving medical products, biologics, medical devices, and special nutritional products (e.g., medical foods, dietary supplements, and infant formulas) to consumers and healthcare professionals. The program distributes alerts on contaminated medical products, such as intravenous solutions, and suspected outbreaks associated with medical devices and products. Safety alerts, recalls, and withdrawals are disseminated via the MedWatch Web site (http://www.fda.gov/medwatch/index.html) and the MedWatch E-list. One can subscribe to the MedWatch E-list at http://www.fda.gov/medwatch/elist.htm.

  2. To collect reports on serious adverse events and suspected product quality problems, such as contamination of a medical device or product. Healthcare providers should report these events to the Adverse Event Reporting Program through links on the MedWatch home page as noted.

- Health Canada's Consumer Product Safety (CPS) division has a program for providing advisories, warnings, and recalls to subscribers via e-mail or RSS feeds (http://www.hc-sc.gc.ca/cps-spc/advisories-avis/index_e.html).

- ProMED-mail—the Program for Monitoring Emerging Diseases was established in 1994 and is now a program of the International Society for Infectious Diseases. According to its Web site, ProMED-mail is "an Internet-based reporting system dedicated to rapid global dissemination of information on outbreaks of infectious diseases and acute exposures to toxins that affect human health . . . By providing early warning of outbreaks of emerging and re-emerging diseases, public health precautions at all levels can be taken in a timely manner to prevent epidemic transmission and to save lives." A team of moderators posts reports to ProMED from various sources, including public health agencies, the media, local observers, and ProMED-mail subscribers. The ProMED program provides a platform for discussion, requests for information, and collaboration in outbreak investigations and prevention efforts. One can subscribe to ProMED-mail at http://www.promedmail.org.

USING INFORMATION TECHNOLOGY FOR LITERATURE AND INFORMATION SEARCHES

One of the first steps in an outbreak investigation is to conduct a search of the literature and other resources. A literature search should provide a review of previous research and experience on a particular disease or infectious agent. For an outbreak investigation, the purpose of the search is to identify the following: if other healthcare organizations have had a similar experience with the implicated organism; risk factors for exposure to the suspected causative agent or disease; sources, reservoirs, and modes of transmission for the agent; potential case definitions; and effective prevention and control measures.[30–32]

Information that can be used when conducting an outbreak investigation can be found in a variety of formats such as medical journals, books, the Internet, electronic databases and indexes, and government and public health agency publications. The most efficient method for doing a literature search is to access the many sources on the Internet by using a personal computer. An advantage of using a computer in a medical or public library is that library personnel can assist the investigator in conducting the literature and information search.

Medical Literature Search Services

Ideally, literature searches should be conducted electronically by using a medical literature search service. General search engines, such as Google and Yahoo!, can also be used to identify relevant information; however, a medical literature search service is more efficient than a general search engine for accessing peer-reviewed medical publications. There are many medical literature search services that provide access to comprehensive databases of information. Some are available free of charge and others are subscription-based. All of the following services described provide information and tutorials at the URL addresses provided.

Examples of search services that are free of charge include PubMed and Google Scholar.

PubMed is a free service of the US National Library of Medicine and the National Institutes of Health that includes over 17 million citations from

MEDLINE (approximately 5000 worldwide journals in 37 languages) and other life science journals for biomedical articles back to the 1950s. PubMed provides abstracts and links to full-text articles and other related resources. Some publishers provide access to full-text articles at no cost through PubMed. An overview of PubMed and a tutorial on how to use the service can be accessed through the PubMed home page (http://www.ncbi.nlm.nih.gov/PubMed). PubMed can provide e-mail alerts to update the user on new articles relating to a query.

Google Scholar is a free service of Google that provides the ability to broadly search for scholarly literature from a variety of sources: peer-reviewed papers, theses, books, abstracts and articles from academic publishers, professional societies, universities, and other organizations. The Google Scholar home page (http://scholar.google.com) provides a Help button to access information on how to use the program.

Subscription-based search services provide access to a broader range of sources for a fee. Examples include Scopus and ISI Web of Knowledge.

Scopus is a subscription-based service that provides an abstract and citation database of research literature and Web sources that offers access to 15,000 peer-reviewed journals from more than 4000 publishers and includes journals, conference proceedings, trade publications, and book series. Scopus can provide e-mail alerts to update the user on new articles relating to a query (http://info.scopus.com).

ISI Web of Knowledge is a subscription-based service that provides access to 22,000 journals and to conference proceedings, Web sites, and books (http://isiwebofknowledge.com).

Journals and Periodicals on the World Wide Web

Many peer-reviewed journals and periodicals that are used by ICPs and healthcare epidemiologists when gathering information on outbreaks and infection prevention and control can be accessed via the Internet.[33] In addition, one can register on each of the Web sites noted here to receive the table of contents of each issue at no cost via e-mail or RSS feed.

Many journals provide links to their table of contents, abstracts, articles in current and past issues, and related information. Although the table of contents, abstracts, and links to related information are available to all at no cost, most of the full-text articles are only available for free to subscribers. Examples of these journals include the following:

- *American Journal of Infection Control*—the official journal of APIC: http://journals.elsevierhealth.com/periodicals/ymic
- *British Journal of Infection Control*—the official journal of the Infection Prevention Society (formerly the Infection Control Nurses Association): http://bji.sagepub.com
- *Clinical Infectious Diseases*—published by the Infectious Diseases Society of America: http://www.journals.uchicago.edu/toc/cid/current
- *Infection Control and Hospital Epidemiology*—the official journal of the Society for Healthcare Epidemiology of America (SHEA): http://www.journals.uchicago.edu/toc/iche/current

- *Journal of Hospital Infections*—the official journal of the Hospital Infection Society (HIS): http://www.elsevier.com/wps/find/journaldescription .cws_home/623052/description#description

Free or open access online journals that are peer-reviewed and provide abstracts, full text of the articles at no cost, and links to related information include:

- *BMJ (British Medical Journal)*—published by BMJ Publishing Group Ltd, a wholly owned subsidary of the British Medical Association: http://www.bmj.com
- *BMC Public Health*—an open access journal published by BioMed Central: http://www.biomedcentral.com/bmcpublichealth
- *BMC Microbiology*—an open access journal published by BioMed Central: http://www.biomedcentral.com/bmcmicrobiol
- *Emerging Infectious Diseases*—published by the CDC: http://www.cdc .gov/NCIDOD/eid

Public health agency periodicals that are available online and provide free subscriptions and electronic notification when each issue is published include:

- *Canada Communicable Disease Report* (CCDR): http://www.phac-aspc .gc.ca/publicat/ccdr-rmtc/index-eng.php
- *Eurosurveillance Report*: http://www.eurosurveillance.org/ew/2007/070621 .asp
- *Morbidity and Mortality Weekly Report* (MMWR): http://www.cdc.gov/ mmwr/

OTHER SOURCES OF INFORMATION ON THE INTERNET

Web sites that provide access to public health and infection prevention and control information have proliferated since the 1990s. This section lists additional examples of resources that are useful for outbreak detection, investigation, reporting, prevention, and control in the healthcare setting.

Centers for Disease Control and Prevention Division of Healthcare Quality and Promotion (DHQP)—The CDC DHQP provides guidelines for preventing infections in patients and healthcare workers, information on organisms of epidemiological importance, such as *Clostridium difficile* and MRSA, and links to a variety of resources.

European Centre for Disease Prevention and Control (ECDC)—The ECDC was established in 2005 to "identify, assess, and communicate current and emerging threats to human health posed by infectious diseases." It works in partnership with national health protection agencies across Europe to strengthen and develop disease surveillance and early warning systems. Links to the various EU surveillance systems are on the ECDC Web site under Activities/Surveillance. A discussion of the EU Disease Surveillance Networks and their Web sites can be found in the May 2006 issue of *Eurosurveillance Report*[34] (http://ecdc.europa.eu/index.html).

Public Health Agency Web Sites—Many state, regional and national public health agencies worldwide develop guidelines for investigating and preventing outbreaks in healthcare settings and post these on their Web sites. Examples include:

- California Department of Public Health—offering their *Healthcare-Associated Infections and Infection Control Guidelines*, including investigating and preventing outbreaks in long-term care and residential facilities: http://www.cdph.ca.gov/pubsforms/Guidelines /Pages/HAIandIC.aspx
- Maryland Department of Health and Mental Hygiene—Epidemiology and Disease Control Program (EDCP). Infection prevention and control guidelines for a variety of settings, including outbreak investigations in LTCFS: http://www.cha.state.md.us /edcp/html/cd_guide.html
- State Government of Victoria, Australia, Department of Human Services—*Guidelines for the Investigation of Gastrointestinal Illness*. Provides guidelines for investigating, controlling, and preventing outbreaks of gastrointestinal illness: http://www.health.vic.gov.au/ideas/diseases/gas_ill_index

Web Search Engines—Web search engines are programs that search, gather, and return information on the World Wide Web in response to a query from a user. *The Spider's Apprentice: A Helpful Guide to Search Engines* describes search engines and their use (http://www.monash.com/spidap.html). Commonly used search engines include Google (http://www.google.com/), Yahoo! (http://www.yahoo .com/), and Ask (http://www.ask.com/).

World Health Organization Epidemic and Pandemic Alert and Response (EPR)—The EPR provides information on, and links to, international alert and response operations, diseases monitored by WHO, the Global Outbreak Alert and Response Network, and the 2005 International Health Regulations (http://www.who.int/csr/en/). It also provides information and links to resources on its Web page "Infection prevention and control in healthcare for preparedness and response to outbreaks" (http://www.who.int/csr/bioriskreduction / infection_control/en/).

WWW Virtual Library: Medicine and Health—Epidemiology—This site is maintained by the Department of Epidemiology and Biostatistics at the University of California, San Francisco. It provides links to government and public health agencies, professional societies and organizations, news and discussion groups, universities, and other related sites worldwide (http://www .epibiostat.ucsf.edu/epidem/epidem.html).

Additional Information—Additional Web-based resources can be found in many of the Suggested Reading and Resources sections at the end of the chapters in this text.

SUMMARY

Events of the past decade, such as the rapid global spread of SARS and its transmission to healthcare providers in several countries, have highlighted the need for accurate surveillance data and rapid transfer of information when responding to outbreaks and other public health emergencies. IT plays a critical role in identifying HAI and in detecting, investigating, and responding to outbreaks in both the healthcare and community settings. ICPs should use the wide variety of IT resources available and should work to automate as many surveillance activities as possible. Using IT to collect, manage, analyze, and report surveillance data reduces the time needed to perform these tasks and subsequently provides more time for infection prevention activities and investigating clusters and potential outbreaks.

REFERENCES

1. Goss LK. Information technology. In: *APIC Text of Infection Control and Epidemiology.* 2nd ed. Washington, DC: Association for Professionals in Infection Control and Epidemiology. 2005;33–2.

2. ProMED-mail. Pneumonia-China (Guangdong). ProMed-mail 2002; 11 February: 20030211.0369. http://www.promedmail.org. Accessed March 29, 2008.

3. Outbreak of severe acute respiratory syndrome—worldwide, 2003. *MMWR.* 2003;52:226–228. [Erratum in: *MMWR Morb Mortal Wkly Rep* 2003;52:284].

4. Bates DW, Evans RS, Murff H, Stetson PD, Pizziferri L, Hripcsak G. Detecting adverse events using information technology. *Am Med Inform Assoc.* 2003;10(2):115–128.

5. Bellini C, Petignat C, Francioloi P, et al. Comparison of automated strategies for surveillance of nosocomial bacteremia. *Infect Control Hosp Epidemiol.* 2007;28:1030–1035.

6. Wisniewski M, Kieszkowski P, Zagorski B, et al. Development of a clinical data warehouse for hospital infection control. *J Am Med Inform Assoc.* 2003;10:454–462.

7. Haas JP, Mendonca EA, Ross B, Friedman C, Larson E. Use of computerized surveillance to detect nosocomial pneumonia in neonatal intensive care unit patients. *Am J Infect Control.* 2005;33:439–443.

8. Farley JE, Srinivasin A, Richards A, Song X, McEachen J, Perl TM. Handheld computer surveillance: shoe-leather epidemiology in the "palm" of your hand. *Am J Infect Control.* 2005;33:444–449.

9. Doherty J, Noirot LA, Mayfield J, et al. Implementing GermWatcher, an enterprise infection control application. *AMIA Annu Symp Proc.* 2006;209–213.

10. Carr JR, Fitzpatrick P, Izzo JL, et al. Changing the infection control paradigm from off-line to real time: the experience at Millard Fillmore Health System. *Infect Control Hosp Epidemiol.* 1997;18(4):255–259.

11. Evans RS, Larsen RA, Burke JP, et al. Computer surveillance of hospital-acquired infections and antibiotic use. *JAMA.* 1986;256:1007–1011.

12. Kahn MG, Steib SA, Fraser VJ, Dunagan WC. An expert system for culture-based infection control surveillance. *Proc Annu Symp Comput Appl Med Care.* 1993;171–175.

13. Pokorny L, Rovira A, Martín-Baranera M, Gimeno C, Alonso-Tarres C, Vilarasau J. Automatic detection of patients with nosocomial infection by a computer-based surveillance system: a validation study in a general hospital. *Infect Control Hosp Epidemiol.* 2006;27:500–503.

14. Peterson D. Automating infection surveillance efforts. Accurate outbreak data can cut costs, antibiotics use. *Mater Manag Health Care.* 2007;16:17–19.

15. Wright MO, Perencevich EN, Novak C, et al. Preliminary assessment of an automated surveillance system for infection control. *Infect Control Hosp Epidemiol.* 2004;25(4):325–332.

16. Muscatello DJ, Churches T, Kaldor J, et al. An automated, broad-based, near real-time public health surveillance system using presentations to hospital emergency departments in New South Wales, Australia. *BMC Public Health.* 2005;5:141. http://www.biomedcentral.com/1471-2458/5/141. Accessed March 30, 2008.

17. Cooper D, Smith G, Baker M, et al. National symptom surveillance using calls to a telephone health advice service—United Kingdom, December 2001–February 2003. *MMWR.* 2004;53(Suppl):179–183.

18. Tsung-Shu Joseph Wu, Fuh-Yuan Frank Shih, Muh-Yong Yen, et al. Establishing a nationwide emergency department-based syndromic surveillance system for better public health responses in Taiwan. *BMC Public Health.* 2008;8:18. http://www.biomedcentral.com/1471-2458/8/18. Accessed March 30, 2008.

19. Lombardo J, Burkom H, Elbert E, et al. A systems overview of the electronic surveillance system for the early notification of community-based epidemics (ESSENCE II). *J Urban Health.* 2003;80(2 Suppl 1):i32–i42.

20. Yuan CM, Love S, Wilson M. Syndromic surveillance at hospital emergency departments–Southeastern Virginia. *MMWR.* 2004;53(Suppl):56–58.

21. Hammond L, Papadopoulos S, Johnson C, Mawhinney S, Nelson B, Todd J. Use of an Internet-based community surveillance network to predict seasonal communicable disease morbidity. *Pediatrics.* 2002;109(3):414–418.

22. Heffernan R, Mostashari F, Das D, et al. New York City syndromic surveillance systems. *MMWR.* 2004;53(Suppl):23–27.

23. Lewis M, Pavlin J, Mansfield J, et al. Disease outbreak detection system using syndromic data in the greater Washington, DC area. *Am J Prev Med.* 2002;23(3):180–186.

24. Tsui F, Espino J, Dato V, Gesteland P, Hutman J, Wagner M. Technical description of RODS: a real-time public health surveillance system. *J Am Med Inform Assoc.* 2003;10:399–408.

25. Dembek Z, Carley K, Siniscalchi A, Hadler J. Hospital admissions syndromic surveillance-Connecticut, September 2001–November 2003. *MMWR.* 2004;53(Suppl):50–52.

26. Platt R, Bocchino C, Caldwell B, et al. Syndromic surveillance using minimum transfer of identifiable data: the example of the national bioterrorism syndromic surveillance demonstration program. *J Urban Health.* 2003;80(2 Suppl 1):i25–i31.

27. Wagner M, Robinson J, Tsui F, Espino J, Hogan W. Design of a national retail data monitor for public health surveillance. *J Am Med Inform Assoc.* 2003;10:409–418.

28. Mandl KD, Overhage M, Wagner MM, et al. Implementing syndromic surveillance: a practical guide informed by the early experience. *J Am Med Inform Assoc.* 2004;11(2):141–150. http://www.pubmedcentral.nih.gov/articlerender.fcgi?tool=pubmed&pubmedid=14633933. Accessed March 30, 2008.

29. Watkins RE, Eagleson S, Hall RG, Dailey L, Plant AJ. Approaches to the evaluation of outbreak detection methods. *BMC Pub Health.* 2006;6:263. http://www.biomedcentral.com/1471-2458/6/263. Accessed March 30, 2008.

30. Gastmeier P, Stamm-Balderjahn S, Hansen S, et al. How outbreaks can contribute to prevention of nosocomial infection: analysis of 1022 outbreaks. *Infect Control Hosp Epidemiol.* 2005;26:357–361.

31. Gastmeier P, Stamm-Balderjahn S, Hansen S, et al. Where should one search when confronted with outbreaks of nosocomial infection? *Am J Infect Control.* 2006;34:603–605.

32. Gastmeier P, Loui A, Stamm-Balderjahn S, et al. Outbreaks in neonatal intensive care units—they are not like others. *Am J Infect Control.* 2007;35:172–176.

33. Abbas UL, Yu VL. Infectious diseases journals on the world wide web: attractions and limitations. *Clin Infect Dis.* 2001;33:817–828. http://www.journals.uchicago.edu/doi/pdf/10.1086/322701. Accessed April 1, 2008.

34. Lenglet A, Hernández Pezzi G. Comparison of the European Union Disease Surveillance Networks' websites. *Euro Surveill.* 2006;11(5):119–122. http://www.eurosurveillance.org/em/v11n05/1105-227.asp. Accessed March 31, 2008.

SUGGESTED READING

Goss LK. Information technology. In: *APIC Text of Infection Control and Epidemiology*. 2nd ed. Washington, DC: Association for Professionals in Infection Control and Epidemiology; 2005.

Woeltje KF. Use of computerized systems in health care epidemiology. In: Jarvis WR, ed.

Bennett and Brachman's Hospital Infections. 5th ed. Philadelphia, PA: Lippincott Williams & Wilkins; 2007;121–128.

CHAPTER 10

Statistical Methods Used in Outbreak Investigation

Deborah Y. Phillips and Kathleen Meehan Arias

> *The source(s) and route(s) of exposure must be determined to understand why an outbreak occurred, how to prevent similar outbreaks in the future, and, if the outbreak is ongoing, how to prevent others from being exposed to the source(s) of infection.*
>
> —Arthur L. Reingold[1]

INTRODUCTION

It can be challenging to have a sense that there is an outbreak occurring and yet have little or no data to substantiate this belief. Basic statistical methods can be used to organize, summarize, and analyze data to determine if there are trends or associations in observations. Statistical methods allow the researcher to find the answers to epidemiologic questions such as the following:

- Are there more cases of a disease than usual or expected? (The term *disease* is used in this chapter to describe an adverse health-related event such as an infection, illness, or injury.)
- Is there a cause-and-effect relationship between an exposure and a disease?
- Could the event be random occurrence?

This chapter includes a basic description of the statistical measures used to describe and analyze an outbreak and is intended to be an introduction to the statistical methods commonly used in healthcare epidemiology, such as frequency measures and measures of central tendency, association, and dispersion. It includes a brief discussion on the use of analytic studies (cohort and case-control studies) and on statistical inference theory (including the concepts of hypothesis testing, probability, and statistical significance). Since a thorough discussion of each of these concepts cannot be accomplished in one chapter, the reader who wishes to obtain more information on these topics is referred to the references noted and to the resources listed in the Suggested Reading and Other Resources sections at the end of this chapter. [2–7]

Numerous computer database and statistical programs are available, and these have virtually eliminated the need to calculate complicated statistical formulas by hand or by using a handheld calculator. Nevertheless, those responsible for implementing infection prevention and control and quality management programs in healthcare settings still need to be familiar with the statistical measures discussed in this chapter and when these measures are to be used.

When investigating an outbreak, the investigator begins by using descriptive statistics to describe the person, place, and time characteristics of the outbreak, as described in Chapter 8. If the most likely risk factors responsible for the outbreak cannot be identified during the descriptive phase, then an analytic study may be designed and conducted. An analytic study attempts to associate potential risk factors or exposures with the development of disease and to determine the strength of that association. Case-control or cohort studies are the analytic study methods that are most frequently used in outbreak investigations to compare rates of disease in various populations in order to determine which exposures or risk factors are most likely responsible for the disease. Although the investigator must be familiar with the use and limitations of these studies, the authors recommend that a statistician be consulted if advanced statistical analysis is necessary when conducting an outbreak investigation.

DESCRIPTIVE STATISTICS

Frequency Measures

Frequency measures are used to characterize the occurrence and risk of disease in a given population during a specified time period. The frequency measures commonly used in healthcare epidemiology are ratios, proportions, and rates. These three measures are based on the same formula:

$$x/y \times 10^n$$

in which x (the numerator) and y (the denominator) are the two groups that are being compared, and 10^n is a constant that is used to transform the result to a convenient number (usually a number that has at least one digit to the left of the decimal place).

Ratios and Proportions

A ratio is a fraction in which the values in the numerator are not necessarily included in the denominator. This means that a ratio can be used to express the relationship between a x and a y when the two have independent values. One may use a ratio to indicate a relationship between two groups. The odds ratio and the risk ratio (or relative risk), which are discussed later in the chapter, are commonly used to measure associations between two groups.

A proportion is a type of ratio in which the values in the numerator are included in the denominator. A proportion is often expressed as a percentage. For example, in a sample of 69 case patients who developed a catheter-associated UTI over a 1-year period, 46 cases are females and 23 cases are males.

To calculate the ratio of female cases to male cases, the following formula is used:

$$x/y \times 10^0$$

in which x is 46 female cases, y is 23 male cases, and the constant is 1 (i.e., $n = 0$ and $10^0 = 1$).

The ratio of females to males would be $46/23 \times 1 = 2/1$. Thus there are two females for each male who developed a catheter-associated UTI. Note that the values in the numerator (the female patients) are not included in the denominator (the male patients).

To calculate the proportion of cases who are males, the following formula is used:

$$x/y \times 10^0$$

in which x is equal to 23 male cases, y is equal to 69 total cases who have a catheter-associated UTI, and 10^0 is equal to 1.

The proportion of cases who are males would be $23/69 \times 1 = 1/3$. This means that one in every three cases is male. If 10^n is 10^2 (100), then the proportion can be expressed as a percentage: $23/69 \times 100 = 33\%$. In this calculation, the values in the numerator (the male cases) are included in the denominator (the total number of cases).

Rates

As Last explains, "Rates describe the frequency with which events occur." In other words, a rate measures the occurrence of an event in a defined population over time. Rates are used to track trends, such as the occurrence of HAIs, over time. The rates most frequently used in healthcare epidemiology are incidence, prevalence, and attack rates. When an increase in a disease or other health-related event is suspected, rates can be calculated and used to determine if there is a change in the occurrence of disease from one period of time to the next.

Incidence rates. Incidence rates are used to measure and compare the frequency of new cases or events in a population. The formula is as follows:

$$\text{Incidence rate} = \frac{\text{the number of new cases that occur in a defined period}}{\text{the population at risk during the same period}} \times 10^n.$$

One type of frequency measure is incidence density, which incorporates time (such as person-years, person-days, or device-days) in the denominator. This gives a more accurate reflection of the population at risk when the likelihood of developing a disease increases as the time of exposure increases. Incidence density is commonly used to calculate the incidence of HAIs because the risk of developing an infection increases as the length of time of exposure to medical devices and the healthcare environment increases, as discussed in

Chapter 2. HAI rates are generally expressed as the number of infections per 1000 person-days (such as patient-days or resident-days) or per 1000 device-days. Incidence density rates used to express the incidence of HAIs that are associated with medical devices, such as mechanical ventilators or intravascular catheters, are commonly expressed as the number of infections per 1000 device-days (such as 3.2 central line-associated bloodstream infections per 1000 central line-days). The formula is as follows:

$$\text{Incidence density} = \frac{\text{the number of new cases that occur in a defined period}}{\substack{\text{the time each person in population at risk is observed,} \\ \text{totaled for all persons}}} \times 10^n$$

in which 10^n is usually 1000 (to provide uniformity of results and to have the final value displayed with at least one digit to the left of the decimal point).

Another type of incidence rate, attack rate, is an incidence rate that is expressed as cases per 100 population (or as a percentage). It is used to describe the new cases of disease that have been observed in a particular group during a limited time period in special circumstances, such as during an epidemic. The formula is as follows:

$$\text{Attack rate} = \frac{\text{the number of new cases in a population in a specified time period}}{\text{the population at risk at the beginning of time period}} \times 100.$$

For example, a newborn nursery reports 17 infants with loose stools in 1 month. During this month, there were 120 patients and 480 patient-days in the newborn nursery. Using the formula above, the incidence rate would be calculated as follows:

$$\frac{\text{17 cases of loose stools in one month}}{\substack{\text{120 patients in newborn nursery} \\ \text{during the month}}} \times 100 = 0.142 \times 100 = 14.2 \text{ cases per 100 patients.}$$

In this example, the incidence rate is expressed as an attack rate (i.e., 14.2% of patients were affected) because $n = 2$ and $10^n = 10^2$ or 100. Using the formula above, the incidence density would be calculated as follows:

$$\frac{\text{17 cases of loose stools in 1 month}}{\substack{\text{480 patient-days in the} \\ \text{same month}}} \times 1000 = 0.0354 \times 1000 = 35.4 \text{ cases per 1000 patient-days}$$

To determine if this incidence is higher than expected, this rate can be compared to the rates for the prior months. Sometimes it may not even be necessary to calculate a rate to determine if an event is unusual; it may be apparent if the disease is rare (such as an HAI with group A streptococcus). For example, during a 2-month period there were 175 patients admitted to the medical/surgical intensive care unit. 40 of the patients subsequently developed an influenza-like illness (ILI). 80 of the patients were medical patients, and the remainder were surgical patients. Of the 40 patients with ILI, 30 were medical patients. The patient-days for this period were 450 for medical patients and 110 for surgical patients.

The overall attack rate for ILI on the unit would be calculated as follows:

$40/175 \times 100 = 22.8\%$.

The ILI attack rate for medical patients would be calculated as follows:

$30/80 \times 100 = 37.5\%$.

The ILI attack rate for surgical patients would be calculated as follows:

$10/95 \times 100 = 10.5\%$

(i.e., 40 total patients with ILI – 30 medical patients with ILI / 175 total patients on unit – 80 medical patients $\times$ 100 = 10.5%).

The incidence density of ILI infection for medical patients would be calculated as follows:

$30/450 \times 1000$ patient-days = 66.7 ILI cases per 1000 patient-days.

The incidence density of ILI infection for surgical patients would be calculated as follows:

$10/110 \times 1000$ patient-days = 90.9 ILI cases per 1000 patient-days.

When analyzing the incidence of infections over time among patients on a healthcare unit, an investigator should calculate the incidence density using patient-days as the denominator, because incidence density (which includes a measurement of risk over time) more accurately reflects the population at risk than the incidence rate.

Finally, in determining incidence rates, numerators and denominators must be chosen with care. As soon as an outbreak is suspected, cases should be identified using a case definition. When calculating incidence rates, the cases are included in the numerator data. Those in the population at risk are placed in the denominator data. It is important that those who are identified as the population at risk (i.e., the denominator) are free of the disease at the beginning of the study period. The selection of an appropriate denominator is one of the most important aspects of measuring disease frequency, as discussed in Chapter 2.

Prevalence rate. Prevalence is a measure of the number of (new and old) cases present in a specified population either during a given period of time (period prevalence) or at a given point in time (point prevalence). The formula for calculating the prevalence rate is as follows:

$$\text{Prevalence rate} = \frac{\text{all new and old cases present for a given period or a given point in time}}{\text{population at risk during same time period}} \times 10^n.$$

A prevalence rate is used to describe the current status of active disease at a particular time in a particular population. It is sometimes helpful to review the incidence and prevalence simultaneously. A low incidence (new cases) may be due to a high prevalence (new and old cases present) in a given population. For instance, if the incidence of infection or colonization with MRSA is relatively low on a patient care unit, but colonized patients remain in this unit for prolonged periods, an explanation for the low incidence (number of new cases) may be the high prevalence. This is because there are very few patients who are at risk, or free of MRSA, to become a new case.

Under stable conditions, that is, when incidence is not changing, the following formula can be used to show the relationship between incidence and prevalence[9]:

$$P = I \times D$$

where P is prevalence, I is incidence, and D is the average duration of disease. A high prevalence of disease in a population can occur if the incidence is high or if the duration of disease is long (such as occurs with chronic diseases or long-term colonization or infection with an infectious agent).

Adjusting rates. The rates of two dissimilar populations should not be compared unless the rates are adjusted for appropriate risk factors, such as age, gender, underlying medical conditions, or other factors that affect the risk of disease. For instance, rates of infection in a population exposed to a medical device are frequently risk-adjusted by incorporating into the denominator the number of days the medical device is in use (e.g., rates of central line-associated bloodstream infections are calculated using central line-days as the denominator). Similarly, rates of ventilator-associated pneumonia are calculated using ventilator-days as the denominator. The CDC's NHSN is an example of a surveillance system in which rates are risk-adjusted to allow for interfacility comparison.[10]

Measures of Central Tendency

Measures of central tendency describe the values around the middle of a set of data. The mean, median, and mode are the principal measures of central tendency.

Mean

The mean is the mathematical average of the values in a set of data. The formula is as follows:

$$\bar{x} = \frac{\Sigma x_i}{n}$$

in which Σx_i is the sum of the individual values in a set and n is the number of values in the set. For example, if the ages among 5 cases in an outbreak are 11, 7, 5, 3, and 4 years, then the mean is:

$$\frac{11 + 7 + 5 + 3 + 4}{5} = 30/5 = 6 \text{ years.}$$

The value of the mean is affected by extreme values in the data set. For example, if a 65 year-old patient is added to the cases in the above data set, the mean, or average, would increase to 15.8 years   [(11 + 7 + 5 + 3 + 4 + 65)/6]. When extreme values are in a data set, the data become skewed and the mean does not give a representative picture of the data, as shown in Figure 10–1. When there are extreme values in a data set, the median should be calculated.

Median

The median is the middle point—the value at which half the measurements lie below the value and half the measurements lie above the value.[8(p80)] The median is useful when there are extreme values in a data set (i.e., the data are skewed).

The median in a data set is calculated as follows:

1. Rank-order the values in either ascending or descending order.
2. Identify the midpoint of the sequence.
   a. If there are an odd number of values, the median is the middle value. For example, in the ranked data set is 11, 7, 5, 4, and 3, the median is the middle value of 5.
   b. If there are an even number of values, then the midpoint between the two middle values is calculated. For example, if the ages in the ranked data set are 11, 7, 6, 5, 4, and 3 years, then the median is the midpoint between the two middle values of the set (6 and 5) or (6 + 5)/2 = 5.5 years.

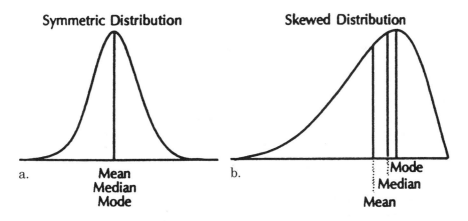

Figure 10–1 Effect of Skewness on the Mean, Median, and Mode

Mode

The mode is the most frequently occurring value in a set of observations. For example, if the ages in a group of controls are 5, 6, 7, 7, 7, 8, and 12, then the mode would be 7.

Some data sets are characterized as bimodal, or having two modes. For example, a sample of ages of cases consisting of the values 3, 4, 4, 5, 5, 5, 5, 5, 5, 6, 7, 8, 9, 9, 9, 9, 9, and 13 would be bimodal, the two modes being 5 and 9 years of age. Some authors have described such a distribution by identifying the major and the minor modes (in this case, the value 5 would be the major mode because it occurs six times, and the value 9 would be the minor mode because it occurs five times). The mode is less affected by skewness (outliers) than is the mean or the median. Mode is infrequently used as a measure of central tendency, particularly in small data sets.

Skewness

In a normal (symmetric) distribution, the mean, median, and mode have the same value as shown in Figure 10–1a. A curve or histogram that is not symmetrical is referred to as skewed or asymmetrical, as shown in Figure 10–1b. A curve that is said to be negatively skewed, as shown in Figure 10–1b, has a tail off to the left and most of the values lie above (to the right of) the mean. The mean is less than the median, which is less than the mode. In contrast, a positively skewed curve would depict a mirror image of this, and the mean is greater than the median, which will be greater than the mode (and the median and mode are to the left of the mean).

Measures of Dispersion

The measures of dispersion describe the distribution of values in a data set around its mean. The most commonly used measures of dispersion are range, deviation, variance, and standard deviation.

Range

The difference between the highest and lowest values in a data set is termed the *range*.[8(p110)] For example, if the length of antibiotic use among cases is 7, 8, 9, 10, and 14 days; the range is 14 − 7 = 7 days.

Deviation

The deviation is the difference between an individual measurement in a data set and the mean value for the set. It is expressed as follows:

$$\text{deviation} = x_i - \bar{x}$$

in which x_i is the ith observation and $\bar{x}$ is the mean.

A measurement may have no deviation (it is equal to the mean), a negative deviation (it is less than the mean), or a positive deviation (it is greater than the mean).

Variance

The variance measures the deviation around the mean of a distribution. It is also called the mean sum of squares or mean square because it is the sum of the squares of deviations from the mean divided by the number of degrees of freedom in the sample set. The variance (s^2) for a sample is expressed as follows:

$$s^2 = \frac{\Sigma(x_i - \bar{x})^2}{n - 1}$$

in which Σ is the sum of, i is the i-th observation (x_1 = first observation, x_2 = second observation, etc.), $\bar{x}$ is the mean, and n is the number of observations.

Standard Deviation

The standard deviation, which may be represented as s or SD, is a measure of dispersion that reflects the distribution of values around the mean. When calculating the standard deviation for a sample, the following formula is used:

$$SD = \sqrt{\frac{\Sigma(x_i - \bar{x})^2}{n - 1}}$$

in which Σ is the sum of, x_i is the ith observation, $\bar{x}$ is the mean, and n is the number of observations.

As can be seen by comparing the two formulas, the standard deviation is the square root of the variance. The standard deviation is always a nonnegative quantity. If the values in a data set are close to the mean, the standard deviation is small (i.e., the values are distributed closely around the mean). If the values in a data set are not close to the mean, the standard deviation is large. For example, the incubation periods for six cases of hepatitis A related to a food-borne outbreak range from 24 to 31 days. Calculate the variance and standard deviation to describe this distribution. Use the data shown in Table 10–1, and the formulas above to calculate the variance and standard deviation.

1. Calculate the mean using the data in the first column (x_i):

   $\bar{x} = \Sigma x_i / n = 168/6 = 28.0$.

2. Subtract the mean from each observation to find the deviations from the mean (shown in the second column). (Note: the sum of the deviations from the mean will always equal zero because the mean is the arithmetic center of the distribution.)

3. Square the deviations from the mean (shown in the third column).

4. Sum the squared deviations (see the third column):

   $\Sigma(x_i - \bar{x})^2 = 40$.

5. Divide the sum of the squared deviations by $n - 1$ to find the variance:

   $\Sigma (x_i - \bar{x})^2 / n - 1 = 40/5 = 8$.

6. Take the square root of the variance to calculate the standard deviation:

   $SD \neq \sqrt{S^2} \neq \sqrt{8} \neq 2.8$.

Table 10–1   Calculating the Variance and Standard Deviation

x_i (observations)	$x_i - \bar{x}$ (deviations from the mean)	$(x_i - \bar{x})^2$ (square of the deviations)
24	$24 - 28.0 = -4.0$	16
25	$25 - 28.0 = -3.0$	9
29	$29 - 28.0 = +1.0$	1
29	$29 - 28.0 = +1.0$	1
30	$30 - 28.0 = +2.0$	4
31	$31 - 28.0 = +3.0$	9
168	$-7.0 + 7.0 = 0$	40

$x_i = i$th observation ; $\bar{x}$ = mean

Source: CDC. *Principles of Epidemiology: An Introduction to Applied Epidemiology and Biostatistics.* 2nd ed. Atlanta, GA: US Department of Health & Human Services; 1992;174–175.

Normal Distribution

A normal distribution represents the natural distribution of values around the mean with progressively fewer observations toward the extremes of the range of values. A normal distribution plotted on a graph shows a bell-shaped curve, in which 68.3 percent of the values will fall within one standard deviation of the mean, 95.5 percent of the values will fall within two standard deviations of the mean, and 99.7 percent of the values will fall within three standard deviations of the mean as shown in Figure 10–2. Statistical inferences about a sample, such as the cases of disease in a population, are frequently based on a normal distribution.

Measures of Association

Measures of association are used during outbreak investigations to evaluate the relationship between exposed and unexposed populations. These statistical measures can express the strength of association between a risk factor (exposure) and an outcome (disease). The measures of association used for outbreak investigations are the risk ratio (or relative risk) and the odds ratio. A two-by-two table (shown in Table 10–2) is used to show comparisons between exposures and outcomes and to calculate risk ratios and odds ratios.

The Risk Ratio (Relative Risk)

The risk ratio (also called the relative risk) is the ratio of the attack rate (or risk of disease) in the exposed population to the attack rate (or risk of disease) in the unexposed population. Using Table 10–2, the attack rate for the exposed population would be $a/a + b$ and the attack rate for the unexposed population would be $c/c + d$. The risk ratio is therefore calculated as follows:

$$\text{Risk ratio} = \frac{a/a + b}{c/c + d}.$$

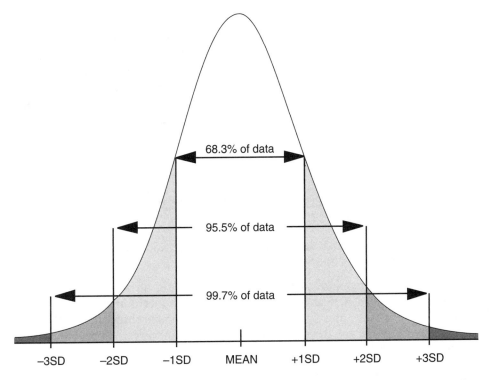

Figure 10–2 Areas Under the Normal Curve that Lie Between 1, 2, and 3 Standard Deviations on Each Side of the Mean

If the value of the risk ratio is equal to 1, the risk is the same in the two groups, and there is no evidence of association between the exposure and outcome. If the risk ratio is greater than 1, the risk is higher for the exposed group, and the exposure may be associated with the outcome. If the risk ratio is less than 1, the risk is lower for the exposed group, and the exposure may possibly protect against the outcome. An investigator can calculate a risk ratio, or relative risk, from the data collected in a cohort study, which is discussed later.

Table 10–2   The Two-by-Two Table

	Disease	No disease	Total
Exposed	a	b	a + b
Unexposed	c	d	c + d
Total	a + c	b + d	N

Note: a = those with exposure and disease; b = those with exposure and no disease; c = those with no exposure and disease; d = those with no exposure and no disease; $a + c$ = total of those with disease; $b + d$ = total of those with no disease; $a + b$ = total of those with exposure; $c + d$ = total of those with no exposure; and $N = a + b + c + d$ = total population in the study.

The Odds Ratio

The odds ratio is similar to the risk ratio except that the odds, instead of the risk (attack rates), are used in the calculation. An odds ratio can be used to approximate the strength of association between an exposure and a disease (outcome). The odds ratio is the ratio of the probability of having a risk factor if the disease is present to the probability of having the risk factor if the disease is absent. Using the two-by-two table, it is calculated as follows:

$$\text{Odds ratio} = \frac{a/b}{c/d} = \frac{a \times d}{b \times c} \quad \text{or}$$

$$\frac{\text{exposed cases/exposed controls}}{\text{unexposed cases/unexposed controls}} = \frac{\text{exposed cases} \times \text{unexposed controls}}{\text{exposed controls} \times \text{unexposed cases}}$$

Those with disease are considered cases (a and c) and those without disease are considered controls (b and d).

If the odds ratio is equal to 1, the odds of disease are the same if the exposure is present and if it is absent (i.e., there is no evidence of association between the exposure and disease). If the odds ratio is greater than 1, the odds of disease are higher for the exposed group, and the exposure is probably associated with the disease.

Confidence Intervals

In an outbreak investigation, if the exposure rates of the cases differ from those of the controls, statistical tests of significance can be done to determine if the difference was likely to have occurred by chance alone or if there may indeed be a causal relationship between the exposure and disease. Probability, or *P*, values traditionally have been used to describe the significance of the findings; however, many authors have recommended that confidence intervals be used, either in place of or in addition to the *P* value to explain the findings.[11–16] A *P* value provides information on statistical significance but does not provide information on the magnitude or precision of the findings. By computing an odds ratio or a risk ratio (which are termed *point estimates*) and a confidence interval, the investigator can provide information on the strength of an association, the precision of the estimate, and the statistical significance.

The confidence interval (CI), sometimes referred to as the margin of error of a study, has been defined as "the computed interval with a stated probability (usually 95%) that the true value of a variable, such as the mean, proportion, or rate, falls within the interval."[17(p26)] In other words, a person using a 95% CI can be confident that if a study were repeated many times, the observed value would fall within the CI in 95 out of 100 studies. Unlike the *P* value, which provides information on statistical significance only, the CI expresses the statistical precision of a point estimate (an observed effect, such as a risk ratio or odds ratio) and the strength of an association. The statistical precision is measured by the size (range) of the confidence interval: the narrower the computed interval, the more precise the estimate. The strength of the association is measured by the magnitude of the difference in the measured outcomes between the two groups (e.g., the higher the numerical value of the risk ratio, the more likely the exposure is related to the outcome).

Confidence intervals provide an alternative to hypothesis testing when ratios of risk or rates are being compared. A 95% CI provides information on whether or not an observation is statistically significant with a P value less than or equal to .05. As noted previously, an odds (or risk) ratio of 1.0 means that the odds (or risk) of disease are the same between the comparison groups whether or not the exposure occurs. If the value of an odds ratio is greater than 1.0, the probability of having a risk factor if the disease is present is greater than the probability of having the risk factor if the disease is absent. If the value of a risk ratio is greater than 1.0, the risk of disease in the exposed population is greater than the risk of disease in the unexposed population. If a ratio's 95% CI does not include 1.0, then statistical significance is implied ($P \leq$ 0.05). If the confidence interval for an odds or risk ratio includes 1.0, then the findings are not statistically significant.

For example, if the odds ratio (the point estimate) for an exposure is said to be 8.2 with a 95% CI of 6.2–10.6, this means: (1) persons with the disease were 8.2 times more likely to have been exposed to the risk factor than those without the disease, and (2) one can be 95% confident (probability of 0.95) that the odds ratio in the population is between the confidence limits of 6.2 and 10.6 (i.e., it may be as low as 6.2 or as high as 10.6). In addition, since the lower limit of this observed CI (6.2) is well above 1.0 (which equals no association), it is implied that the results are statistically significant at the 0.05 level.

As another example, if an odds ratio is 1.6 with a 95% CI of 0.8–2.4, then the findings are considered not statistically significant because 1.0 is included in the confidence interval.

Although P values traditionally have been used to show the statistical significance between disease and risk factors in outbreaks, odds or risk ratios and 95% CIs are now usually used. For example, in a 2007 report of an outbreak of *Salmonella oranienburg* infections that was found to be associated with eating fruit salad served in healthcare facilities, the CDC presented the following data[18]:

> 14 (70%) of 20 case-patients, compared with four (13%) of 30 controls, ate fruit salad [matched odds ratio (mOR) = 8.9; 95% CI = 2.3–35.5].
> Illness was associated with eating fruit salad in a health-care facility.

As illustrated by this report, when a point estimate (odds ratio) and CI are given, the reader has more information with which to interpret the results than if a P value alone is reported because the magnitude of the odds ratio provides an estimate of the strength of association between a disease and a risk factor, and the CI provides an estimate of the statistical significance and the precision of this finding. For instance, in this report, the odds ratio for fruit salad was 8.9, which means that those who were ill were 8.9 times more likely to have eaten fruit salad than those who were not ill. The CI of 2.3 to 35.5 infers that these findings are statistically significant because the lower confidence limit of 2.3 is above 1.0.

Confidence intervals can be computed using computer programs, formulas, tables, or graphs, and the method varies according to the type of data. Because the methods used to calculate them are complex, a discussion of the computation of confidence intervals is beyond the scope of this chapter. For more information, the reader should refer to the references given[11–16] or to one of the statistics texts listed in the Suggested Reading list at the end of this chapter. In practice, an investigator should consult a statistician to ensure that the correct method will be used to compute any confidence intervals used to describe the findings of an outbreak investigation.

ANALYTIC STUDIES

Analytic studies are used to compare rates of disease between two groups. This comparison allows an investigator (1) to quantify relationships between risk factors and disease, and (2) to determine the strength of association in these causal relationships. Analytic studies are used to test the hypotheses proposed to explain the occurrence of an outbreak.

The two major categories of epidemiologic studies used to examine cause and effect are experimental and observational. In experimental studies, the investigator controls the exposures to specific factors and then follows the subjects to determine the effect of the exposure (e.g., a clinical trial of a new drug). In observational studies, the investigator observes the natural course of events. Observational studies are used to analyze outbreaks because the investigator is observing the outcomes to prior exposures over which the investigator has no control. The two types of observational studies most commonly used in outbreak investigations are the retrospective cohort study and the case-control study.

Cohort Studies and the Risk Ratio (Relative Risk)

In a cohort study, subjects are categorized based on their *exposure* to a specific factor and then they are observed to see if they develop a disease. A cohort study may be conducted prospectively or retrospectively. In a prospective cohort study, subjects may be observed over a prolonged period of time in order to examine the natural history or incidence (risk) of a disease. The Nurses' Health Study is an example of a long-term (over 30 years) prospective cohort study and is among the largest prospective investigations into the risk factors for major chronic diseases in women.[19] Using a retrospective cohort study, an event that has already occurred (such as an outbreak) can be analyzed by reconstructing records of exposures and studying their outcomes. A retrospective cohort study can be used only when studying a well-defined population, such as the attendees of a luncheon or the patients of a surgeon. It cannot be used if the true population at risk cannot be identified (such as an outbreak associated with a widely distributed commercial product because it would not be possible to identify all the users of the product).

When conducting a cohort study, it is helpful to develop a spreadsheet listing potential risk factors and attack rates, as shown in the example in Table 10–3. The investigator can then scan the data to look for three characteristics[20(p375)]:

1. A high attack rate in those exposed to the factor
2. A low attack rate in those not exposed to the factor
3. A factor to which most of the cases were exposed (so that exposure could possibly be implicated as a risk factor responsible for the outbreak)

For example, residents, personnel, and visitors developed acute gastroenteritis after attending a Sunday luncheon at an LTCF that provides assisted living and nursing care. Of the 90 persons who attended the luncheon, 86 were available for interview, and 41 met the case definition for acute gastroenteritis. Attack rates for those who did and those who did not eat particular food items are shown in Table 10–3.

According to the data in Table 10–3: (1) the ice cream is the item that has the highest attack rate (88%), (2) the attack rate is low among those who did not eat ice cream (9.1%), and (3) most of those who met the case definition for gastroenteritis ate ice cream (37/41). Therefore, it is likely that the ice cream was the vehicle.

The risk ratio (relative risk) can be calculated to show the association between eating ice cream and developing gastroenteritis. The relative risk is the ratio of the attack rate in the exposed population to the attack rate in the unexposed population. A two-by-two table (Table 10–4) can be used to demonstrate the comparison of attack rates between the exposed (ate ice cream) and unexposed (did not eat ice cream) groups. Using the data in Table 10–4, the risk ratio would be the attack rate for those who ate ice cream (88) divided by the attack rate for those who did not eat ice cream (9.1), or 88/9.1 = 9.7.

Table 10–3 Attack Rates by Items Served at a Luncheon at a Long-Term Care Facility.

	Number of Persons Who Ate Item				Number of Persons Who Did Not Eat Item			
	Ill	*Well*	*Total*	*Attack rate (%)*	*Ill*	*Well*	*Total*	*Attack rate (%)*
Egg salad	20	17	37	54	18	27	45	40
Ham sandwich	23	18	41	56	19	36	55	35
Turkey sandwich	22	18	40	55	8	40	48	17
Ice cream	37	5	42	88	4	40	44	9.1
Water	27	17	44	61	22	20	42	52
Milk	18	25	43	42	17	26	43	40
Coffee	17	32	49	35	21	16	37	57

Table 10–4   Attack Rate by Consumption of Ice Cream.

	Ill	Well	Total	Attack rate (%)
Ate ice cream	37	5	42	88
Did not eat ice cream	4	40	44	9.1
Total	41	45	86	48

Once a measure of association, such as a risk ratio, has been computed to quantify a relationship between exposure and outcome, the investigator can use a statistical test of significance, such as a chi-square test, to determine the likelihood of this relationship occurring by chance alone. In practice, a combination of cohort and case-control studies are frequently used when investigating clusters and outbreaks. Exhibit 10–1 demonstrates the use of rates and the risk ratio to identify an apparent risk factor for developing an MRSA infection. A case-control study could then be designed to further delineate risk factors associated with developing disease (in this example, a case-control study could be designed to identify risk factors that may exist on a trauma service but not on a surgical service).

Exhibit 10–1   Using Rates and Ratios (Measures of Association) to Identify Risk Factors

The following information was collected during an investigation of an outbreak of infections caused by MRSA in a surgical intensive care unit (SICU): During a three-month period, 180 patients were admitted to the SICU and 15 patients developed an MRSA infection. Twenty-five patients were on the trauma service, and the other patients were on the surgical service. Of the 15 patients who developed MRSA infection, 10 were on the trauma service. From the information presented, it appears that being on the trauma service may be a risk factor for developing an MRSA infection. An investigator can use a two-by-two table to display this data and to calculate attack rates (incidence or risk of disease) and a risk ratio:

Number of Cases of MRSA and Attack Rates, by Service, in the SICU
During a three-Month Period

	MRSA infection present	MRSA infection absent	Total	Attack rate(%)
Trauma service	$a = 10$	$b = 15$	$a + b = 25$	40
Surgical service	$c = 5$	$d = 150$	$c + d = 155$	3.2
Total	$a + c = 15$	$b + d = 165$	$a + b + c + d = 180$	8.3

Calculate the following rates:
1. Overall attack rate of MRSA infection in the SICU: $a + c/a + b + c + d \times 100 = 15/180 \times 100 = 8.3\%$

2. Attack rate for patients on the trauma service: $a/a + b \times 100 = 10/25 \times 100 = 40\%$
3. Attack rate for patients on the surgical service: $c/c + d \times 100 = 5/155 \times 100 = 3.2\%$

Calculate the risk ratio between patients on the trauma service and those on the surgical service:

risk ratio = attack rate for trauma service/attack rate for surgical service

risk ratio = $(a/a + b) / (c/c + d) = 40/3.2 = 12.5$

Interpretation: The risk for MRSA infection for patients on the trauma service (40%) appears to be 12.5 times higher than the risk for patients on the surgical service (3.2%). Therefore, being a patient on the trauma service appears to be a risk factor for developing an MRSA infection.

As discussed in the previous section, confidence intervals of the risk ratio are frequently determined and presented in the final report of an outbreak investigation. This is illustrated in a report of an outbreak of gram-negative bacterial bloodstream infections (BSIs) associated with contamination of the waste drain port in hemodialysis machines[21]:

> Results of a cohort study of all patients receiving dialysis at the center during the two-month epidemic period indicated that the risk for gram-negative BSI was associated with exposure to any of three particular dialysis machines (seven BSIs in 20 patients who were exposed to one or more of the three machines versus three BSIs in 64 patients who were exposed to the other machines; relative risk = 7.5; 95% CI = 2.1–26.2).

The interpretation of this report is that persons who were exposed to the particular dialysis machines were 7.5 times more likely to develop a gram-negative BSI than those who were not exposed to the machines. This finding is considered statistically significant at $P \leq .05$ because the CI does not include 1.0.

The Case-Control Study and the Odds Ratio

The case-control study is used to demonstrate whether or not an association exists between a disease (outcome) and a risk factor (exposure) in an outbreak investigation. A case-control study begins with the identification of persons with the *disease* being studied (the cases). A suitable comparison group of persons without the disease (the controls) is then chosen, and the two groups are compared in relation to their exposures. As in the cohort study, associations and quantitative comparisons of risk are made through the use of two-by-two tables, as shown in Table 10–2. A cohort study allows the computation of a risk ratio; however, a case-control study yields an odds ratio. This is because attack rates (needed to compute the risk ratio) cannot always be calculated in a case-control study because the entire population at risk may not be defined. Once the strength of association is measured (i.e., the odds ratio is calculated), the investigator can use statistical tests of significance and confidence intervals to evaluate the likelihood of the association occurring by chance.

The case-control study is the method most commonly used to investigate outbreaks because it is relatively inexpensive to conduct, is usually of short duration, can be used for rare diseases, requires relatively few study subjects, and allows for testing of multiple hypotheses.[17,22] A case-control study can be used when the population at risk (the cohort) cannot be adequately defined or cannot be fully identified (such as may occur in a multistate outbreak of salmonellosis associated with a contaminated food).

(Note: A case-control study differs from a cohort study in that the subjects are enrolled into a case-control study based on whether or not they have a *disease*. In a cohort study, subjects are included in the study based on their *exposure* and are then followed for the development of disease.)

In an outbreak investigation, the magnitude of an odds ratio is indicative of the strength of an association between an exposure and a disease. As in a cohort study, it has become common practice to compute the confidence intervals of the odds ratio as shown in this report of an outbreak of SARS in an apartment complex[23(p1734)]:

> For building E, apartment units (not persons) on the middle and upper floors had higher probabilities of infection than did units on lower floors, with an odds ratio of 5.15 (95% CI, 2.6–10.3; $P < 0.001$) for the middle floors and 3.1 (95% CI, 1.6–6.2; $P < 0.01$) for the upper floors.

An odds ratio of 5.15 for the middle floors implies that those apartments on the middle floors were 5 times more likely to be infected than those on the lower floors. A 95% CI of 2.6–10.3 means that these odds could be as low as 2.6 or as high as 10.3 Since the CI does not include 1.0, the findings are considered statistically significant at a P value less than or equal to 0.05. The calculated P value for the middle floors was less than .001.

Designing and Conducting a Case-Control Study

Case-control studies must be carefully designed and conducted in order to ensure valid results. Although a detailed explanation of the design of a case-control study is beyond the scope of this chapter, the reader should be aware of several methodological problems that can affect the study results: improper or biased selection of cases or controls, information bias, confounding, and too small a sample size.

The reader who wishes detailed information on designing and conducting a case-control study may refer to the text by Schlesselman in the Suggested Reading section of this chapter or to the articles by Wacholder et al. in the references listed.[24–26] In practice, a statistician should be consulted before conducting a case-control study to ensure that the study is appropriately designed.

Bias

Bias is "the deviation of results or inferences from the truth, or processes leading to such deviation."[8] Bias can lead to conclusions that are distorted (different from the truth). Some types of bias may occur in either a case-control or cohort study. Selection bias can occur when the cases selected for study do not represent the entire population at risk. This can occur if a nonrandom method is used to select study subjects (e.g., the selection is unconsciously or consciously influenced in some way) or if some of the study subjects are unavailable (e.g., they refuse to participate, their records are missing, their disease is mild and they do not seek medical care and are therefore not detected, or they seek medical care and their disease is undiagnosed or misdiagnosed). Information bias can occur if the information collected is incorrect because of inaccurate recall (e.g., a participant at a luncheon does not correctly remember what he ate) or because it is inconsistently collected (observer bias). Observer bias occurs when collection or interpretation of data about exposures is systematically different for persons who have the disease than those who do not or data about outcomes is systematically different for persons who are exposed than for persons who are not exposed.

Selecting Cases

Cases are selected based on a case definition, as discussed in Chapter 8. A case-control study conducted as part of an outbreak investigation differs from other case-control studies in that the case definition in an outbreak investigation frequently changes during the course of the investigation. In the initial stages, a case definition may be broad in order to identify all potential cases (e.g., all persons who developed gastroenteritis from April 10 through 17). The case definition may be refined as the investigation progresses and potential risk factors are identified (e.g., all persons who developed gastroenteritis from April 11 through April 15 and who ate food prepared by the hospital kitchen).

In many outbreaks in healthcare facilities, the number of cases is small, and it is possible to include all of them in a case-control study. All of the cases should be included whenever possible to avoid the need to select a sample and introduce biases. In a large outbreak, however, it may not be practical, or possible, to identify or include all of the cases. In this instance, cases may be selected (sampled) from those who are ill. Care must be taken to ensure that the cases sampled are representative of the entire population with disease so that the study findings can be validly extrapolated to the whole population. To help eliminate some sampling biases, additional cases should be sought out during an outbreak to determine the magnitude of the problem.

Selecting Controls

Controls must come from the same environment where the cases' exposures occurred (i.e., they must be from the same population at risk for exposure and must be at the same risk of acquiring the disease).[24] Controls should be similar to the cases in many respects except for the presence of the disease being studied. For instance, if a case-control study is being designed to investigate an outbreak of group A streptococcal infections in postpartum patients, then the controls should be selected from postpartum patients who were hospitalized at the same time as the cases but who did not develop a group A streptococcal infection. Ideally, controls should be randomly selected from the population at risk to avoid selection bias.

Confounding Variables

"Comparisons may differ from the truth and therefore be biased when the association between exposure and the health problem varies because a third factor confounds the association."[17(p24)] This difference can happen when a third factor is associated with both the exposure and the disease. Confounding factors that can bias results include age, sex, length of stay in a healthcare facility, or underlying disease. For example, confounding could occur if there were a community outbreak of gastroenteritis and the investigators selected only those cases who were seen in a hospital. If most of the cases seen at a hospital were elderly, it could be inferred that the illness had struck the elderly population when in fact this population may be more likely to become clinically ill and then go to a hospital for treatment. One method of reducing confounding errors is to choose controls that are the same age and sex as each case.

Sample Size

A case-control study must contain a sufficiently large number of study subjects in order to be able to detect an association, if one exists, between an exposure and a disease. Multiple mathematical formulas are available to determine an appropriate sample size, and these can be found in many statistics textbooks and articles.[27–30] However, it is advisable to consult a trained statistician to assist with this task. As the number of study subjects (cases) increases, the power to detect a statistically significant association increases. One control for each case is generally sufficient if there are more than 50 cases in an outbreak[31] Since outbreaks in healthcare facilities generally involve fewer than 50 cases, two controls are frequently selected for each case whenever possible.

For example, if investigating an outbreak of six cases of aspergillosis that occurred among patients on a bone marrow transplant unit, the investigator would want to select at least two controls for each case, and the controls would be chosen from the population of patients who were on the bone marrow transplant unit at the same time as the cases but who did not develop aspergillosis.

HYPOTHESIS TESTING (INFERENTIAL STATISTICS)

The following is a simplified explanation of statistical significance testing as it is used for investigating an outbreak. The reader is referred to one of many statistics textbooks, including the Suggested Reading and Other Resources at the end of this chapter, for a detailed discussion of the concepts noted here.

During an outbreak investigation, descriptive studies are used to describe those who are ill, when they became ill, and where they were when they became ill. From this information, the population at risk can generally be identified. Although this information may be enough to allow the investigator to identify potential risk factors and implement control measures that will interrupt the outbreak, it may sometimes be necessary, or desirable, to more specifically pinpoint the exposure that resulted in the disease. This is done by conducting an analytic epidemiologic study (usually a case-control or retrospective cohort study). Before conducting an analytic study, the investigator must first formulate a hypothesis (a statement that says a specific exposure results in disease) and then design the analytic study to test this hypothesis (i.e., use tests of statistical significance to assess the relationship between the specific exposure and the disease being studied). Statistical significance testing helps the investigator evaluate the role of chance by determining the probability that an association between an exposure and a disease actually exists.

There are six steps in the statistical significance testing process[32(p22)]:

1. State the hypothesis
2. Formulate the null hypothesis
3. Choose a statistical significance cutoff level
4. Conduct an analytic study
5. Apply statistical significance test
6. Reject, or fail to reject, the null hypothesis

State the Hypothesis

To generate a hypothesis about the likely causative risk factor(s) or exposure(s) responsible for disease in an outbreak situation, the investigator should carefully review the existing epidemiologic and laboratory data and conduct a literature search, as discussed in Chapter 8. The hypothesis states that a difference exists between the study group and the control group. Care must be taken when generating the hypothesis. Although the source of an outbreak may appear to be obvious, it is prudent to hold an open mind and look for answers that may not have been considered. For example, an investigation of an outbreak of nosocomial legionellosis at a hospital in Rhode Island revealed that *Legionella pneumophila* was in the hospital potable water supply and this was the likely source for the outbreak. When a sudden increase in new cases occurred, it was believed to be related to the potable water; however, an extensive epidemiologic investigation demonstrated that a new cooling tower at the hospital was the source of the second outbreak.[33]

Formulate the Null Hypothesis

A null hypothesis is generated before testing for statistical significance. The null hypothesis states that no difference exists between the study group and the control group (i.e., the results observed in a study are no different from what might have occurred by chance alone). In other words, the null hypothesis states that the proportion of disease in the exposed group is the same as the proportion of disease in the nonexposed group (i.e., the exposure has no effect on the development of disease). It should be noted that an investigator can never "prove" an association between a factor (exposure) and an outcome (disease); however, inferences can be made based on statistical testing.

For example, if investigating an outbreak of group A streptococcal surgical site infections, an investigator could state that a likely risk factor for developing disease would be exposure to a colonized or infected health care provider. A possible study hypothesis would be "Patients exposed to surgeon N are more likely to develop a group A streptococcal surgical site infection than patients not exposed to surgeon N." This hypothesis is based on published reports of investigations of outbreaks of group A streptococcal surgical site infections in which a colonized or infected member of the surgical team was found to be the most likely source of the organism. The null hypothesis for this study hypothesis could be "There is no difference in group A streptococcal surgical site infection rates between patients who were exposed to surgeon N and patients who were not exposed to surgeon N."

Choose a Statistical Significance Cutoff Level

In outbreak investigations, a 5% chance of occurrence is traditionally used as the statistical cutoff level. This means that the investigator will accept the fact that an association that is found between an exposure and the disease being studied may occur by chance alone 5% of the time. This also means that the P value must be less than .05 in order for the investigator to be able to reject the null hypothesis.

Conduct an Analytic Study

As previously discussed, when conducting an investigation of an outbreak in a healthcare setting, a case-control or retrospective cohort study is usually used to allow the investigator to collect data on a study group (the cases or the cohort) and a control group so the two groups can be compared in relationship to their exposures and the presence or absence of disease.

Apply a Statistical Significance Test

Tests of statistical significance are then used to determine the probability that the results of comparison testing could have occurred by chance alone if the exposure is not related to the disease. If differences are found between the study group and the control group, the investigator must choose which test of statistical significance to use to determine the probability that these differences would occur if no true difference exists (i.e., if the null hypothesis were true). In outbreak investigations in healthcare settings, the most commonly used tests of significance are the chi-square and Fisher exact tests, which will be discussed later.

Reject, or Fail to Reject, the Null Hypothesis

If 5% is used as the statistical cutoff level, the investigator can reject the null hypothesis (and thus can accept the study hypothesis) if the statistical test shows that the association is likely to occur less than 5% of the time by chance alone (i.e., the P value is less than .05).

Type I and Type II Errors

An investigator's inference about an association can be wrong if the findings are due to bias or confounding in the study or to chance alone. A type I error

Table 10–5 The Four Possible Outcomes of Statistical Significance Testing

	Association Between Factor and Outcome Exists (Null Hypothesis Is Not True)	No Association Between Factor and Outcome Exists (Null Hypothesis Is True)
Reject null hypothesis	Correct	Type I error
Fail to reject null hypothesis	Type II error	Correct

occurs when an investigator states that there is an association when in fact there is no association (i.e., the investigator rejects a null hypothesis that is actually true). A type II error occurs when the investigator states that there is no association when, in fact, there is an association (i.e., the investigator fails to reject a null hypothesis that is actually false). Table 10–5 uses a two-by-two table to illustrate the four possible outcomes of statistical significance testing.

Although these errors are not always avoidable, the likelihood of making a type II error can be minimized by using a larger sample size. By choosing the statistical cutoff level, the investigator decides before beginning the study what probability of committing a type I error can be accepted (usually 5%).

TESTS OF STATISTICAL SIGNIFICANCE

The Chi-Square Test

The chi-square test is commonly used in outbreak investigations to evaluate the probability that observed differences between two populations, such as cases and controls, could have occurred by chance alone if an exposure is not truly associated with disease. There are several variations of the chi-square test.[6] Since a detailed explanation of this test is beyond the scope of this chapter, the reader is referred to the article by Gaddis and Gaddis[6] or to one of the statistics references noted in the Suggested Reading section at the end of the chapter.

Using the two-by-two table shown in Table 10–2, a frequently used formula for calculating chi-square is as follows[20(p377)]:

$$\text{Chi-square} = \frac{N[\,|ad - bc| - N/2\,]^2}{(a + b)(c + d)(a + c)(b + d)}.$$

Once the value for chi-square has been calculated, the investigator then uses a table of chi-squares (found in a textbook of statistical tables) to look up the associated *P* value. An example of a table of chi-squares is shown in Table 10–6.

Table 10–6 Table of Chi-Squares

Degree of Freedom	Probability						
	0.50	0.20	0.10	0.05	0.02	0.01	0.001
1	.455	1.642	2.706	3.841	5.412	6.635	10.827
2	1.386	3.219	4.605	5.991	7.824	9.210	13.815
3	2.366	4.642	6.251	7.815	9.837	11.345	16.268
4	3.357	5.989	7.779	9.488	11.668	13.277	18.465
5	4.351	7.289	9.236	11.070	13.388	15.086	20.517
10	9.342	13.442	15.987	18.307	21.161	23.209	29.588
15	14.339	19.311	22.307	24.996	28.259	30.578	37.697
20	19.337	25.038	28.412	31.410	35.020	37.566	43.315
25	24.337	30.675	34.382	37.652	41.566	44.314	52.620
30	29.336	36.250	40.256	43.773	47.962	50.892	59.703

Source: Reprinted from *Principles of Epidemiology: An Introduction to Applied Epidemiology and Biostatistics*, 2nd ed. Atlanta, GA: CDC; 1992:378.

To use a table of chi-squares, the degrees of freedom, defined as the number of independent comparisons that can be made between the members of a sample, must be known. A two-by-two table has one degree of freedom. Using Table 10–6 and a statistical cutoff point of 0.05, if the computed chi-square value is greater than 3.841, then the probability, or *P* value, would be less than 0.05, and the null hypothesis can be rejected.

Because it can be quite time consuming to calculate chi-square by hand, most investigators opt to use a computer with a statistical software package.

The chi-square test can be used if the number of subjects in a study is approximately 30 or more.[31(p6–44)] For smaller populations, or if the value of any of the cells in a two-by-two table is less than 5, Fisher's exact test should be used.[6]

Fisher's Exact Test

Fisher's exact test, which is used for evaluating data in two-by-two contingency tables, is a variant of the chi-square test. Fisher's exact test is the preferred test for studies with few subjects. The formula for Fisher's exact test calculates the *P* value directly, so a table of chi-squares is not needed. Since calculating Fisher's exact test manually or with a calculator is arduous, a computer program should be used for calculating this test statistic.

USING COMPUTERS TO MAKE LIFE EASIER

Computers have greatly enhanced accuracy and reduced the time it takes to calculate complex mathematical formulas; however, the investigator still needs to understand which statistical methods to use and when to use them. There are two basic types of software programs that can be used to manage epidemiologic data: database managers, which store and organize data, and statistical packages, which can analyze it. There are many computer software programs that can be used to store, manage, and analyze epidemiologic data. Examples are SPSS (SPSS, Inc., Chicago, IL), SAS (SAS Institute, Cary, NC), Epi Info, and infection control-specific programs such as AICE (Automated Infection Control Expert) (Infection Control and Prevention Analysts, Inc., Austin, TX). Epi Info is a software program that was developed by the CDC to manage and analyze data collected during an epidemiologic investigation. Epi Info, which can be used to calculate odds ratios, relative risk, 95% CIs, chi-squares, P values, and so on, can be downloaded free of charge from the CDC Web site at http://www.cdc.gov/epiinfo. Epi Info Tutorials and training resources are also available on the CDC Web site.

Examples of other programs and resources for performing statistical tests can be found in the Resources section at the end of this chapter.

INTERPRETING RESULTS: THE MEANING OF STATISTICAL SIGNIFICANCE

A result is said to be statistically significant if the computed P value is lower than the significance level chosen for the study because this means that it is highly unlikely that the observed association occurred by chance alone. If an investigator is using a significance level of $P = .05$, and the computed P value is lower than .05, this result is said to be statistically significant because the probability that the findings occurred by chance alone are less than 1 in 20. As discussed earlier in the chapter, many researchers recommend calculating the P value and/or the confidence intervals in addition to a measurement of association, such as an odds ratio, when analyzing the findings of an epidemiologic study.

The results of statistical significance tests and other statistical measurements, such as rates, ratios, and proportions, must be interpreted with caution. As discussed in Chapter 1, two important concepts in analytic epidemiology are cause and association. A cause is a factor that directly influences the occurrence of a disease. An association is a statistical relationship between two or more variables, such as an exposure and a disease. While an investigator cannot use statistics to prove that a particular factor caused a disease, if statistical testing shows that a group of people with exposure to a specified factor are more likely to have a disease than a group of people who are not exposed to that factor, then the factor is said to be associated with the disease. It is important to keep in mind that findings may be statistically significant but clinically irrelevant. This is because a statistically significant finding may be artifactual or spurious (i.e., a type I error, which is a false association due to chance or some bias in the study) or may be the result of confounding (e.g., a third factor may account for an apparent association). The following criteria can be used to judge whether or not an association is causal (i.e., the suspected factor is the likely cause of the event)[17(p27)]:

1. Strength of association: The prevalence of disease is higher in the exposed group than in the nonexposed group.

2. Dose–response relationship: There is a quantitative relationship between the amount of exposure to the factor and the frequency of disease.

3. Consistency of association: The findings have been confirmed by different investigators in different populations.

4. Chronological relationship: Exposure to the factor precedes the onset of disease.

5. Biologically plausible: The findings are coherent with existing information; they are acceptable in light of current knowledge.

SUMMARY

When investigating an outbreak, the investigator should conduct a literature search to gather clues about the possible risk factors associated with the disease or condition. Data should be collected to describe the characteristics of the cases so that potential risk factors can be identified and analyzed and a hypothesis explaining the occurrence of an outbreak can be generated. In many outbreak investigations, the information gathered in a descriptive epidemiologic study will be sufficient to identify likely risk factors so that effective control measures can be implemented to interrupt the outbreak. Further statistical analysis will be needed to pinpoint the associated risk factors more precisely if the problem continues or recurs, if the disease or condition involves significant morbidity or mortality, or if the outbreak is unique and the investigator wishes to publish the findings of the investigation. The authors strongly recommend that those who are investigating an outbreak consult a statistician before conducting an analytic epidemiologic study, such as a case-control or cohort study, and use computers as much as possible for managing data and performing statistical tests.

REFERENCES

1. Reingold AL. Outbreak investigations—a perspective. *Emer Infect Dis.* 1998;4:24.
2. Gaddis ML, Gaddis GM. Introduction to biostatistics: part 1, basic concepts. *Ann Emerg Med.* 1990;19:86–89.
3. Gaddis ML, Gaddis GM. Introduction to biostatistics: part 2, descriptive statistics. *Ann Emerg Med.* 1990;19:309–315.
4. Gaddis ML, Gaddis GM. Introduction to biostatistics: part 3, sensitivity, specificity, predictive value, and hypothesis testing. *Ann Emerg Med.* 1990;19:591–596.
5. Gaddis ML, Gaddis GM. Introduction to biostatistics: part 4, statistical inference techniques in hypothesis testing. *Ann Emerg Med.* 1990;19:820–825.
6. Gaddis ML, Gaddis GM. Introduction to biostatistics: part 5, statistical inference techniques for hypothesis testing with nonparametric data. *Ann Emerg Med.* 1990;19:1054–1059.
7. Gaddis ML, Gaddis GM. Introduction to biostatistics: part 6, correlation and regression. *Ann Emerg Med.* 1990;19:1462–1468.
8. Last JM, Spasoff RA, Harris S, Thuriaux M. *A Dictionary of Epidemiology.* International Epidemiological Association. New York, NY: Oxford University Press; 2000.

9. Freeman J, Hitchison GB. Prevalence, incidence and duration. *Am J Epidemiol.* 1980; 112:707–723.

10. Edwards JR, Peterson KD, Andrus ML, et al. National Healthcare Safety Network (NHSN) report, data summary for 2006, issued June 2007. *Am J Infect Control.* 2007;35:290–301.

11. Young KD, Lewis RJ. What is confidence? Part 1: the use and interpretation of confidence intervals. *Ann Emerg Med.* 1997;30:307–310.

12. Young KD, Lewis RJ. What is confidence? Part 2: detailed definition and determination of confidence intervals. *Ann Emerg Med.* 1997;30:311–318.

13. Gardner MJ, Altman DG. Confidence intervals rather than *P* values: estimation rather than hypothesis testing. *Br Med J.* 1986;292:746–750.

14. Morris JA, Gardner MJ. Calculating confidence intervals for relative risks (odds ratios) and standardized ratios and rates. *Br Med J.* 1988;296:1313–1316.

15. Birnbaum D, Sheps SB. The merits of confidence intervals relative to hypothesis testing. *Infect Control Hosp Epidemiol.* 1992;13:553–555.

16. Woolson RF, Kleinman JC. Perspectives on statistical significance testing. *Ann Rev Public Health.* 1989;10:423–440.

17. Last JM, Tyler CW. Epidemiology. In: Wallace RB, ed. *Maxcy-Rosenau-Last Public Health and Preventive Medicine.* 14th ed. Stamford, CT: Appleton & Lange; 1998:5–33.

18. Centers for Disease Control and Prevention. *Salmonella oranienburg* infections associated with fruit salad served in health-care facilities—Northeastern United States and Canada, 2006. *MMWR.* 2007;56(39):1025–1028.

19. Harvard School of Public Health. Nurses' Health Study. http://www.channing.harvard.edu/nhs/index.html. Accessed March 14, 2008.

20. Centers for Disease Control and Prevention. *Principles of Epidemiology: An Introduction to Applied Epidemiology and Biostatistics.* Atlanta, GA: CDC; 1992.

21. Centers for Disease Control and Prevention. Outbreaks of gram-negative bacterial bloodstream infections traced to probable contamination of hemodialysis machines—Canada, 1995, United States, 1997, and Israel, 1997. *MMWR.* 1998;47:55–58.

22. Dwyer DM, Strickler H, Goodman RA, Armenian HK. Use of case-control studies in outbreak investigations. *Epidemiol Rev.* 1994;16:109–123.

23. Yu ITS, Li Y, Wong TW, et al. Evidence of airborne transmission of the severe acute respiratory syndrome virus. *N Engl J Med.* 2004;350:1731–1739.

24. Wacholder S, McLaughlin JK, Silverman DT, Mandel JS. Selection of controls in case-control studies. I. Principles. *Am J Epidemiol.* 1992;135:1019–1028.

25. Wacholder S, McLaughlin JK, Silverman DT, Mandel JS. Selection of controls in case-control studies. II. Types of controls. *Am J Epidemiol.* 1992;135:1029–1041.

26. Wacholder S, McLaughlin JK, Silverman DT, Mandel JS. Selection of controls in case-control studies. III. Design options. *Am J Epidemiol.* 1992;135:1042–1050.

27. Kelsey JL, Thompson WD, Evans AS. *Methods in Observational Epidemiology.* New York, NY: Oxford University Press; 1986.

28. Kleinbaum D, Rosner B. *Fundamentals of Biostatistics.* Boston, MA: Duxbury Press; 1982.

29. Hennekens CH, Buring J. *Epidemiology in Medicine.* Boston, MA: Little, Brown and Company; 1987:260.

30. Edmiston CE, Josephson A, Pottinger J, Ciasco-Tsivitis M, Palenik C. The numbers game: sample-size determination. *Am J Infect Control.* 1993;21:151–154.

31. Centers for Disease Control and Prevention. *Principles of Epidemiology in Public Health Practice.* 3rd ed. Atlanta, GA: US Department of Health and Human Services; 2004.

32. Riegelman RK, Hirsch RP. Analysis. In: *Studying a Study and Testing a Test: How to Read the Health Science Literature.* 3rd ed. Philadelphia: Lippincott-Raven Publishers; 1996:22–39.

33. Garbe PL, Davis BJ, Weisfeld JS. Nosocomial Legionnaires' disease: epidemiologic demonstration of cooling towers as a source. *JAMA.* 1985;254:521–524.

SUGGESTED READING AND RESOURCES

Campbell MJ, Machin D. *Medical Statistics: A Common Sense Approach.* Chichester, UK: John Wiley & Sons; 1990.

Centers for Disease Control and Prevention. *Principles of Epidemiology in Public Health Practice.* 3rd ed. Atlanta, GA: US Department of Health and Human Services; 2004.

Dwyer DM, Strickler H, Goodman RA, Armenian HK. Use of case-control studies in outbreak investigations. *Epidemiol Rev.* 1994;16:109–123.

Fletcher RH, Fletcher SW, Wagner EH. *Clinical Epidemiology: The Essentials.* Baltimore, MD: Williams & Wilkins; 1996.

Hennekens CH, Buring J. *Epidemiology in Medicine.* Boston/Toronto: Little, Brown and Company; 1987.

Hulley SB, Cummings SR. *Designing Clinical Research: An Epidemiologic Approach.* Baltimore, MD: Williams & Wilkins; 1988.

Kleinbaum D, Kupper L, Morgenstern H. *Epidemiologic Research: Principles and Quantitative Methods.* Belmont, CA: Lifetime Learning Publications; 1982.

Muñoz A, Townsend T. Design and analytical issues in studies of infectious diseases. In: Wenzel RP. *Prevention and Control of Nosocomial Infections.* Baltimore, MD: Williams & Wilkins; 1997:215–230.

Ning L. Statistics in infection control studies. In: Wenzel RP. *Prevention and Control of Nosocomial Infections.* Baltimore, MD: Williams & Wilkins; 1997:231–240.

Reingold AL. Outbreak investigations—a perspective. *Emerg Infect Dis.* 1998;4:21–27.

Riegelman RK, Hirsch RP. *Studying a Study and Testing a Test: How to Read the Health Science Literature.* 3rd ed. Philadelphia, PA: Lippincott-Raven; 1996.

Schlesselman JJ. *Case-Control Studies: Design, Conduct, Analysis.* New York, NY: Oxford University Press, 1982.

Zar JH. *Biostatistical Analysis.* Englewood Cliffs, NJ: Prentice-Hall, Inc; 1981.

Resources

Epi Info was developed by the CDC in Atlanta, Georgia, in the 1970s to allow public health personnel to efficiently manage data collected on site during an outbreak investigation. Epi Info can be used to create data collection forms; store and analyze data; perform a variety of statistical calculations; and produce tables, graphs, and maps. Although Epi Info is a CDC trademark, the programs, documentation, and teaching materials are in the public domain and may be freely copied, distributed, and translated. Information, tutorials, and the Microsoft Windows version are available at http://www.cdc.gov/epiinfo/. A DOS version, including user manual, frequently asked questions, and tutorials, is still available at http://www.cdc.gov/epiinfo/Epi6/ei6.htm.

Principles of Epidemiology in Public Health Practice, 3rd ed, Course Number SS1000, is a training course that is available from the CDC. It is a print-based self-study course covering basic epidemiology principles, concepts, and procedures generally used in the surveillance and investigation of health-related events. It includes information on the applications of descriptive and analytic epidemiology and addresses how to calculate and interpret frequency measures (ratios, proportions, and rates) and measures of central tendency. This course may be accessed through the Public Health Training Network of the CDC at http://www2a.cdc.gov/PHTN/alpha.asp. The print text for the course is *Principles of Epidemiology in Public Health Practice: An Introduction to Applied Epidemiology and Biostatistics.* 3rd ed. Atlanta, GA: Centers for Disease Control and Prevention, Office of Workforce and Career Development; 2005. It can be downloaded free of charge at http://www2a.cdc.gov/TCEOnline/registration/detailpage.asp?res_id=1394.

Lane, D. National Science Foundation's division of undergraduate education Rice virtual lab in statistics. http://onlinestatbook.com/rvls.html. Contains an online statistics book, demonstrations, case studies and an analysis lab to assist the user with statistical calculations.

SISA (Simple Interactive Statistics Analysis). http://home.clara.net/sisa. Allows the user to do statistical analysis directly on the Internet.

STATS—STeve's Attempt to Teach Statistics. Children's Mercy Hospital and Clinics. http://www.childrens-mercy.org/stats/index.asp. This is an online resource offering basic and advanced statistics lessons with a Q&A option; answers are posted online by a statistician, in a personable manner.

Swinscow TDV. Revised by Campbell MJ. *Statistics at Square One.* 9th ed.

BMJ Publishing Group; 1997. http://www.bmj.com/collections/statsbk/index.dtl. Accessed March 14, 2008. Contains definitions and descriptions of basic statistics terms and formulas.

CHAPTER 11

The Role of the Laboratory in Outbreak Detection, Prevention, and Investigation

Kathleen Meehan Arias

> The microbiology laboratory's rapid and consistent identification of nosocomial pathogens is a keystone in the surveillance and control of hospital-acquired infections.
>
> —R. A. Weinstein, 1978[1]

INTRODUCTION

With their elusive epidemiology, infectious diseases present new threats and increasingly complex challenges for healthcare systems. Ecological changes, global warming, and the massive increases in movements of people and foodstuffs around the globe facilitate the dispersion of microbial pathogens. Emerging infections as well as increasing antimicrobial resistance in community- and hospital-acquired infections demand close monitoring and continuous revision of diagnosis, management and control strategies.[2(pg1)]

The clinical microbiology laboratory plays an essential role in the detection, prevention, and control of infectious diseases. Through the analysis of specimens for bacteria, viruses, fungi, and other pathogens, clinical microbiology laboratory personnel contribute to the diagnosis and treatment of infectious diseases. By actively participating in the infection surveillance, prevention, and control (ISPC) programs in healthcare facilities, they assist in the identification and prevention of HAI and outbreaks.[1,3–8] Through data collection and reporting, microbiology laboratories support infection surveillance programs at the local, national, and international levels.[9–12]

This chapter discusses the critical role that the clinical microbiology laboratory plays in outbreak detection, prevention, and investigation and specifically addresses how the laboratory participates in the following:

- ISPC programs
- Providing timely and accurate identification of microorganisms
- Detecting antimicrobial resistance
- Addressing challenges presented by emerging and reemerging infectious diseases
- Infection surveillance
- Identifying clusters and outbreaks

- Outbreak investigation and response
- Meeting reporting needs and requirements
- Public health activities
- Consultation and education
- Supporting employee and personnel health programs

INFECTION SURVEILLANCE, PREVENTION, AND CONTROL PROGRAMS

The clinical microbiology lab is an essential partner in a healthcare organization's ISPC.[1,3-8] ICPs use laboratory and clinical data to detect patients with HAI, determine the site of infection, and identify risk factors so that infection prevention measures can be implemented. Since most HAIs are initially detected through microbiology laboratory data, the clinical microbiology laboratory plays an essential role in preventing infections by providing these data.

The microbiology laboratory should identify a microbiologist who is interested in infection prevention and control and select that person to serve as its liaison to the ISPC program and its representative on the infection control committee. Active participation on the infection control committee provides opportunities for the clinical microbiologist to explain laboratory tests and practices to the committee members, inform the committee members about new developments in identifying microorganisms and detecting antimicrobial resistance, learn about the types and incidence of HAIs in the organization, discuss surveillance findings, understand the scope and role of the ISPC program, and identify microbiologic approaches that could be used to solve ISPC problems.

IDENTIFICATION OF MICROORGANISMS

The clinical microbiology laboratory is responsible for providing timely and accurate detection and identification of an ever-expanding variety of microorganisms.[3-5,11,13] Technological developments in the past two decades have greatly aided the recovery and identification of infectious agents.[3,5,11,13-20] However, the development of new and often costly microbiological testing methods challenges the clinical microbiology laboratory to identify and adopt those methods that are appropriate for the clinical setting and patient populations that it serves.[17]

Rapid Test Methods and Molecular Procedures for Detecting and Identifying Microorganisms

There are many diagnostic tests that can provide rapid (same-day) identification of microorganisms. Commercial biochemical and immunological tests, such as those that detect *Staphylococcus aureus* in positive blood cultures, and direct antigen screens for *Neisseria meningitidis, Streptococcus pneumoniae,* and group B streptococcus in cerebral spinal fluid, have long been used. The biotechnology boom of the 1990s provided new technology and molecular test methods for detecting, identifying, and characterizing microorganisms, including many agents that do not grow in culture media.[3,13–18] Examples of molecular tests for identifying microorganisms that frequently cause outbreaks in healthcare settings include the following[3,14,17,21–23]:

- PCR for identification of MRSA and varicella-zoster virus in clinical specimens

- PCR and transcription-mediated amplification (TMA) for detection of *Mycobacterium tuberculosis* in clinical specimens and cultures

- PCR for detection of *Bordetella pertussis* in nasopharyngeal secretions, norovirus in stool specimens, and influenza A virus in respiratory specimens

Molecular typing methods for characterizing microorganisms are discussed later in this chapter under "Outbreak Investigation."

Clinical microbiology laboratory personnel should work with clinicians and members of the infection prevention and control team to determine which microbiologic tests are appropriate for use.[3,17] Since the sensitivity and specificity of laboratory test methods differ, the clinical microbiologist should educate healthcare providers and ICP personnel on the use, advantages, and limitations of the various tests and the interpretation of test results.[14] For instance, pertussis (whooping cough) is characterized by nonspecific signs and symptoms that makes early and accurate diagnosis challenging. There are several laboratory methods for diagnosing or screening for pertussis, including culture, serology, direct fluorescent antibody stain, and PCR; however, these tests vary in sensitivity and specificity.[22,24–26] There are currently no standard protocols for pertussis PCR testing, and false-positive results and subsequent misdiagnoses have been documented with PCR.[24–26]

DETECTION OF ANTIMICROBIAL RESISTANCE

The laboratory plays a critical role in detecting and reporting antimicrobial-resistant organisms and resistance trends.[3,7] Antimicrobial resistance can be detected using a variety of methods, including traditional disc diffusion and broth dilution, automated systems, the E test, and molecular tests.[27] Molecular methods for detecting antimicrobial resistance are available for many organisms, including MRSA, VRE, *M. tuberculosis*, and extended spectrum beta-lactamase (ESBL) producing *E. coli* and *K. pneumoniae* as shown in Table 11–1.[14,17]

Each of these methods has advantages and disadvantages, and they differ in sensitivity. The clinical microbiologist should explain the methods used for determining antimicrobial resistance, and how to interpret the results, to clinicians and the infection prevention and control team.

The microbiology laboratory should provide cumulative antimicrobial susceptibility data (antibiograms) to clinicians and the infection control committee. When compiling an antibiogram, the laboratory should follow the guidelines published by the National Committee for Clinical Laboratory Standards (NCCLS) (now the Clinical and Laboratory Standards Institute).[28]

Table 11–1 Molecular Methods for Detecting Antimicrobial Resistance

Organism(s)	Antimicrobial Agent(s)	Gene	Detection Method
Staphylococci	Methicillin Oxacillin	$mecA$[a]	Standard DNA probe Branched-chain DNA probe; PCR
Enterococci	Vancomycin	$vanA, B, C, D$[b]	Standard DNA probe PCR
Enterobacteriaceae *Haemophilus influenzae*; *Neisseria gonorrhoeae*	Beta-lactams	bla_{TEM} and bla_{SHV}[c]	Standard probe PCR and RFLP PCR and sequencing
Enterobacteriaceae and gram-positive cocci	Quinolones	Point mutations in $gyrA, gyrB, parC,$ and $parE$	PCR and sequencing
Mycobacterium tuberculosis[d]	Rifampin Isoniazid Ethambutol Streptomycin	Point mutations in $rpoB$ Point mutations in $katG, inhA,$ and $ahpC$ Point mutations in $embB$; Point mutations in $rpsL$ and rrs	PCR and SSCP PCR and sequencing PCR and SSCP PCR and sequencing PCR and RFLP
Herpes viruses[e]	Acyclovir and related drugs Foscarnet	Mutations or deletions in the TK gene Point mutations in DNA polymerase gene	PCR and sequencing PCR and sequencing
HIV[f]	Nucleoside reverse transcriptase inhibitors; Protease inhibitors	Point mutations in RT gene Point mutations in PROT gene	PCR and sequencing PCR and LIPA PCR and sequencing

[a] $mecA$ encodes for the altered penicillin-binding protein PBP2a'; phenotypic methods may require 48 hours incubation or more to detect resistance and are less than 100% sensitive. Detection of $mecA$ has potential for clinical application in specific circumstances.

[b] Vancomycin resistance in enterococci may be related to one of four distinct resistance genotypes of which $vanA$ and $vanB$ are most important. Genotypic detection of resistance is useful in validation of phenotypic methods.

[c] The genetic basis of resistance to beta-lactam antibiotics is extremely complex. The bla_{TEM} and bla_{SHV} genes are the two most common sets of plasmid encoded beta-lactamases. The presence of either a bla_{TEM} or bla_{SHV} gene implies ampicillin resistance. Variants of the bla_{TEM} and bla_{SHV} genes (ESBL) may also encode for resistance to a range of third-generation cephalosporins and to monobactams.

[d] *M. tuberculosis* is very slow growing. Four weeks or more may be required to obtain phenotypic susceptibility test results. Detection of resistance genes in *M. tuberculosis* has potential for clinical application in the short term.

[e] There are no phenotypic methods sufficiently practical for routine clinical detection of resistance to antiviral agents. Genotypic methods represent a practical method for routine detection of antiviral resistance.

[f] Abbreviations not defined in text: RFLP, restriction fragment length polymorphism; SSCP, single-stranded conformational polymorphism; LIPA, line probe assay; TK, thymidine kinase; RT, reverse transcriptase; PROT, protease.

Source: Pfaller MA. Molecular approaches to diagnosing and managing infectious diseases: practicality and costs. *Emerg Infect Dis.* 2001;7:312–318. http://www.cdc.gov/ncidod/eid/vol7no2/pfaller.htm. Accessed May 29, 2008.

CHALLENGES PRESENTED BY EMERGING AND REEMERGING DISEASES AND BIOTERRORISM

In addition to providing timely and accurate identification of known pathogens in routine clinical specimens, clinical microbiology laboratory personnel must be able to recognize the occurrence of new diseases and the biological agents thought to be most likely used in a bioterrorist event.[29] Since the 1970s, over 35 new human pathogens have been identified, and many known pathogens have emerged or reemerged.[30–39] Examples of pathogenic microbes and infectious diseases recognized since 1973 are shown in Table 11–2,[34–39] and a list of microbes identified as potential biological terrorism agents is in Table 11–3.[40]

Table 11–2   Examples of Pathogenic Microbes and Infectious Diseases Recognized Since 1973

Year	Microbe	Type	Disease
1973	Rotavirus	Virus	Major cause of infantile diarrhea worldwide
1975	Parvovirus B19	Virus	Aplastic crisis in chronic hemolytic anemia
1976	*Cryptosporidium parvum*	Parasite	Acute and chronic diarrhea
1977	Ebola virus	Virus	Ebola hemorrhagic fever
1977	*Legionella pneumophila*	Bacteria	Legionnaires' disease
1977	Hantaan virus	Virus	Hemorrhagic fever with renal syndrome (HFRS)
1977	*Campylobacter jejuni*	Bacteria	Enteric pathogens distributed globally
1980	Human T-lymphotropic virus I (HTLV-1)	Virus	T-cell lymphoma-leukemia
1981	Toxin-producing strains of *Staphylococcus aureus*	Bacteria	Toxic shock syndrome (tampon use)
1982	*Escherichia coli* O157:H7	Bacteria	Hemorrhagic colitis; hemolytic uremic syndrome
1982	HTLV-II	Virus	Hairy cell leukemia
1982	*Borrelia burgdorferi*	Bacteria	Lyme disease
1983	Human immunodeficiency virus (HIV)	Virus	Acquired immunodeficiency syndrome (AIDS)
1983	*Helicobacter pylori*	Bacteria	Peptic ulcer disease
1985	*Enterocytozoon bieneusi*	Parasite	Persistent diarrhea
1986	*Cyclospora cayetanensis*	Parasite	Persistent diarrhea
1988	Human herpes-virus-6 (HHV-6)	Virus	Roseola subitum
1988	Hepatitis E	Virus	Enterically transmitted non-A, non-B hepatitis

continues

Table 11–2   *(Continued)*

Year	Microbe	Type	Disease
1989	*Ehrlichia chafeensis*	Bacteria	Human ehrlichiosis
1989	Hepatitis C	Virus	Parenterally transmitted non-A, non-B liver infection
1991	Guanarito virus	Virus	Venezuelan hemorrhagic fever
1991	*Encephalitozoon hellem*	Parasite	Conjunctivitis, disseminated disease
1991	New species of *Babesia*	Parasite	Atypical babesiosis
1992	*Vibrio cholerae* O139	Bacteria	New strain associated with epidemic cholera
1992	*Bartonella henselae*	Bacteria	Cat-scratch disease; bacillary angiomatosis
1993	Sin Nombre virus	Virus	Adult respiratory distress syndrome
1993	*Encephalitozoon cuniculi*	Parasite	Disseminated disease
1994	Sabia virus	Virus	Brazilian hemorrhagic fever
1994	Hendra virus	Virus	Acute respiratory syndrome
1995	HHV-8	Virus	Associated with Kaposi sarcoma in AIDS patients
1996	Australian bat lyssavirus	Virus	Encephalitis
1998	Nipah virus	Virus	Encephalitis
2001	Human metapneumovirus	Virus	Respiratory disease
2003	Sudden acute respiratory syndrome (SARS) coronavirus (SARS CoV)	Virus	Sudden acute respiratory syndrome

Source: Adapted from Lederberg J. Infectious disease as an evolutionary paradigm. *Emerg Infect Dis.* 1997;3(4): 417–423. http://www.cdc.gov/ncidod/EID/vol3no4/adobe/lederber.pdf. Accessed May 20, 2008.

Many of these new and reemerging pathogens, such as the noroviruses, *Legionella pneumophila*, the hepatitis B and C viruses, *Clostridium difficile*, multidrug-resistant *Mycobacterium tuberculosis*, influenza virus, and MRSA, have caused outbreaks in hospitals and other healthcare settings and are discussed elsewhere in this book. Outbreaks will continue to occur as new diseases emerge and known pathogens evolve. Human-to-human transmission of avian influenza A H5N1 has been documented, and a pandemic with this or another influenza virus is likely to occur.[33]

The ability of a previously unrecognized human pathogen to emerge and rapidly cause a pandemic was demonstrated by the outbreak of SARS that began in late 2002 in the People's Republic of China and spread to more than 25 countries on five continents before it was brought under control in July 2003.[32] Clinical, research, and public health laboratories played a critical role in diagnosing and investigating this new disease even before the etiologic agent was identified. To diagnose patients who fit the clinical picture of SARS, laboratories performed bacterial and viral cultures, direct microscopic examinations using Gram stain, electron microscopy, and a variety of serologic and molecular tests to detect a respiratory pathogen.[41] When all of these tests were negative, the likelihood that a suspected case patient had SARS increased, treatable infections could be ruled out, and isolation precautions and contact tracing could be done to interrupt further transmission. Clinical and public health laboratories collaborated to isolate the causative agent of SARS and in March 2003, a novel coronavirus, SARS CoV, was identified and specific diagnostic tests were quickly developed.[32]

When *Bacillus anthracis* spores were mailed in letters via the United States postal system in September 2001, some of the resulting anthrax cases were

Table 11–3　Critical Biological Agent Categories for Public Health Preparedness

Biological Agent(s)	*Disease*
Category A	
Variola major	Smallpox
Bacillus anthracis	Anthrax
Yersinia pestis	Plague
Clostridium botulinum (botulinum toxins)	Botulism
Francisella tularensis	Tularemia
Filoviruses and arenaviruses (e.g., Ebola virus, Lassa virus)	Viral hemorrhagic fevers
Category B	
Coxiella burnetii	Q fever
Brucella spp.	Brucellosis
Burkholderia mallei	Glanders
Burkholderia pseudomallei	Melioidosis
Alphaviruses (VEE, EEE, WEE[a])	Encephalitis
Rickettsia prowazekii	Typhus fever
Toxins (e.g., ricin, staphylococcal enterotoxin B)	Toxic syndromes
Chlamydia psittaci	Psittacosis
Food safety threats (e.g., *Salmonella* spp., *Escherichia* coli O157:H7)	
Water safety threats (e.g., *Vibrio cholerae*, *Cryptosporidium parvum*)	
Category C	
Emerging threat agents (e.g., Nipah virus, hantavirus)	

[a] Venezuelan equine (VEE), eastern equine (EEE), and western equine encephalomyelitis (WEE) viruses

Source: Rotz LD, Khan AS, Lillibridge SR, Ostroff SM, Hughes JM. Public health assessment of potential biological terrorism agents. *Emerg Infect Dis.* 2002;8(2):226. http://www.cdc.gov/ncidod/eid/vol8no2/pdf/01-0164.pdf. Accessed May 20, 2008.

detected and reported by clinical microbiology laboratory personnel.[42] Micro-biology laboratories nationwide were notified of the intentional release of an-thrax spores and conducted surveillance for cases. However, clinical microbiology laboratories in hospitals near the sites that received or processed the contaminated mail were inundated with requests to culture clinical speci-mens, environmental samples, and powder for *B. anthracis*. These laboratories had to work quickly to implement an emergency response to effectively meet the challenge. By working with clinicians and public health and law enforce-ment personnel, they played an integral role in detecting cases so that inter-ventions could be taken to prevent additional exposures.[42]

INFECTION SURVEILLANCE

The microbiologist and the ICP should collaborate to identify the informa-tion and data sources that are needed for HAI surveillance, such as results of cultures, acid-fast bacilli smears, antimicrobial susceptibility testing, tests for epidemiologically significant organisms, and serologic tests.[3,4,43] These results should be made readily available to the ICP and should be provided electroni-cally rather than on paper. When possible, the data should be downloaded into a retrievable database in the ISPC department. Although most clinical micro-biology laboratories have automated data collection, management, and report-ing processes, many ISPC programs do not effectively use computerized systems. ICPs can greatly benefit by working with lab personnel to identify how already available data and reports can be provided directly to the personal computer in their office and what special reports can readily be produced by a few keystrokes. Many clinical microbiology laboratory data management sys-tems can provide epidemiologic reports, such as trends of pathogens identified in a particular patient care unit or type of specimen, and antibiotic suscepti-bility patterns for specific isolates and antimicrobials. The ICP, clinical micro-biology laboratory, and infection control committee should collaborate to determine what reports are available, which would be beneficial for clinicians and the ISPC program, and how they could be provided.

The laboratory should maintain a list of epidemiologically important organ-isms and test results, such as positive tests for *Bordetella pertussis* and *Neisse-ria meningitidis* and sputum smears that contain acid-fast bacilli, that should be immediately reported to the patient care unit and the ICP. Clinical microbi-ology laboratory personnel play an important role in outbreak prevention by reporting epidemiologically significant findings such as a positive pertussis test result to the ICP and the patient's health care providers so that measures promptly can be taken to prevent disease transmission.

Infectious disease surveillance is not limited to the hospital inpatient set-ting. In the past few decades much health care has moved from inpatient to outpatient, home care, and long-term care settings.[7,44] Many hospital-based ICPs are responsible for the ISPC programs in hospital-affiliated ambulatory care services such as same-day surgery centers, dialysis units, and clinics. Since diagnostic testing for the patients in these settings may be performed through the hospital laboratory, clinical microbiology laboratory personnel play an important part in detecting healthcare- and community-associated infections and outbreaks in nonhospital healthcare settings.[7]

Identification of Clusters and Outbreaks

Because microbiology laboratory personnel are familiar with the microorganisms commonly isolated from the clinical specimens that they receive, they are frequently among the first to detect an unusual organism, cluster of infections, or unique antimicrobial resistance pattern.[3,4] By reporting these findings immediately to the ICP and healthcare providers, they serve as an early warning system for outbreaks and multidrug-resistant organisms. For instance, laboratory personnel in the author's hospital notified the ISPC department about the admission of two patients who had gastroenteritis and presumptive *Salmonella* species isolated from stool cultures. The ICP discovered that the patients were friends who had attended a wedding reception the day prior to developing diarrhea and who knew that a few more attendees were also ill. The ICP notified the health department about the two cases and the subsequent investigation uncovered a community *Salmonella* outbreak that was traced to contaminated meat.

OUTBREAK INVESTIGATION AND RESPONSE

The clinical microbiology laboratory plays an integral role in outbreak investigation by doing the following:

- Participating as an active member of the outbreak investigation team
- Providing and analyzing data on the usual or endemic occurrence of organisms[3,4]
- Identifying and storing microbial isolates that are involved in a suspected cluster or outbreak so they will be available for further testing[3,4]
- Conducting supplemental studies such as serologic tests for immunity or cultures of specimens from patients, personnel, or environmental sources[3,4,43]
- Identifying the need for selective or other specialized culture media to isolate the etiologic agent involved in the outbreak[4,27,46]
- Providing information and guidance on the type of specimens needed for special studies and the methods for collecting and transporting specimens[27,46]
- Identifying the appropriate typing tests that should be used to determine if the isolates are related and whether the tests can be done on site or the isolates should be sent to a reference laboratory[14–16]

The ICP should immediately notify the laboratory when an outbreak is suspected so that isolates of possible etiologic agents can be saved in case further analysis is needed. Since outbreaks result in much fear and confusion, the laboratory and infection control committee should prepare an action plan in advance to guide response activities should an outbreak occur.

Special Studies

Supplemental cultures or other diagnostic tests may be needed during the course of an outbreak investigation to identify (1) persons who are infected or colonized, (2) potential sources or reservoirs of an etiologic agent, (3) the likely modes of transmission of an organism, (4) if transmission is still occurring, or (5) the immune status of exposed persons. The laboratory should only perform supplemental studies under the direction of the outbreak investigation team and only after the team has determined why the studies are being done and how the results will be interpreted and used.

Microbiologic Cultures

"Microbiologic sampling of air, water, and inanimate surfaces (i.e., environmental sampling) is an expensive and time-consuming process that is complicated by many variables in protocol, analysis, and interpretation."[47(p88)] Supplemental cultures should only be done as part of an outbreak investigation when a person or environmental source is implicated epidemiologically in the transmission of an infectious agent.[45,47] Extensive microbiologic culturing of personnel or the environment is generally not warranted and should not be done unless a full-scale epidemiologic study is conducted and the study implicates a personnel carrier or an environmental source and the significant isolates are typed for evidence of strain relatedness.[45,47] Neither environmental nor personnel cultures should be done unless there is a plan for interpreting and acting on the results obtained.[47] Microorganisms isolated from personnel or environmental cultures should be linked to clinical isolates by molecular strain typing whenever possible.[47]

It is important to remember that a person, item, or surface is not necessarily the source of an outbreak just because it is culture positive; any of these may have become contaminated by the true source or by an infected or colonized person. As discussed in Chapter 8, if microbiologic culturing of personnel, patients, residents, or the environment is to be done, arrangements should be made with the laboratory, with personnel in areas where testing will occur, and with the organization's administrator, who must determine how to cover the expenses involved.

Culturing Personnel

If culturing of personnel is done, specimens should be labeled with a code, rather than with a person's name, to protect the identity of anyone who is culture positive for the organism being studied. Only one person should hold the key connecting the codes and names. Culturing creates substantial anxiety among personnel because they will be concerned that they may be involved in causing the outbreak. Therefore, the decision to culture personnel must be made carefully, based on epidemiologic evidence, and personnel should be assured that the results of testing will remain confidential—to allay concerns that they will be blamed for the outbreak if they are culture positive.

If an infectious agent has a carrier state or can cause colonization, it may sometimes be desirable to culture patients or residents to determine the extent of the spread in the population at risk. Culture surveys should not be done on persons or the environment unless the significant organisms that are isolated are typed or otherwise characterized to determine if they are related strains.

Specimen Collection

If special studies are to be done, the laboratory should identify the appropriate specimen needed to identify or isolate the etiologic agent and how to collect and transport it.[48] The lab should provide instructions to those who will collect the specimens and those who will be tested, as needed. The types of specimens, the sites to be cultured, and the collection methods will depend on the agent being studied. For instance, *S. aureus* is usually best detected in nares and wound cultures[49] and viruses and enteric bacilli causing gastroenteritis in stool samples or rectal swabs.[50,51]

Protocols for determining what types of specimens are needed and how to collect and transport specimens have been developed by the CDC,[50,51] the American Society for Microbiology,[46] and many state health departments.[52-55]

EPIDEMIOLOGIC TYPING METHODS

When used as an adjunct to an epidemiologic investigation, the characterization or typing of microorganisms is a powerful tool for investigating outbreaks of healthcare-associated infection.[14-17,45,47,56] There are many methods for typing microbial isolates.[3,15,16] Phenotypic techniques, which detect characteristics that are expressed by an organism, include biotyping, serotyping, antimicrobial susceptibility, bacteriophage and bacteriocin typing, PAGE, MLEE, and immuno-blotting.[3,16] Genotypic (or molecular) techniques, which examine an organism's genetic content, include plasmid analysis, REA, ribotyping, PFGE, and PCR.[3,15,16] Examples of genotypic methods for epidemiologic typing of microorganisms are shown in Table 11–4. Molecular typing can be used for a variety of purposes, including to demonstrate the occurrence of an outbreak,[56-58] the transmission of organisms from patient to patient[17,59,61] and between patients and health care providers,[59-61] and to identify likely environmental sources and reservoirs of microorganisms.[47,58]

The results of typing tests must be used and interpreted with caution to avoid erroneous conclusions.[14,16] As noted by van Belkum et al. "It must be emphasized that typing results can never stand alone and need to be interpreted in the context of all available epidemiological, clinical, and demographic data relating to the infectious disease under investigation."[16(p1)]

For instance, the finding that there is only one strain circulating in a healthcare setting does not necessarily mean that all of the infections are related—there may be only a single strain circulating in the community even though there may be many reservoirs or sources. Conversely, if multiple strains are found, there may still be an outbreak, as multiple strains have been found to cause an outbreak (based on epidemiologic evidence). For additional information on

Table 11–4   Genotypic Methods for Epidemiologic Typing of Microorganisms*

Method	Examples	Comments
Plasmid analysis	Staphylococci Enterobacteriaceae	Plasmids may be digested with restriction endonucleases Only useful when organisms carry plasmids
Restriction endonuclease analysis of chromosomal DNA with conventional electrophoresis	Enterococci *Staphylococcus aureus* *Clostridium difficile* *Candida* spp.	Large number of bands Difficult to interpret Not amenable to computer analysis
PFGE	Enterobacteriaceae Staphylococci Enterococci *Candida* spp.	Fewer bands Amenable to computer analysis Very broad application
Genome restriction fragment length polymorphism analysis: ribotyping, insertion sequence, probe finger-printing	Enterobacteriaceae Staphylococci *Pseudomonas aeruginosa* *Mycobacterium tuberculosis*; *Candida* spp.	Fewer bands Computer analysis Sequence-based profiles Automated
PCR-based methods: repetitive elements PCR spacer typing, selective amplification of genome restriction fragments, multilocus allelic sequence-based typing	Enterobacteriaceae *Acinetobacter* spp. Staphylococci *M. tuberculosis* Hepatitis C virus	Crude extracts and small amounts of DNA may suffice
Library probe genotypic hybridization schemes: multilocus probe dot-blot patterns, high-density oligonucleotide patterns	*Burkholderia cepacia* *S. aureus* *M. tuberculosis*	Unambiguous yes-no result Less discrimination than other methods Couple with DNA chip technology

* The table contains examples of available methods and applications and is not intended to be all-inclusive.

Source: Pfaller MA. Molecular approaches to diagnosing and managing infectious diseases: practicality and costs. *Emerg Infect Dis.* 2001;7:312–318. http://www.cdc.gov/ncidod/eid/vol7no2/pfaller.htm. Accessed May 29, 2008.

typing systems, the reader is referred to the guidelines by van Belkum et al.[16] and the review by Singh et al.[15]

REPORTING REQUIREMENTS

In the United States, every state has notifiable disease requirements mandating laboratories to report specific diseases and conditions to state and local health departments.[62,63] The diseases and conditions that laboratories must report to the state health department varies by state. State health departments subsequently transmit data to the CDC's National Notifiable Diseases Surveillance System (NNDSS). The list of nationally notifiable infectious diseases can be found in Chapter 2 (Exhibit 2–2) and on the CDC Web site (http://www.cdc.gov/ncphi/disss/nndss/phs/infdis.htm). Local, state, and national public health agencies use data collected at the local level to monitor trends and detect outbreaks so that prevention and control measures can be implemented. Public health reporting requirements and case definitions for notifiable diseases are discussed in Appendix B (Appendix B is available for download at this text's web site: http://www.jbpub.com/catalog/9780763757793/). The clinical microbiology laboratory should work with the ISPC program personnel to implement procedures that ensure the reporting of notifiable diseases.

As a result of pressure from legislators, regulators, health care payers, accreditation agencies, and others to reduce the occurrence of HAIs, data reporting requirements for infectious diseases and HAI-related information have increased significantly since 2000. In addition to notifiable diseases, many states require laboratories and/or health care facilities to report data on the incidence of specific organisms, such as MRSA, VRE, and *Clostridium difficile*, and on specific HAIs such as central line-associated bloodstream infections.[64–66] Because these mandates will increase as the Centers for Medicare and Medicaid Services (CMS) phases in its HAI reporting requirements,[67] the clinical microbiology lab and ISPC personnel should collaborate to keep up with the changing requirements and identify the most efficient methods for reporting these data.

ADDITIONAL PUBLIC HEALTH ACTIVITIES

Clinical microbiology laboratory personnel should subscribe to public health electronic communication networks such as the ProMED-mail (http://www.promedmail.org) and the CDC Clinician Updates (http://www.bt.cdc.gov/clinregistry) as discussed in Chapter 9. These networks support the early detection and response to outbreaks of common and unusual pathogens and the measurement of the effectiveness of public health interventions.

When applicable, clinical microbiology laboratories should serve as sentinel laboratories in the CDC's Laboratory Response Network (LRN). Information on sentinel laboratories and the LRN can be found on the CDC (http://www.bt.cdc.gov/lrn/biological.asp) and American Society for Microbiology (ASM) (http://www.asm.org/policy/index.asp?bid=6342) Web sites. The emergence and reemergence of infectious diseases, the demands of increasing regulatory requirements and economic constraints, and the occurrence of multistate and international food-borne outbreaks have served as an impetus for public health and clinical laboratories to "communicate, cooperate, and collaborate as never before to seek the common ground where knowledge and resources can be shared."[68(p9)]

EMERGENCY PREPAREDNESS

As demonstrated by SARS and the anthrax bioterrorist event in the United States, laboratories play a critical role in the response to natural and man-made outbreaks.[32,41,42] Education and training on emerging infectious diseases, emergency response, and likely bioterrorism agents (Table 11–3) should be provided to laboratory personnel who should be prepared for the influx of specimens that will occur during a widespread community, regional, or national outbreak; a pandemic; or a bioterrorist event.[29,69–72] The clinical microbiology laboratory should have an emergency preparedness plan that addresses bioterrorism, other infectious disease emergencies, and surge capacity.[29,69–72] The plan should include "event recognition, access to and interaction with the various LRN level laboratories, communication protocols, safety guidelines, training of personnel to ensure competence and awareness, packaging and shipment of infectious substances, and laboratory security."[69(p4)] It should be integrated into the hospital's institutional emergency preparedness plan and coordinated with local and state public health and emergency response agencies, the public health laboratory system, law enforcement agencies, and other stakeholders. The ASM provides a template that can be used for a clinical laboratory bioterrorism readiness plan.[71]

Emergency preparedness and bioterrorism information is available from the ASM,[71–72] CDC,[73] academic institutions,[74] professional organizations,[75] and state and local health departments.

EMPLOYEE (PERSONNEL) HEALTH

The clinical laboratory supports occupational health programs in health care settings by doing the following:

- Providing timely and accurate testing for routine preemployment screening, such as immunity for hepatitis B and varicella zoster virus (VZV)[76,77] and latent tuberculosis (TB) infection using a blood assay test for *Mycobacterium tuberculosis* (BAMT).[78] Accurate screening can prevent infections in personnel and subsequent outbreaks.[76]
- Assisting in the follow-up of personnel exposed to communicable diseases such as measles, chickenpox, and tuberculosis (Appendix C)
- Implementing safety practices in the laboratory to prevent exposure of personnel to infectious agents[27,46,69,77,79]

Laboratory personnel that handle clinical specimens, cultures, and infectious materials are at risk for exposure to human pathogens and laboratory-acquired infections.[77,80–82] Laboratory-acquired infections have been caused by a wide variety of bacteria, viruses, fungi, and parasites, and exposure has occurred through ingestion, inoculation, inhalation, and contamination of skin or mucous membranes.[77,80,81] Clinical microbiology laboratories should ensure that personnel are trained in, and use, safe work practices (such as safe sharps handling and no food or drink consumption in the laboratory), safety equipment (such as biological safety cabinets), and personnel protective equipment (such as gloves, masks, face shields, and lab coats).[80] Guidelines for safe work practices in the laboratory have been written by the CDC and NIH,[79] the NCCLS,[83] the WHO,[84] and others.[80]

QUALITY ASSURANCE AND PSEUDO-OUTBREAKS

Pseudo-outbreaks, or clusters of false infections, occur frequently in health care settings, as discussed in Chapter 6. Many pseudo-outbreaks are related to cross-contamination and technical errors in the laboratory. Pseudo-outbreaks have been traced to the introduction of new laboratory procedures[85] and equipment,[86,87] specimen cross-contamination due to faulty ventilation in the laboratory,[88] contaminated saline used as dilutent in processing specimens,[89,90] laboratory errors in processing respiratory specimens,[91] contaminated instruments,[92,93] and cross-contamination during processing specimens.[94] Pseudo-outbreaks may result in much time spent by those who are investigating the outbreak, and pseudo-infections may result in unnecessary treatment or prophylaxis of patients, residents, or staff and the loss of confidence in medical personnel and the laboratory. Laboratory personnel should ensure that good routine microbiological techniques are used at all times to reduce the risk of specimen and culture contamination and the occurrence of a pseudo-outbreak.

The reader is referred to Chapter 6 for additional information on pseudo-outbreaks related to the laboratory and measures to prevent them from occurring.

SUMMARY

The clinical microbiology laboratory plays a critical role in health care and public health by contributing to the diagnosis and treatment of infectious diseases, identifying antimicrobial resistance and epidemiologically important organisms, and detecting and responding to outbreaks. At the local level, the clinical microbiology laboratory provides information used to identify, treat, and prevent community- and health care-associated infections and forms the backbone of ISPC programs in health care facilities. At the national and international levels, the laboratory supports the public health infrastructure needed to rapidly detect, prevent, and contain the spread of infectious diseases.

Advances in clinical microbiology laboratory testing methodology and automation, molecular epidemiology, and information technology have enhanced the ability of the clinical microbiology laboratory to support ISPC programs at many levels. These advances place clinical microbiology laboratory personnel on the front line of efforts to identify, prevent, and control the spread of infectious agents in health care and community settings.

REFERENCES

1. Weinstein RA, Mallison GF. The role of the microbiology laboratory in surveillance and control of nosocomial infections. *Am J Clin Pathol.* 1978;69(2):130–136.

2. Struelens MJ, Van Elder J, and participants in the workshop. Introduction: progress towards meeting the challenges in clinical microbiology and infectious diseases. *Clin Micro Infect Dis.* 2005;11(Suppl. 1):1–2.

3. Pfaller MA, Herwaldt LA. The clinical microbiology laboratory and infection control: emerging pathogens, antimicrobial resistance, and new technology. *Clin Infect Dis.* 1997;25(4):858–870. http://www.journals.uchicago.edu/doi/pdf/10.1086/515557. Accessed May 6, 2008.

4. Emori G, Gaynes RP. An overview of nosocomial infections, including the role of the microbiology laboratory. *Clin Microbiol Rev.* 1993;6(4):428–442. http://cmr.asm.org/cgi/reprint/6/4/428?view=long&pmid=8269394. Accessed May 6, 2008.

5. Diekema DJ, Pfaller MA. Chapter 10. Infection control epidemiology and clinical microbiology. In: Murray PR, Baron EJ, Jorgensen JH, Landry ML, Pfaller MA. eds. *Manual of Clinical Microbiology*. 9th ed. Washington, DC: ASM Press. 2007.

6. Kolmos HJ. Interaction between the microbiology laboratory and clinician: what the microbiologist can provide. *J Hosp Infect*. 1999;43(Suppl:S)285–291.

7. Simor AE. The role of the laboratory in infection prevention and control programs in long-term care facilities for the elderly. *Infect Control Hosp Epidemiol*. 2001;22:459–463.

8. Boyce J. Hospital epidemiology in smaller hospitals. *Infect Control Hosp Epidemiol*. 1995; 16:600–606.

9. Dato V, Wagner MM, Fapohunda A. How outbreaks of infectious disease are detected: a review of surveillance systems and outbreaks. *Pub Health Rep*. 2004;119:464–471. http://www.public healthreports.org/userfiles/119_5/119464.pdf. Accessed May 16, 2008.

10. Weinberg J. Surveillance and control of infectious diseases at local, national and international levels. *Clin Microbiol Infect*. 2005;11(Suppl. 1):12–14. http://www.blackwell-synergy .com/doi/full/10.1111/j.1469-0691.2005.01083.x. Accessed May 16, 2008.

11. Canton R. Role of the microbiology laboratory in infectious disease surveillance, alert, and response. *Clin Micro Infect*. 2005;11(Suppl. 1):3–8. http://www.blackwell-synergy.com/doi/full/ 10.1111/j.1469-0691.2005.01081.x. Accessed May 16, 2008.

12. Panackal AA, M'ikanatha NM, Tsui FC, et al. Automatic electronic laboratory-based reporting of notifiable infectious diseases at a large health system. *Emerg Infect Dis*. 2002;8:685–691. http://www.cdc.gov/ncidod/EID/vol8no7/01-0493.htm. Accessed May 16, 2008.

13. Cockerill FR III, Smith TF. Response of the clinical microbiology laboratory to emerging (new) and reemerging infectious diseases. *J Clin Microbiol*. 2004;42:2359–2365. http://www.pubmed central.nih.gov/picrender.fcgi?artid=1390794&blobtype=pdf. Accessed May 7, 2008.

14. Speers DJ. Clinical applications of molecular biology for infectious diseases. *Clin Biochem Rev*. 2006;27:39–51. http://www.pubmedcentral.nih.gov/picrender.fcgi?artid=1390794&blobtype= pdf. Accessed May 7, 2008.

15. Singh A, Goering RV, Simjee S, Foley SL, Zervos MJ. Application of molecular techniques to the study of hospital infection. *Clin Microbiol Rev*. 2006;19(3):512–530. http://cmr.asm.org/ cgi/reprint/19/3/512. Accessed May 20, 2008.

16. van Belkum A, Tassios PT, Dojksoom L, et al for the European Society of Clinical Microbiology and Infectious Diseases (ESCMID) Study Group on Epidemiological Markers (ESGEM). Guidelines for the validation and application of typing methods for use in bacterial epidemiology. *Clin Microbiol Infect*. 2007;13(Suppl 3):1–46. http://www.blackwell-synergy.com/toc/ clm/13/s3. Accessed May 6, 2008.

17. Pfaller MA. Molecular approaches to diagnosing and managing infectious diseases: practicality and costs. *Emerg Infect Dis*. 2001;7:312–318. http://www.cdc.gov/ncidod/eid/vol7no2/pfaller .htm. Accessed May 29, 2008.

18. Weber S, Pfaller MA, Herwaldt LA. Role of molecular epidemiology in infection control. *Infect Dis Clin North Am*. 1997;11(2):257–278.

19. Espy MJ, Uhl JR, Sloan M, et al. Real-time PCR in clinical microbiology: applications for routine laboratory testing. *Clin Micro Rev*. 2006;19(1):165–256. http://cmr.asm.org/cgi/reprint/ 19/1/165. Accessed May 30, 2008.

20. Pfaller MA. Diagnosis and management of infectious diseases: molecular methods for the new millennium. *Clinical Laboratory News*. 2000;26:10–13.

21. Harbarth S, Masuet-Aumatell C, Schrenzel J, et al. Evaluation of rapid screening and preemptive contact isolation for detecting and controlling methicillin-resistant *Staphylococcus aureus* in critical care: an interventional cohort study. *Crit Care*. 2006;10:128. http://ccforum .com/content/10/2/128. Accessed May 29, 2008.

22. Sotir MJ, Cappozzo DL, Warshauer DM, et al. Evaluation of polymerase chain reaction and culture for diagnosis of pertussis in the control of a county-wide outbreak focused among adolescents and adults. *Clin Infect Dis*. 2007;44:1216–1219.

23. Centers for Disease Control and Prevention. Norovirus activity—United States, 2002. *MMWR*. 2003;52(03):41–45. http://www.cdc.gov/mmwr/preview/mmwrhtml/mm5203a1.htm. Accessed May 29, 2008.

24. Lievano FA, Reynolds MA, Waring AL, et al. Issues associated with and recommendations for using PCR to detect outbreaks of pertussis. *J Clin Micro.* 2002;40(8):2801–2805. http://jcm .asm.org/cgi/reprint/40/8/2801. Accessed May 28, 2008.

25. Fry NK, Tzivra O, Ting Li Y, et al. Laboratory diagnosis of pertussis infections: the role of PCR and serology. *J Med Microbiol.* 2004;53:519–525.

26. Outbreaks of respiratory illness mistakenly attributed to pertussis—New Hampshire, Massachusetts, and Tennessee, 2004–2006. *MMWR.* 2007;56(33):837–842. http://iier.isciii.es/ mmwr/preview/mmwrhtml/mm5633a1.htm. Accessed May 7, 2008.

27. Murray PR, Baron EJ, Jorgensen JH, Landry ML, Pfaller MA, eds. *Manual of Clinical Microbiology.* 9th ed. Washington, DC: ASM Press; 2007.

28. National Committee for Clinical Laboratory Standards (NCCLS). Analysis and presentation of cumulative antimicrobial susceptibility test data: approved standard. NCCLS document M39-A. Wayne, PA: NCCLS; 2002.

29. Kleitman WF, Ruoff KL. Bioterrorism: implications for the clinical microbiologist. *Clin Microbiol Rev.* 2001;14(2):364–381. http://cmr.asm.org/cgi/content/full/14/2/364. Accessed May 19, 2008.

30. Merrell DS, Falkow S. Frontal and stealth attack strategies in microbial pathogenesis. *Nature.* 2004;430:250–256.

31. Lederberg J, Shope R, Oaks S, eds. Emerging infections: microbial threats to health in the United States. Washington, DC: National Academy Press; 1992:36–41. http://www.nap.edu/ catalog.php?record_id=2008. Accessed April 21, 2008.

32. Peiris JSM, Guan Y. Confronting SARS: a view from Hong Kong. *Philos Trans R Soc Lond B Biol Sci.* 2004;29;359:1075–1079. http://www.pubmedcentral.nih.gov/articlerender.fcgi?artid= 1693390. Accessed May 18, 2008.

33. Yuen KY, Wong SSY. Human infection by avian influenza A H5N1. *Hong Kong Med J.* 2005;11(3)189–199. http://www.hkmj.org/article_pdfs/hkm0506p189.pdf. Accessed May 19, 2008.

34. Fauci AS, Touchette NA, Folkers GK. Emerging infectious diseases: a 10-year perspective from the National Institute of Allergy and Infectious Diseases. *Emerg Infect Dis.* 2005;11:519–524. http://www.cdc.gov/Ncidod/eid/vol11no04/04-1167.htm. Accessed May 29, 2008.

35. Lederberg J. Infectious disease as an evolutionary paradigm. *Emerg Infect Dis.* 1997;3(4):417–423. http://www.cdc.gov/ncidod/EID/vol3no4/adobe/lederber.pdf. Accessed May 20, 2008.

36. Smolinski MS, Hamburg MA, Lederberg J, eds. *Microbial Threats to Health: Emergence, Detection, and Response.* Washington, DC: National Academies Press; 2003:1. http://www .nap.edu/catalog.php?record_id=10636. Accessed April 21, 2008.

37. Fauci AS. Infectious diseases: considerations for the 21st century. *Clin Infect Dis.* 2001;32(5):675–685. http://www.journals.uchicago.edu/doi/pdf/10.1086/319235. Accessed September 27, 2008.

38. Mackenzie JS, Chua KB, Daniels PW, et al. Emerging viral diseases of southeast Asia and the western pacific. *Emerg Infect Dis.* 2001;7(Suppl.3):497–504. http://www.cdc.gov/ncidod/eid/ vol7no3_supp/pdf/mackenzie.pdf. Accessed May 20, 2008.

39. van den Hoogen BG, deJong JC, Groen J, et al. A newly discovered human pneumovirus isolated from young children with respiratory tract disease. *Nat Med.* 2001;7:719–724.

40. Rotz LD, Khan AS, Lillibridge SR, Ostroff SM, Hughes JM. Public health assessment of potential biological terrorism agents. *Emerg Infect Dis.* 2002;8(2):226. http://www.cdc.gov/ncidod/ eid/vol8no2/pdf/01-0164.pdf. Accessed May 20, 2008.

41. Health Canada. Epidemiology, clinical presentation and laboratory investigation of severe acute respiratory syndrome (SARS) in Canada, March 2003. *Can Comm Dis Report.* 2003;29:71–75. http://www.phac-aspc.gc.ca/publicat/ccdr-rmtc/03pdf/cdr2908.pdf. Accessed May 18, 2008.

42. Jenigan DB, Raghunathan PL, Bell BP, et al. Investigation of bioterrorism-related anthrax, United States, 2001: epidemiologic findings. *Emerg Infect Dis.* 2002;8:1019–1028. http://www .cdc.gov/ncidod/EID/vol8no10/02-0353.htm. Accessed May 29, 2008.

43. McGowan JE Jr, Metchock BG. Basic microbiology support for hospital epidemiology. *Infect Control Hosp Epidemiol.* 1996;17:298–303.

44. Jarvis WR. Infection control and changing health-care delivery systems. *Emerg Infect Dis.* 2001;7:171–173.

45. Beck-Sague C, Jarvis WR, Martone WJ. Outbreak investigations. *Infect Control Hosp Epidemiol.* 1997;18:138–145.

46. Garcia LS. *Clinical Microbiology Procedures Handbook.* 2nd ed. Washington, DC: ASM Press. 2004/2007.

47. Sehulster LM, Chinn RYW, Arduino MJ, et al. *Guidelines for Environmental Infection Control in Health-Care Facilities. Recommendations from CDC and the Healthcare Infection Control Practices Advisory Committee (HICPAC).* Chicago IL:American Society for Healthcare Engineering/American Hospital Association; 2004. http://www.cdc.gov/ncidod/dhqp/gl_environ infection.html. Accessed May 30, 2008.

48. Miller JM, Krisher K, Holmes HT. General principles of specimen collection and handling. In: Murray PR, Baron EJ, Jorgensen JH, Landry ML, Pfaller MA, eds. *Manual of Clinical Microbiology.* 9th ed. Washington, DC: ASM Press; 2007.

49. Wenzel RP, Reagan DR, Bertino JS, Baron EJ, Arias K. Methicillin-resistant *Staphylococcus aureus* outbreak: a consensus panel's definition and management guidelines. *Am J Infect Control.* 1998;26:102–110.

50. Centers for Disease Control and Prevention. Norwalk-like viruses. Public health consequences and outbreak management. *MMWR.* 2001;50(No.RR-9):1–17.

51. Centers for Disease Control and Prevention. Outbreak Response and Surveillance Team (ORST): foodborne disease surveillance and outbreak investigation toolkit. http://www.cdc .gov/foodborneoutbreaks/toolkit.htm. Accessed May 30, 2008.

52. Maryland Department of Health and Mental Hygiene. Guidelines for the epidemiological investigation of gastroenteritis outbreaks in long-term care facilities, 2001. http://www .cha.state.md.us/edcp/guidelines/ge96.html. Accessed May 30, 2008.

53. Maryland Department of Health and Mental Hygiene. Guidelines for the prevention and control of upper and lower acute respiratory illnesses (including influenza and pneumonia) in long-term care facilities, 2000. http://www.cha.state.md.us/edcp/guidelines/resp97.html. Accessed May 30, 2008.

54. Maryland Department of Health and Mental Hygiene. Guidelines for control of scabies in long-term Care Facilities. http://www.cha.state.md.us/edcp/guidelines/scabies96.html. Accessed May 30, 2008.

55. California Department of Health Services Division of Communicable Disease Control. Prevention and control of gastroenteritis in California long-term care facilities. 2000. http:// www.dhs.ca.gov/ps/dcdc/disb/pdf/PCofGE0900_ms.pdf. Accessed May 30, 2008.

56. Jarvis WR. Usefulness of molecular epidemiology for outbreak investigations. *Infect Control Hosp Epidemiol.* 1994;15:500–503.

57. Lopman BA, Gallimore C, Gray JJ, et al. Linking healthcare associated norovirus outbreaks: a molecular epidemiologic method for investigating transmission. *BMC Infect Dis.* 2006;6:108–118.

58. Ganeswire R, Thongi KL, Puthuchearly SD. Nosocomial outbreak of *Enterobacter gergoviae* bacteremia in a neonatal intensive care unit. *J Hosp Infect.* 2003;53:292–296.

59. Huang WL, Jou R, Yeh PF, Huang A, and the Outbreak Investigation Team. Laboratory investigation of a nosocomial transmission of tuberculosis at a district general hospital. *J Formos Med Assoc.* 2007;106:520–527.

60. Sheretz RJ, Reagan DR, Hampton KD, et al. A cloud adult: the *Staphylococcus aureus*-virus interaction revisited. *Ann Intern Med.* 1996;124:539–547.

61. Milisavljevic V, Wu F, Larson E, et al. Molecular epidemiology of *Serratia marcescens* outbreaks in two neonatal intensive care units. *Infect Control Hosp Epidemiol.* 2004;9:719–721.

62. Roush S, Birkhead G, Koo D, Cobb A, Fleming D. Mandatory reporting of diseases and conditions by health care professionals and laboratories. *JAMA.* 1999;282(2):164–170. http://jama .ama-assn.org/cgi/content/full/282/2/164. Accessed May 16, 2008.

63. Centers for Disease Control and Prevention. Mandatory reporting of infectious diseases by clinicians. *MMWR.* 1990;39(9):1–11,16–17. http://www.cdc.gov/mmwR/preview/mmwrhtml/ 00001665.htm. Accessed May 16, 2008.

64. Weinstein RA, Siegel JD, Brennan PJ. Infection-control report cards—securing patient safety. *N Engl J Med.* 2005;353(3):225–227.

65. McKibben L, Horan TC, Tokars JI, et al. Guidance on public reporting of healthcare-associated infections: recommendations of the Healthcare Infection Control Practices Advisory Committee. *Am J Infect Control.* 2005;33:217–226.

66. Lindenauer PK, Remus D, Roman S, et al. Public reporting and pay for performance in hospital quality improvement. *N Engl J Med.* 2007;356:486–496.

67. Department of Health and Human Services. Centers for Medicare & Medicaid Services. 42 CFR Parts 411, 412, 413, and 489. Medicare program; proposed changes to the hospital inpatient prospective payment systems and fiscal year 2008 rates. Proposed rule. http://www.cms .hhs.gov/AcuteInpatientPPS/downloads/CMS-1533-P.pdf. Accessed May 30, 2008.

68. Beebe JL. Public health and clinical laboratories: partners in the age of emerging infections. *Clin Micro Newsletter.* 2006;28(2):9–12.

69. Snyder JW. Role of the hospital-based microbiology laboratory in preparation for and response to a bioterrorism event. *J Clin Micro.* 2003;41:1–4. http://jcm.asm.org/cgi/content/full/41/1/1. Accessed May 31, 2008.

70. Shapiro DS. Surge capacity for response to bioterrorism in hospital clinical microbiology laboratories. *J Clin Microbiol.* 2003;41(12):5372–5376. http://www.pubmedcentral.nih.gov/article render.fcgi?artid=308964. Accessed May 31, 2008.

71. American Society for Microbiology. Sentinel laboratory guidelines for suspected agents of bioterrorism. Clinical laboratory bioterrorism readiness plan. Revised August, 2006. http://www.asm.org/ASM/files/LeftMarginHeaderList/DOWNLOADFILENAME/ 000000001206/BTtemplateRevised8-10-6.doc. Accessed May 30, 2008.

72. Snyder JW, Check W. *American Bioterrorism Threats to Our Future. The Role of the Clinical Microbiology Laboratory in Detection, Identification, and Confirmation of Biological Agents.* A report from the American Academy of Microbiology and the American College of Microbiology. 2001. http://www.asm.org/ASM/files/CCLIBRARYFILES/FILENAME/0000000672/bioterrorism-bw.pdf. Accessed May 31, 2008.

73. Centers for Disease Control and Prevention. *Emergency Preparedness and Response— Bioterrorism.* http://www.bt.cdc.gov/bioterrorism/. Accessed May 31, 2008.

74. Saint Louis University School of Public Health. Institute for Biosecurity. http://bioterrorism .slu.edu/bt/internet.htm. Accessed May 31, 2008.

75. Infectious Disease Society of America. *Biodefense Information and Resources.* http://www .idsociety.org/BT/ToC.htm. Accessed May 31, 2008.

76. Behrman A, Schmidt S, Crivaro A, Watson B. A cluster of primary varicella cases among healthcare workers with false-positive varicella virus titers. *Infect Control Hosp Epidemiol.* 2003;24:202–206. http://www.cdc.gov/mmwr/pdf/rr/rr5415.pdr. Accessed May 30, 2008.

77. Bolyard EA, Tablan OC, Willams WW, et al. *Guideline for Infection Control in Health Care Personnel, 1998.* http://www.cdc.gov/ncidod/dhqp/gl_hcpersonnel.html. Accessed May 30, 2008.

78. Guidelines for using the QuantiFERON®-TB gold test for detecting *Mycobacterium tuberculosis* infection, United States. *MMWR.* 2005;54(15):49–55.

79. Centers for Disease Control and Prevention and National Institutes of Health. *Biosafety in Microbiological and Biomedical Laboratories.* 5th ed. Washington, DC: United States Government Printing Office. 2007. http://www.cdc.gov/od/ohs/biosfty/bmbl5/bmbl5toc.htm. Accessed May 30, 2008.

80. Sewell DL. Laboratory-associated infections and biosafety. *Clin Microbiol Rev.* 1995;8(3):389–405. http://www.pubmedcentral.nih.gov/picrender.fcgi?artid=174631&blobtype=pdf. Accessed May 30, 2008.

81. Herwaldt BL. Laboratory-acquired parasitic infections from accidental exposures. *Clin Microbiol Rev.* 2001;14(4):659–688. http://cmr.highwire.org/cgi/content/full/14/4/659. Accessed May 30, 2008.

82. Yagupsky P, Baron EJ. Laboratory exposures to *Brucellae* and implications for bioterrorism. *Emerg Infect Dis.* 2005;11(8):1180–1184.

83. Clinical Laboratory Standards Institute. *Protection of Laboratory Workers from Occupationally Acquired Infections,* 2nd ed. Wayne, PA: Clinical Laboratory Standards Institute. 2005.

84. World Health Organization. *Laboratory Biosafety Manual.* 2nd ed. (revised). Interim guidelines. Geneva, Switzerland: World Health Organization. 2003. http://www.who.int/csr/resources/publications/biosafety/who_cds_csr_lyo_20034/en/. Accessed May 30, 2008.

85. Apisarnthanarak A, Kiratisin P, Thongphubeth K, Yuakyen C, Mundy LM. Pseudo-outbreak of *Acinetobacter lwoffii* infection in a tertiary care center in Thailand. *Infect Control Hosp Epidemiol.* 2007;28(5):637–639.

86. Diederen BM, Verhulst C, van't Veen A, van Keulen PH, Kluytmans JA. Pseudo-outbreak of hepatitis B virus infection associated with contamination of a semiautomatic cap remover. *Infect Control Hosp Epidemiol.* 2006;27(11):1258–1260.

87. Pearson ML, Pegues DA, Carson LA, et al. Cluster of *Enterobacter cloacae* pseudobacteremias associated with use of an agar slant blood culturing system. *J Clin Microbiol.* 1993;31:2599–2603.

88. Segal-Maurer S, Kreiswirth BN, Burns JM, et al. *Mycobacterium tuberculosis* specimen contamination revisited: the role of laboratory environmental control in a pseudo-outbreak. *Infect Control Hosp Epidemiol.* 1998;19:101–105.

89. Gravowitz EV, Keenholtz SL. A pseudoepidemic of *Alcaligenes xylosoxidans* attributable to contaminated saline. *Am J Infect Control.* 1998;26:146–148.

90. Forman W, Axelrod P, St John K, et al. Investigation of a pseudo-outbreak of orthopedic infections caused by *Pseudomonas aeruginosa. Infect Control Hosp Epidemiol.* 1994;15:652–657.

91. Sule O, Ludlam HA, Walker CW, Brown DFJ, Kauffman ME. A pseudo-outbreak of respiratory infection with *Acinetobacter* species. *Infect Control Hosp Epidemiol.* 1997;18:510–512.

92. Gravel-Topper D, Sample ML, Oxley C, Toye B, Woods DE, Garber GE. Three-year outbreak of pseudobacteremia with *Burkholderia cepacia* traced to a contaminated blood gas analyzer. *Infect Control Hosp Epidemiol.* 1996;17:737–740.

93. Bradley SF, Wilson KH, Rosloniec MA, Kauffman CA. Recurrent pseudobacteremias traced to a radiometric blood culture device. *Infect Control.* 1987;8:281–283.

94. Budnick LD, Moll ME, Hull HF, Mann JM, Kendal AP. A pseudo-outbreak of influenza A associated with use of laboratory stock strain. *Am J Public Health.* 1984;76:607–609.

RESOURCES

Print

Garcia LS. 2007 Update: *Clinical Microbiology Procedures Handbook.* 2nd ed. Washington, DC: ASM Press; 2007.

Murray PR, Baron EJ, Jorgensen JH, Landry ML, Pfaller MA, eds. *Manual of Clinical Microbiology.* 9th ed. Washington, DC: ASM Press; 2007.

National Committee for Clinical Laboratory Standards (NCCLS). Analysis and presentation of cumulative antimicrobial susceptibility test data: approved standard. NCCLS document M39-A. Wayne, PA: NCCLS; 2002.

van Belkum A, Tassios PT, Dojksoom L, et al., for the European Society of Clinical Microbiology and Infectious Diseases (ESCMID) Study Group on Epidemiological Markers (ESGEM). Guidelines for the validation and application of typing methods for use in bacterial epidemiology. *Clin Microbiol Infect.* 2007;13(Suppl 3):1–46. http://www.blackwell-synergy.com/toc/clm/13/s3. Accessed May 6, 2008.

Online

CDC Biosafety in the Laboratory Training Module. http://www.cdc.gov/od/ohs/pdffiles/Module%202%20-%20Biosafety.pdf. Accessed May 30, 2008.

CDC Biosecurity in the Laboratory Training Module. http://www.cdc.gov/od/ohs/biosfty/biosfty.htm.

CDC Seasonal Flu Web site: Clinical Description and Lab Diagnosis of Influenza. http://www.cdc.gov/flu/professionals/diagnosis/index.htm. Accessed May 31, 2008.

CDC Manual for the Surveillance of Vaccine-Preventable Diseases. 3rd ed. 2002. Contains information on available diagnostic test methods and specimen collection methods for a variety of vaccine-preventable diseases. http://www.cdc.gov/vaccines/pubs/surv-manual/default.htm. Accessed May 31, 2008.

Photo Gallery of Bacterial Pathogens. http://www.geocities.com/CapeCanaveral/3504/gallery.htm. Accessed May 31, 2008.

Procedure Manuals Online

Some commercial laboratories, public health agencies, and other organizations have clinical microbiology laboratory manuals online. An example is the *Online Microbiology Lab Manual* of the Mount Sinai Hospital in Toronto, Canada. http://microbiology.mtsinai.on.ca/manual/default .asp#general. Accessed May 31, 2008.

CHAPTER 12

Collecting, Organizing, and Displaying Epidemiologic Data

Kathleen Meehan Arias

> Excellence in statistical graphics consists of complex ideas communicated with clarity, precision, and efficiency.
>
> —Edward R. Tufte[1(p13)]

INTRODUCTION

Surveillance is an integral part of any healthcare organization's infection prevention and control program. Because surveillance involves the ongoing collection, analysis, interpretation, and dissemination of large amounts of data, ICP personnel should be familiar with the tools and methods used to process this data and communicate their findings to others. The purpose of this chapter is to discuss practical tools that can be used to collect, organize, and display epidemiologic data, including:

- Forms and databases to collect and organize data
- Tables, graphs, and charts to organize and display data
- Computers to manage data

COLLECTING AND ORGANIZING EPIDEMIOLOGIC DATA

Using Forms and Databases

To detect an outbreak or a cluster of events, data must be compared over time; therefore, the data must be collected accurately and consistently and then collated. This can be accomplished by creating data collection forms and simple databases tailored to fit individual needs, as discussed in Chapter 2. Forms and databases should be used for routine surveillance activities, special studies, and outbreak investigations. These forms and databases should be carefully designed to include only those data points that are likely to be used in the final analysis so that the user does not waste valuable time and resources collecting unnecessary information.

One of the most common methods used to store and collate epidemiologic data is a rectangular database that consists of rows and columns. Each row contains information on one individual, and each column contains information on one characteristic or variable. The first two columns usually contain the case's name or initials and a medical record number or other unique identifier since two cases may have the same name. The size of the database depends on the number of individuals (or cases) and variables being studied (e.g., age, sex, location, surgery, procedures, symptoms, medications, food eaten, and other exposures).

The Line List

One of the initial steps in investigating a possible outbreak or a cluster of events is the creation of a rectangular database known as a line list. Whether created by hand or on a computer, each row in a line list represents a case, usually a person with a disease or an adverse outcome, and each column contains information on variables relevant to the event being studied. A line list allows data to be visually inspected to see if any one factor stands out. When conducting an outbreak investigation, a data collection form should be created and used for recording information on each case. This form may be paper or electronic. Using a form allows information to be collected consistently and efficiently. The information on the data collection form is then transferred to the line list for inspection. Examples of a data collection form and its corresponding line list are shown in Exhibits 12–1 and 12–2, respectively. Information on creating line lists and data collection forms can be found in Chapter 2.

Using Computers

Hospitals and other healthcare facilities have various computer systems for managing client information such as demographics, billing, diagnostic test results, and treatment provided. These systems should be used whenever pos-

---

Exhibit 12–1   Data Collection Form

Necrotizing Enterocolitis (NEC) Surveillance

Name _____   Unit # _____

DOB _____   Weight _____

Gestation _____   APGAR _____

NEC	Confirmatory test(s)	Hemorrhagic gastroenteritis (if not NEC)	Date onset	Outcome
Yes No	___ Clinical ___ Histopathologic ___ Roentgenographic	Yes No		Resolved Fatal

C. difficile		
Pos	Neg	Not done

Rotavirus		
Pos	Neg	Not done

Culture data for the week prior to NEC

Date	Source	Organism(s) isolated

Procedures, treatment, etc., prior to NEC

Transfusions	Yes	No
PDA diagnosed	Yes	No
Type feeding	Breastmilk	Formula

Medications

Indocin	Yes	No
Theophylline	Yes	No
Furosemide	Yes	No

Feeding (in the five days prior to NEC)

Date	Feeding	cc/kg/day

DOB = date of birth; PDA = patent ductus arteriosis

Source: Author.

sible to access data needed for surveillance (e.g., name, age, sex, unit/ward, admission and discharge dates, diagnosis, diagnostic test results, and medications given). Some microbiology laboratories use programs that can provide epidemiologic reports, such as the names or numbers of patients on a specific nursing unit from whom a particular organism was isolated over a specified period of time. Some programs can provide lists of names and locations of individuals for whom isolation precautions were ordered or lists of patients or residents and their admission diagnoses. These pieces of information can be used to identify clusters of infection or colonization; persons admitted with infections that can be transmitted to others, such as tuberculosis; or patients readmitted with infections that were acquired from a previous hospitalization, such as surgical site infections.

Exhibit 12–2   Patients with Necrotizing Enterocolitis (NEC)

Name	Medical Record	DOB	Weight	Apgar	Gestation (wks)	C. difficile		Rotavirus		Other infectious agent	Transfusion		PDA		Type feeding		Indocin		Theoph.		Furosemide	
						y	n	y	n		y	n	y	n	b	f	y	n	y	n	y	n

NOTE: DOB = date of birth; PDA = patent ductus arteriosis; type feeding: b = breastmilk, f = formula; theoph. = theophylline; y = yes; n = no.

The various computer programs and systems used in an institution are frequently incompatible and may not share data over a network. This often hinders the seamless flow of data and exchange of information between departments. Infection prevention and control personnel should discuss their data management needs with personnel who are familiar with the information systems in their facility. This will help to identify the following:

- Reports generated for other departments that could also be useful for infection surveillance, such as lists of admission diagnoses or surgical procedures
- Reports that can be produced specifically for the infection control or quality management departments (such as positive microbiology culture reports, positive and negative wound culture reports, viral hepatitis serology results, and *Clostridium difficile* toxin results)
- Mainframe systems containing patient or resident data and how to obtain access to that data or have it downloaded to a readily retrievable database such as Microsoft Excel
- Programs that connect to medical literature databases and the Internet, and how to obtain access
- Information on how to obtain access to a personal computer (PC) if one is not readily available

Infection control and quality management personnel in many healthcare settings in the United States use a PC. Some have found portable notebook or palm computers to be a valuable tool for collecting and storing epidemiologic data as these computers allow the user to enter data while making rounds anywhere in a facility, thus decreasing the need for paper forms. Although a PC allows large amounts of information to be processed quickly, it is important to keep in mind that it is only a tool. The user, not the computer, should determine how to manage the data. In many cases, surveillance data can be managed easily by using paper forms to collect data, and spreadsheets or simple databases to store, sort, and report it. There are many word-processing, spreadsheet, statistics, database, graphics, and commercial infection surveillance software programs from which to choose. To avoid costly mistakes, it is important to identify the needs of the healthcare organization and setting before purchasing software.[2]

Refer to Chapter 9 for more information on the use of technology in infection prevention and control programs and outbreak investigation.

DISPLAYING EPIDEMIOLOGIC DATA

Using Tables, Graphs, and Charts

Tables, graphs, and charts can be used to organize, summarize, and visually display epidemiologic data. While computers have certainly made it easier to prepare these visual displays, it is still necessary to understand their proper design and function in order to use them appropriately and effectively. This section defines and describes the features of tables, graphs, and charts; demonstrates how to correctly construct a table, graph, or chart; and explains when to use each of these tools.

Once data has been collected and checked for accuracy and completeness, it should be collated and analyzed to identify the frequency of occurrence of disease and any patterns, trends, and relationships. The findings must then be communicated to others. Although line lists and other databases are indispensable tools for collating and examining raw data, they usually contain too much information to be useful for presenting it to others. Therefore, tables, graphs, and charts are usually used to illustrate data.

Tables

A table is a display of data that is arranged in rows and columns. In healthcare epidemiology, tables are frequently used to present quantitative data, such as the rates of infection on patient care units. The information in a table is often used to prepare a graph or chart. Figure 12–1 shows the features of a properly constructed table used to present epidemiologic data. The first column shows the classes into which the data are grouped (here it is age group in years) and the second column lists the frequencies of events in each class (here it is the number of cases of TB).

Each table should be self-explanatory (i.e., it should contain all of the information needed for the reader to understand what is being presented) and should contain the following features[2(p207)]:

- A clear title that describes the data presented: what, where, and when. The title is generally placed at the top of the table. When showing more than one table, each title should be preceded with a table number (e.g., Table 1, Table 2).
- A label for each row and column. The units of measurement should be included (e.g., age in years; percent; rate per 1000 device-days; number of cases; number of records reviewed; number of incidents).

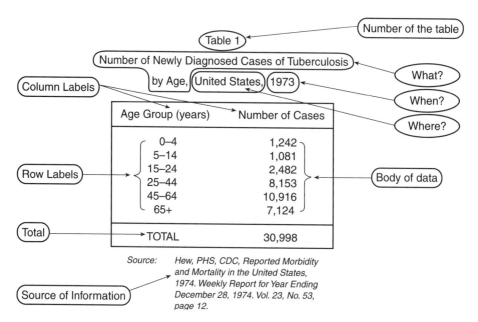

Figure 12–1 Features of a Properly Constructed Table

Source: Reprinted from Homestudy Course 3030-G: Principles of Epidemiology, Manual 4, Methods for Organizing Epidemiologic Data, pg 3, 1977. Centers for Disease Control and Prevention.

- Totals for rows and columns, as appropriate
- Footnotes to explain any abbreviations, codes, or explanations (e.g., SSI = surgical site infection; percentages do not add up to 100% due to rounding) or any exclusions (e.g., three patients excluded because charts not available).

The one-variable table. The most basic table shows data distributed by one variable, as shown in Figure 12–1. In this type of table, known as a simple frequency distribution, the first column shows the categories of the data being displayed, and the second column lists the number, or frequency, of persons or events in each category. Additional columns can be added to show the numbers of the population at risk and the incidence rates in each category. Data such as this can be used to identify potential problems and to target areas for improvement.

For example, Table 12–1 displays a simple frequency distribution in which the category (column 1) is the residential units in the Greentree Nursing Home and the variable, or event, being studied (column 2) is the number of residents who sustained a fall. Column 3 displays the resident-days for the population at risk in each unit, and column 4 shows the incidence rate in each unit. The data displayed in Table 12–1 suggests a possible problem on 1 East, where the incidence rate of 17.5 falls per 1000 resident-days is considerably higher than any other unit. An investigation of the resident population in each unit shows that 1 East is a unit for residents with Alzheimer's disease and other dementias that may put this population at higher risk for falls than the

Table 12–1   Incidence of Resident Falls, by Unit, June 2008, Greentree Nursing Home

Unit	No. Residents Experiencing a Fall	No. Resident-Days	Fall Rate (No. Falls per 1000 Resident-Days)
1 East	6	342	17.5
1 West	1	465	2.2
1 North	2	644	3.1
2 East	3	450	6.7
2 West	2	330	6.1
2 North	3	620	4.8
Total	17	2851	6.0

Source: Author.

residents of the other units. This information could possibly be used to target 1 East for a falls risk-reduction program.

Two- and three-variable tables. Data can also be cross-tabulated to show numbers distributed by a second or third variable. Table 12–2 shows the same data as in Table 12–1 except that it is cross-tabulated by a second variable, age. The data in Table 12–2 illustrates that the incidence of falls in those over 70 years of age is three times greater (7.5 versus 2.3) than the incidence of falls in those equal to or less than 70 years of age. This information could be used to focus efforts on reducing the risk of falls for those residents over 70 years of age.

The data in Table 12–2 could also be shown distributed by a third variable, such as sex. The maximum number of variables that should be used in a table

Table 12–2   Incidence of Resident Falls, by Unit and Age, June 2008, Greentree Nursing Home

Unit	≤ 70 years			> 70 years		
	No. residents experiencing a fall	No. resident-days	Rate (No. falls per 1000 resident-days)	No. residents experiencing a fall	No. resident-days	Rate (No. falls per 1000 resident-days
1 East	1	54	18.5	5	288	17.4
1 West	0	87	0	1	378	2.6
1 North	0	343	0	2	301	6.6
2 East	1	150	6.7	1	300	6.7
2 West	0	112	0	2	218	9.2
2 North	0	117	0	3	503	6.0
Total	2	863	2.3	15	1988	7.5

Source: Author.

is three, so that it does not appear too busy.[2(p210)] It is better to use several small tables than to try to compress data into one large table.

The two-by-two table. This type of table is used to study the association between two variables. In an outbreak investigation the two-by-two table is used to study the association between an exposure to a risk factor and the presence or absence of a disease. It is called a "two-by-two" table because it contains two variables that are cross-tabulated into two categories. Exhibit 12–3 is an illustration of the usual format of a two-by-two table. The use of these tables is explained in Chapter 10.

Although tables are excellent tools for showing quantitative data, they are generally not useful for identifying trends and showing comparisons. Graphs and charts are better suited for this purpose. Graphs and charts are frequently used to display the data that is organized in tables. Many computer programs, especially spreadsheet programs, allow the user to generate graphs and charts from the data in tables without having to reenter the data.

Graphs

A graph is a method used for visually displaying quantitative data. The types of graphs explained here are arithmetic-scale line graphs and histograms. Both of these graphs are rectangular coordinate graphs that consist of two lines, one horizontal and one vertical, that intersect at a right angle. The horizontal line is known as the x-axis and the vertical line is known as the y-axis.

Arithmetic-scale line graphs. In healthcare epidemiology, the arithmetic-scale line graph is commonly used to show trends, patterns, or differences over time, as shown in Figure 12–2. Time is shown on the x-axis, and the frequency of the event monitored, such as rate, percent, or numbers of cases, is shown on the y-axis. An arithmetic-scale line graph has equal intervals (tick marks) along each axis. This type of graph can be used to show one series of data or to compare several series, such as in Figure 12–2. Each series of data is plotted as a line. An arithmetic-scale line graph should be used when illustrating trends in numbers or rates over time.[2(p227)]

Histograms. A histogram is used to graph a frequency distribution of a set of continuous data (i.e., the number of times an event occurs in each interval).[2(p236)] A continuous data set consists of a series of measurements for which there are an infinite number of possible values between the lowest value and the high-

---

Exhibit 12–3   General Format for a Two-by-Two Table

	Disease	*No Disease*	*Total*
Exposed	a	b	a + b
Unexposed	c	d	c + d
Total	a + c	b + d	a + b + c + d

Source: Author.

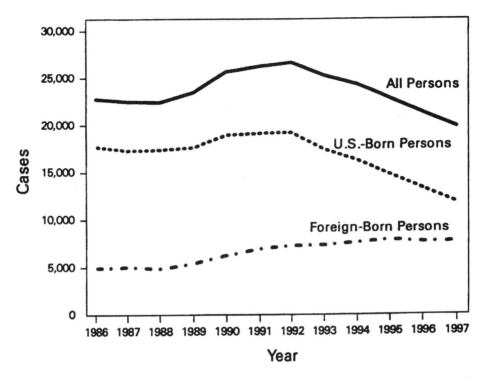

Figure 12–2 Number of Persons with Reported Cases of Tuberculosis, by Country of Birth—United States, 1986–1997

Source: CDC. Tuberculosis morbidity—United States, 1997. *MMWR*. 1998;47(13):255. http://www.cdc.gov/mmwr/preview/mmwrhtml/00051957.htm

est value in the set (such as time, weight, age, volume, or concentration). When plotted on a histogram, the data should appear as adjoining columns with the height of each column being proportional to the frequency of events in that interval (Figure 12–3). A histogram should be used to display the number of cases (not rates) over time.

When conducting an outbreak investigation, one of the initial steps is to create an epidemic curve. The epidemic curve is actually a histogram that shows the number of cases of disease in an outbreak on the y-axis and the time of onset on the x-axis. The time interval on the x-axis should be appropriate for the disease or event being depicted. The interval may be hours for diseases with a short incubation period, such as staphylococcal food poisoning, or weeks for those with a long incubation period, such as hepatitis A. When drawing an epidemic curve, the columns may be shown as stacks of squares, with each square representing one case, as shown in Figure 12–3, although many computer programs will not construct this type of graph. It is also perfectly acceptable to omit the horizontal lines between each of the cases, as shown in Figure 12–4.

The following guidelines should be used when constructing a graph:

- The title should clearly describe the data being presented: what, where, and when. The title can be placed at the top or bottom of the graph.

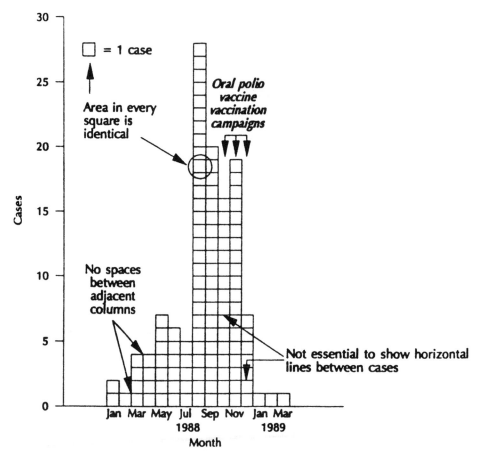

Figure 12–3 Reported Cases of Paralytic Poliomyelitis by Month of Occurrence

Source: CDC. *Principles of Epidemiology: An Introduction to Applied Epidemiology and Biostatistics.* 2nd ed. Atlanta, GA: CDC; 1992:266.

- The graph should be kept simple—it will be easier to read and will present the data more effectively.
- The independent variable (the method of classification), such as time, should be plotted on the *x*-axis (horizontal).
- The dependent variable should be plotted on the *y*-axis (vertical). This variable is usually a measure of frequency, such as the number of incidents, rate of disease, or number of cases.
- When plotting more than one variable, each should be clearly differentiated by using a legend or key. If black-and-white copies of the report are likely to be made, the lines or the areas representing the different variables on a graph should be made sufficiently dissimilar so that the reader can tell them apart. For example, lines should be solid, dotted, and so on, as shown in Figure 12–2, and columns should be solid, shaded, hatched, and so on, as shown in Figure 12–4.
- The *x*- and *y*-axes should be labeled with the appropriate units of measurement.

- Each graph should be self-explanatory and should contain all of the information needed for the reader to understand what is being presented.
- The *y*-axis should begin with 0. The largest value to appear on the *y*-axis is selected by identifying the largest value in the set and rounding up to a slightly higher number. For instance, in Figure 12–2, the cases are shown in intervals of 5000, and the highest value in the set of numbers plotted on the graph is slightly more than 25,000; therefore, 30,000 was chosen as the highest value in the range shown on the *y*-axis.
- The date of preparation should be noted because the data may change over time. For instance, when an arithmetic-scale line graph is used to display surgical site infection rates, the data may change as new cases are reported, and when drawing a histogram for an epidemic curve, the data may change as new cases are identified during the course of an outbreak investigation.
- The source of the data should be placed in a footnote, especially if the data are not original.

Charts

The three types of charts used in healthcare epidemiology are bar charts, pie charts, and maps (geographic coordinate charts).

Bar charts. Figure 12–5 shows the components of a bar chart.

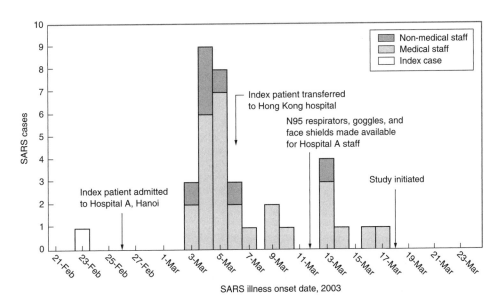

Figure 12–4 Epidemic Curve (Histogram) of the SARS Outbreak Among Hospital A Staff, Hanoi, 2003

Source: Reynolds et al. Factors associated with nosocomial SARS-CoV transmission among healthcare workers in Hanoi, Vietnam, 2003. *BMC Public Health.* 2006;6:207. http://www.biomedcentral.com/1471-2458/6/207. Accessed September 28, 2008.

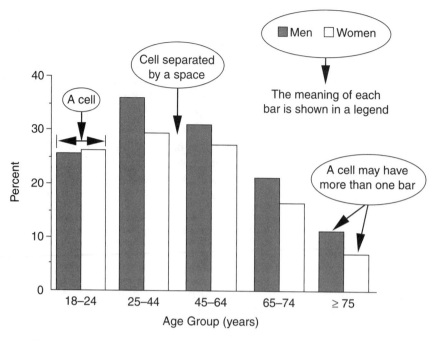

Figure 12–5 Example of a Vertical Bar Chart with Annotation

Bar charts can be used to show frequency distributions of a set of discrete data, as in Figure 12–6 (a simple bar chart), or to compare magnitudes of several sets of data, as in Figure 12–7 (a grouped bar chart). In these charts, each category of a variable (i.e., set of data) is represented by a bar, which may be displayed either vertically, as in Figures 12–6 and 12–7, or horizontally, as in Figure 12–8. The height or length of the bar is proportional to the values in

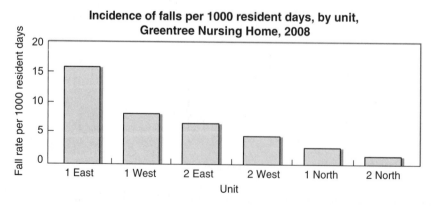

Figure 12–6 Frequency Distribution Shown as a Bar Chart: Incidence of Falls per 1000 Resident-Days, by Unit, Greentree Nursing Home, 2008

Source: Author.

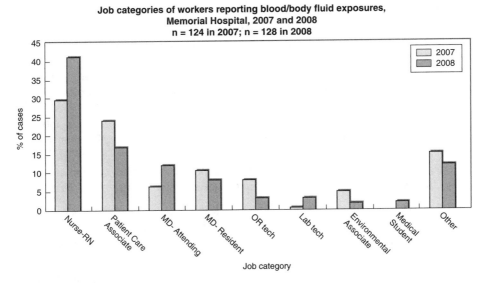

Figure 12–7 Grouped Bar Chart Showing Comparison of Two Sets of Data. Job Categories of Workers Reporting Blood/Body Fluid Exposures, Memorial Hospital, 2007 and 2008

Source: Author.

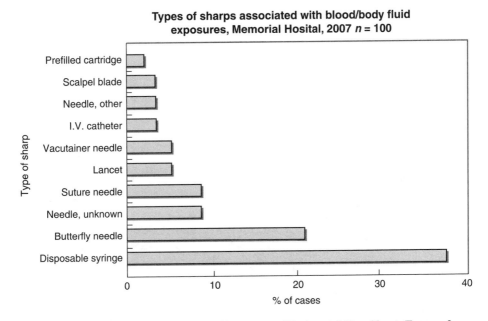

Figure 12–8 Frequency Distribution Shown as a Horizontal Bar Chart: Types of Sharps Associated with Blood/Body Fluid Exposures, Memorial Hospital, 2007

Source: Author.

that category. A stacked bar chart can also be used to display several sets of data, as in Figure 12–9, which displays the same data as that in Figure 12–7. Note that the grouped bar chart is more effective for comparing the numbers in the two years displayed in Figures 12–7 and 12–9.

Vertical bar charts (Figures 12–6 and 12–7) differ from histograms (Figures 12–3 and 12–4) in that each bar or cell in a vertical bar chart is separated by a space, whereas in a histogram the bars are adjoining. A bar chart is used to display information that is discrete and noncontinuous, such as sex, race, job category or location, or that is shown as being discrete and noncontinuous, such as age groups, as shown in Figure 12–5. By contrast, a histogram is used to display the frequency distribution of a set of continuous data (such as time or age).

The following guidelines should be used when constructing a bar chart:

- The title should clearly describe the data presented: what, where, and when. In an epidemiological report, the title is placed at the top of the chart.
- When creating a chart that has more than one bar in a cell, each bar should be clearly differentiated by using a legend or key as in Figure 12–7.
- The categories in a stacked bar chart should be clearly differentiated by using a legend or key, as in Figure 12–9. If black-and-white copies of the report are likely to be made, the areas representing each bar or each component should have clearly discernible shades or patterns.
- When possible, the categories that define the bars should be positioned in such a way that the length or height of the bars is in ascending or descending order.

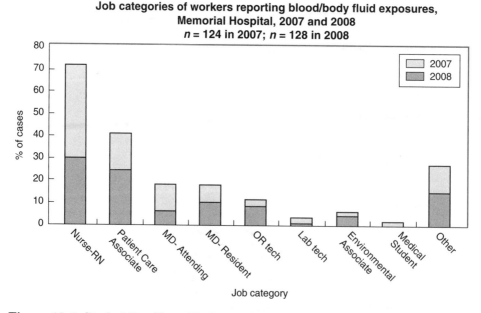

Figure 12–9 Stacked Bar Chart Displaying Two Sets of Data. Job Categories of Workers Reporting Blood/Body Fluid Exposures, Memorial Hospital, 2007 and 2008

Source: Author.

- All of the bars should be the same width.
- The length or height of each bar should be proportional to the values in each category.
- There should be a space between each bar or each cell (group of bars).
- The *x*- and *y*-axes should be labeled.
- As in a table or a graph, a bar chart should be self-explanatory and should contain all of the information needed for the reader to understand what is being presented.
- The source of the data should be placed in a footnote, especially if the data are not original.

Pie charts. Pie charts are used for showing the component parts of a set of data, as in Figure 12–10. Each slice of the pie represents a proportion of the whole. The following guidelines should be used when constructing a pie chart:

- The title should clearly describe the data presented: what, where and when. The title may be placed at the top or the bottom of the chart.

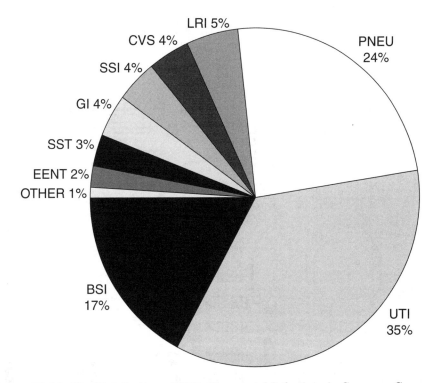

Figure 12–10 Site Distribution of 2321 Nosocomial Infections in Coronary Care Units, NNIS System, 1992–1997. PNEU, pneumonia; UTI, urinary tract infection; BSI, primary bloodstream infection; EENT, eye, ear, nose, and throat infection; SST, skin and soft tissue infection; GI, gastrointestinal infection; SSI, surgical site infection; CVS, cardiovascular system infection; LRI, lower respiratory tract infection other than pneumonia; OTHER, other.

Source: National Nosocomial Infections Surveillance (NNIS) System Report, Data Summary from October 1986–April 1998. CDC. http://www.cdc.gov/ncidod/dhqp/nnis_pubs.html.

- Each slice should be labeled with the percentage that it represents. The label can be placed either inside the slice or outside and next to it.
- Each piece of the pie should be differentiated clearly by using a legend or key. The chart is easier to read if the components are different colors or, when using black and white, clearly discernible shades or patterns.
- The total number of cases or events (the number that represents 100 percent) should be noted somewhere on the chart.
- The chart should be self-explanatory and should contain all of the information needed for the reader to understand what is being presented.
- The source of the data should be placed in a footnote, especially if the data are not original.

Maps

Maps can be used to show where a disease or event occurred. Two types of maps used to display epidemiological data are spot maps and area maps.

Spot maps. Spot maps are constructed by drawing a dot or some other symbol at each location where an event occurred, as in Figure 12–11. When investigating an outbreak or a cluster of infections, a spot map can be used to illustrate the geographic distribution of the cases and may be useful in forming a hypothesis on how a disease may have spread.

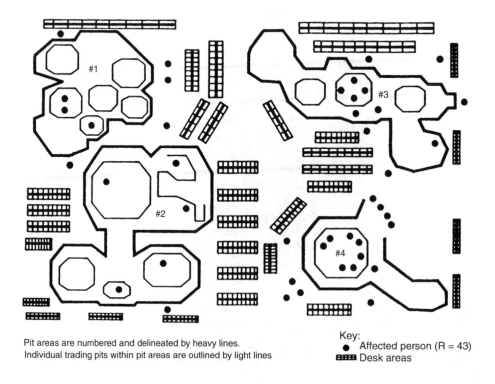

Pit areas are numbered and delineated by heavy lines.
Individual trading pits within pit areas are outlined by light lines

Key:
● Affected person (R = 43)
▦ Desk areas

Figure 12–11 Spot Map Illustrating the Occurrence of Mumps Cases in Trading Pits of Exchange A, Chicago, Illinois, August 18–December 25, 1987

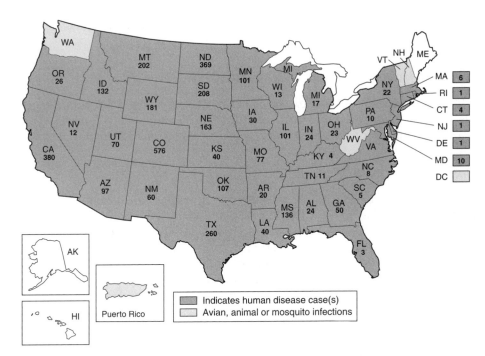

Figure 12–12 Area Map Illustrating 2007 West Nile Virus Activity in Humans, Animals, and Mosquitoes in the United States, by State, Reported to the CDC as of March 4, 2008

Source: Division of Vector-Borne Disease, CDC. http://www.cdc.gov/ncidod/dvbid/westnile/Mapsactivity/ surv&control07Maps.htm

Area maps. Area maps are used to show the geographic distribution of a disease or an event. The distribution can be shown as a rate, such as the incidence of a disease, or as the number of events or cases. Figure 12–12 shows both number of reported cases of human disease and avian, animal, and mosquito infections with West Nile Virus in 2007 in the United States. Area maps are frequently used by health departments to show patterns of infectious diseases and are useful for evaluating the occurrence of a specific disease, such as tuberculosis or influenza, in a community.

USING COMPUTERS TO CREATE GRAPHS AND CHARTS

Histograms vs. Bar Charts

Computers are generally used to prepare reports of outbreak investigations. When choosing a software program, it is important to select one that can create the types of charts and graphs that are needed for preparing epidemiology reports. When constructing an epidemic curve (the number of cases occurring over time in an outbreak), one should use a histogram—a graph that has adjoining columns, rather than a bar chart that has spaces between each column. Some commonly used spreadsheet and graphics programs easily can be used to produce bar charts, but to create a histogram the gaps between the bars must be set to zero.

Selecting the Best Method to Illustrate Data

It is important to choose the method of illustrating epidemiologic data that is best suited for conveying that particular data easily and quickly. Table 12–3 provides a guideline for selecting a graph or chart to illustrate epidemiologic data.

Avoiding "Chartjunk"

Many computer programs produce three-dimensional bar charts and pie charts. Which is better—a three-dimensional or a two-dimensional graphic? The pie charts in Figure 12–13 display the same information; however, one chart is two-dimensional and the other is three-dimensional. As a rule, a two-dimensional chart should be used, especially when information must be communicated quickly in a short presentation, because it is easier to judge the relative sizes of the component parts in the two-dimensional version of the pie than in the three-dimensional version.

The bar charts in Figure 12–14 contain the same data, a comparison of rates in two different years; however, one is two-dimensional and the other contains gridlines and three-dimensional bars. Which chart gets the message across more quickly? Graphs and charts are used to communicate information to others—it is important to keep them simple and avoid the glitter.[3] The "third dimension" in three-dimensional charts contains no additional information. Graphic activity that is unrelated to data information, such as three-dimensional

---

Table 12–3   Guideline for Selecting a Graph or Chart to Illustrate Epidemiologic Data

Type of Graph or Chart	When to Use
Arithmetic-scale line graph	Display trends in numbers or rates over time
Histogram	1. Show frequency distribution of a continuous variable 2. Show number of cases over time during an epidemic (epidemic curve)
Simple bar chart	Compare size or frequency of different categories of a single variable
Grouped bar chart	Compare size or frequency of different categories of two to four series of data
Stacked bar chart	Compare totals and illustrate component parts of the total among different groups
Pie chart	Show components of a whole
Spot map	Show location of cases or events
Area map	Display events or rates geographically

Source: Adapted from *Principles of Epidemiology: An Introduction to Applied Epidemiology and Biostatistics.* 2nd ed. Atlanta, GA: CDC; 1992:263.

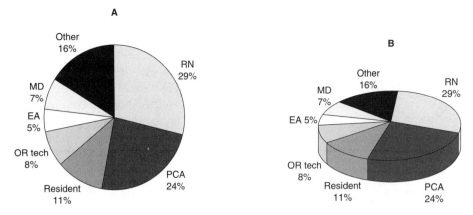

Figure 12–13 Job Category Distribution of 58 Personnel with Needlesticks, St. Anne's Hospital, 2007

Source: Author.

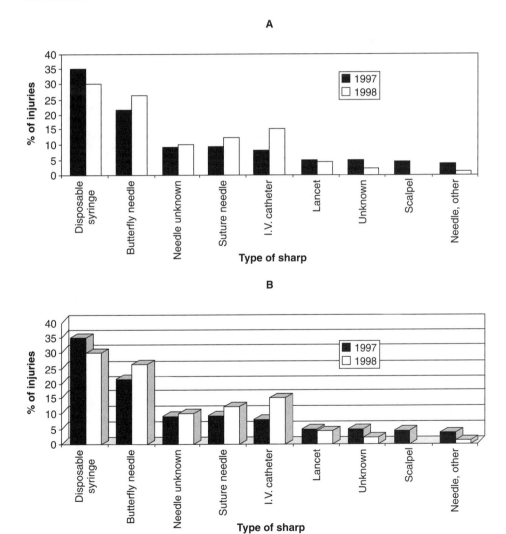

Figure 12–14 Types of Sharps Associated with Injuries, Community Hospital, 2006 and 2007

graphics, gridlines, and excessive cross-hatching, has been called "chartjunk"[1] and should be avoided. As stated by Tufte, "Graphical excellence is that which gives to the viewer the greatest number of ideas in the shortest time with the least ink in the smallest space."[1(p51)]

REFERENCES

1. Tufte ER. *The Visual Display of Quantitative Information*. Cheshire, CT: Graphics Press; 1983.
2. Centers for Disease Control and Prevention. *Principles of Epidemiology: An Introduction to Applied Epidemiology and Biostatistics*. 2nd ed. Atlanta, GA: Centers for Disease Control and Prevention, Epidemiology Program Office; 1992.
3. Jolley D. The glitter of the t table. *Lancet*. 1993;342:27–29.

SUGGESTED READING AND RESOURCES

Centers for Disease Control and Prevention. *Principles of Epidemiology in Public Health Practice: An Introduction to Applied Epidemiology and Biostatistics*. 3rd ed. Atlanta, GA: Centers for Disease Control and Prevention, Office of Workforce and Career Development; 2005. http://www2a.cdc.gov/TCEOnline/registration/detailpage.asp?res_id=1394. Accessed March 11, 2008.

Tufte ER. *The Visual Display of Quantitative Information*. Cheshire, CT: Graphics Press; 1983.

Tufte ER. *The Visual Display of Quantitative Information*. 2nd ed. Cheshire, CT: Graphics Press; 2001.

Glossary

The terms in this glossary have been adapted for use in the healthcare setting. Many of the definitions are taken or adapted from the glossaries in (1) the CDC Home Study Course 3030-G, Principles of Epidemiology, US Department of Health and Human Services, Centers for Disease Control. Atlanta, GA; 1985; and (2) the Centers for Disease Control and Prevention. Principles of Epidemiology: An Introduction to Applied Epidemiology and Biostatistics. 2nd ed. Centers for Disease Control and Prevention. Atlanta, GA; 1992.

Agent. A biological, physical, or chemical entity capable of causing disease.

Antiseptic. A chemical germicide formulated to inactivate microbial agents on skin or tissue.

Attack rate. A measure of the frequency of new cases of a disease or condition in a specified population during a specified period of time; usually expressed as a percent.

Bar chart. A visual display of quantitative data in which each category or value of a variable is represented by a bar.

Bias. Deviation of results from the truth.

Baseline. A number or value used as a base for measurement or comparison.

Carrier. A person who has no apparent clinical disease but harbors a specific infectious agent and is capable of transmitting the agent to others; a carrier is a potential source of infection.

Case. A person who has a particular disease or condition under investigation.

Case-control study. A type of observational analytic study. Enrollment into the study is based on presence ("case") or absence ("control") of a particular disease or condition. Characteristics such as previous exposure to particular agents are then compared between cases and controls.

Case definition. Standard criteria used for deciding whether a person has a particular disease or condition, by specifying clinical, laboratory, and epidemiologic characteristics (such as time, place, and person).

Chain of infection. A process that begins when an agent leaves its reservoir or host through a portal of exit, and is conveyed by some mode of transmission, then enters through an appropriate portal of entry to infect a susceptible host.

Cleaning. The process of physically removing foreign material, such as dirt, blood, microorganisms, and body fluids, from a surface.

Cluster. A group of cases of a disease or other health-related event that occurs closely related in time and place. The number of cases may or may not exceed the expected number; frequently the expected number is not known.

Cohort. A well-defined group of persons selected for a study. Persons in the group have had a common exposure, and are then followed up for the occurrence of disease.

Cohort study. A type of observational analytic study. Also known as a prospective study.

Colonization. Presence and growth of a micro-organism on a host that has no symptoms or cellular injury. A colonized host may serve as a source of infection.

Common source outbreak. An outbreak that results from a group of persons being exposed to a common noxious influence, such as an infectious agent or toxin. If the group is exposed over a relatively brief period of time, so that all cases occur within one incubation period, then the common source outbreak is further classified as a point source outbreak. In some common source outbreaks, persons may be exposed over a period of days, weeks, or longer, with the exposure being either intermittent or continuous.

Communicable. May be transmitted directly or indirectly from one person to another.

Contact. (1) Exposure to a source of infection; (2) a person that has been exposed to a source of infection.

Contagious. Able to easily transmit an infectious agent from one person to another.

Contingency table. A two-variable table with cross-tabulated data.

Control. In a case-control study, the person or group of persons without the disease or condition being studied; the group to which the cases (those with the disease or condition) are compared.

Data, continuous. Data consisting of measurements of things for which there are an infinite number of possible values between the minimum and the maximum values in the data set (e.g., age, weight, height, and temperature).

Data, discrete. Data consisting of measurements of things that can be counted or measured only in whole units (e.g., the number of persons with a specific disease or condition).

Demographic information. Those characteristics of a person, such as age, sex, and race, that are used in descriptive epidemiology to characterize the population at risk.

Denominator. The lower portion of a fraction; contains the data used to calculate a rate or ratio. In a rate, the denominator is usually the population at risk.

Dependent variable. In a statistical analysis, the outcome variable(s), or the variable(s), whose values are a function of other variable(s) called independent variable(s) in the relationship under study.

Descriptive epidemiology. The aspect of epidemiology concerned with organizing and summarizing health-related data according to time, place, and person.

Direct transmission. The immediate transfer of an agent from a reservoir to a susceptible host by direct contact or droplet spread.

Disease. A condition that represents a deviation from normal health and is associated with characteristic signs and symptoms.

Disinfectant. A chemical germicide formulated to inactivate microbial agents on inanimate surfaces.

Disinfection. A process that eliminates pathogenic microorganisms, except bacterial spores, from a surface.

Droplets. Liquid particles expelled into the air when a person talks, sings, coughs, or sneezes.

Droplet nuclei. The residue of dried droplets that may remain suspended in the air for long periods, may be carried over great distances, and are easily inhaled into the lungs.

Droplet spread. The direct transmission of an infectious agent from a reservoir to a susceptible host by spray with relatively large, short-ranged aerosols produced by sneezing, coughing, or talking.

Endemic. The usual presence of a disease or infectious agent within a given geographic area or population group.

Endogenous. Originating or growing from within.

Exogenous. Originating from an external source.

Environmental factor. An extrinsic factor (geology, climate, insects, sanitation, health services, etc.) that affects the agent and the opportunity for exposure.

Epidemic. The occurrence of more cases of a disease or event than expected during a specified period of time in a given area or among a specific group of people.

Epidemic curve. A histogram that shows the course of a disease outbreak or epidemic by plotting the number of cases by time of onset.

Epidemic period. A time period when the number of cases of disease or events reported is greater than expected.

Epidemiology. The study of the distribution and determinants of health-related states or events in specified populations, and the application of this study to the control of health problems.

Experimental study. A study in which the investigator specifies the exposure category for each individual in the study and then follows the individual to determined the effects of the exposure (e.g., a clinical trial)

Etiology. The cause of a specific disease.

Etiologic agent. An agent that causes a specific disease.

Fomite. An inanimate object that can become contaminated and transmit infectious agents.

Frequency distribution. A tabulation of the number of times an event occurs in each class interval or category; often displayed in a two-column table in which the left column lists the individual values or categories and the right column indicates the number of events in each category.

Graph. A visual display of quantitative data that uses a system of coordinates.

Histogram. A graph that displays the frequency distribution of a continuous variable. Rectangles are drawn in such a way that their bases lie on a linear scale representing different intervals, and their heights are proportional to the frequencies of the values within each of the intervals.

Host. A person or animal that can be infected by an infectious agent under natural conditions.

Hypothesis. A supposition, arrived at from observation or reflection, that leads to refutable predictions. Any conjecture cast in a form that will allow it to be tested and refuted.

Hypothesis, null. The first step in testing for statistical significance in which it is assumed that an exposure is not related to a disease or other health-related event.

Iatrogenic. Related to a medical intervention.

Immunity, active. Resistance developed in response to stimulus by an antigen (infecting agent or vaccine) and usually characterized by the presence of antibody produced by the host.

Immunity, herd. The resistance of a group to invasion and spread of an infectious agent, based on the resistance to infection of a high proportion of individual members of the group. The resistance is a product of the number of susceptible persons and the probability that those who are susceptible will come into contact with an infected person.

Immunity, passive. Immunity conferred by an antibody produced in another host and acquired either naturally by an infant from its mother or artificially by administration of an antibody-containing preparation (antiserum or immune globulin).

Incidence rate. A measure of the frequency that an event, such as a new case of illness, occurs in a population over a period of time. When calculating an incidence rate, the numerator is the number of new cases occurring during a given time period and the denominator is the population at risk during that time period.

Incubation period. The interval between the effective exposure of a susceptible host to an infectious agent and the onset of signs and symptoms of disease.

Independent variable. An exposure, risk factor, or other characteristic being observed or measured that is hypothesized to influence an event or manifestation (i.e., the dependent variable).

Index case. The first recognized case having a specific disease or attribute.

Indirect transmission. The transmission of an agent carried from a reservoir to a susceptible host either by suspended air particles or by an animate (vector) or inanimate (vehicle) intermediary.

Infection. The entry and multiplication of an infectious agent into the body of man resulting in a reaction.

Infectivity. The ability of an agent to infect a host.

Infestation. The lodgment, development, and reproduction of arthropods on the body or in the clothes.

Isolation. The separation of infected persons from those who are not infected for the purpose of preventing the spread of an infectious agent to others.

Line-listing. A rectangular database in which each row represents a case, usually a person with a disease or health-related condition, and each column contains information on variables relevant to the event being studied.

Mean, arithmetic. The measure of central location commonly called the average; it is calculated by adding together all of the individual values in a data set and dividing by the number of values in the set.

Measure of association. A quantified relationship between exposure and disease; examples of measures of association include relative risk, rate ratio, and odds ratio.

Measure of central location. A measure of central tendency; a central value that represents a distribution of data. Measures of central location include the mean, median, and mode.

Measure of dispersion. A measure of the spread of a distribution out from its central value. Measures of dispersion used in epidemiology include the variance and the standard deviation.

Median. The measure of central location that divides a set of data into two equal parts.

Mode. A measure of central location; the value that occurs most frequently in a set of observations.

Mode of transmission. The mechanism by which an agent is spread from person to person.

Morbidity. Any departure, subjective or objective, from a state of physiological or psychological well-being.

Natural history of disease. The temporal course of disease from onset (inception) to resolution.

Necessary cause. A causal factor whose presence is required for the occurrence of a disease or health-related event.

Normal curve. A bell-shaped curve that results when a normal distribution is graphed.

Normal distribution. The symmetrical clustering of values around a central location. The properties of a normal distribution include the following. (1) It is a continuous, symmetrical distribution in which both tails extend to infinity; (2) the arithmetic mean, median, and mode are identical; and (3) its shape is determined by the mean and standard deviation.

Nosocomial infection. An infection resulting from exposure to a source within a healthcare facility; may occur in patients, personnel, or visitors.

Numerator. The upper portion of a fraction. In epidemiology, it is usually the number of cases of a disease or event being studied.

Observational study. An epidemiological study in which nature is allowed to take its course. Changes or differences in one characteristic are studied in relation to changes or differences in others, without the intervention of the investigator.

Odds ratio. A measure of association that quantifies the relationship between an exposure and health outcome from a comparative study.

Outbreak. Synonymous with *epidemic*.

Pandemic. An epidemic that occurs over a very wide area, such as several countries or continents, and which usually affects a large proportion of the population.

Pathogenicity. The capacity of an agent to cause disease.

Pie chart. A circular chart in which the size of each slice of the pie is proportional to the frequency of each category of a variable.

Population. The total number of persons in a specified place or area.

Prevalence. The number or proportion of cases or events in a given population.

Prevalence rate. The proportion of persons in a population who have a particular disease or attribute at a given point in time (i.e., point prevalence) or over a given time interval (i.e., period prevalence).

Propagated outbreak. An outbreak that spreads from person to person rather than originating from a common source.

Proportion. A type of ratio in which the numerator is included in the denominator.

Pseudoepidemic. A real cluster or increase in false infections or an artificial cluster or increase in true infections.

Pseudo-outbreak. See *pseudoepidemic*.

Random sample. A sample derived by selecting individuals such that each individual has the same probability of being selected.

Range. In statistics, the difference between the largest and the smallest values in a distribution. In common use, the span of values from smallest to largest.

Rate. An expression of the frequency with which an illness or event occurs in a defined population.

Ratio. The value obtained by dividing one quantity by another.

Relative risk. A comparison of the risk of some health-related event, such as disease, in two groups.

Reservoir. The habitat in which an infectious agent normally lives, grows, and multiplies; reservoirs may be human, animal, or environmental.

Risk. The probability that an event will occur (e.g., that a person will develop a specific disease).

Risk factor. A characteristic that is associated with an increased occurrence of disease or other health-related event (e. g., exposure to a therapeutic or diagnostic procedure).

Risk ratio. A comparison of the risk of some health-related event, such as disease, in two groups.

Sample. A selected subset of a population.

Secondary attack rate. A measure of the frequency of new cases of a disease among the contacts of known cases.

Sensitivity. The ability of a system to detect epidemics and other changes in disease occurrence. The proportion of persons with disease who are correctly identified by a screening test or case definition as having disease.

Skewed. A distribution that is asymmetrical.

Source of infection. A person, animal, or inanimate object from which an infectious agent is transmitted to a host.

Specificity. The proportion of persons without disease who are correctly identified by a screening test or case definition as not having disease.

Sporadic. A disease that occurs infrequently and irregularly.

Spot map. A map that indicates the location of each case of a disease or event.

Standard deviation. The most widely used measure of dispersion of a frequency distribution, equal to the positive square root of the variance.

Standard error of the mean. The standard deviation of a theoretical distribution of sample means about the true population mean.

Standard precautions. An infection prevention and control strategy designed to reduce the risk of transmission of microorganisms from both recognized and unrecognized sources of infection in healthcare settings. These precautions are applied to all patients regardless of their diagnosis or presumed infection status.

Sterilization. A process that eliminates or destroys all forms of microorganisms.

Surveillance. The systematic collection, analysis, interpretation, and dissemination of data on an ongoing basis, to gain knowledge of the pattern of disease or event occurrence in a population in order to control and prevent disease in that population.

Susceptible. A person who does not have sufficient resistance to an infectious agent to prevent infection if exposure occurs.

Validity. The degree to which a measurement actually measures or detects what it is supposed to measure.

Variable. Any characteristic or attribute that can be measured.

Variance. A measure of the dispersion shown by a set of observations, defined by the sum of the squares of deviations from the mean, divided by the number of degrees of freedom in the set of observations.

Vector. An animate intermediary, frequently an arthropod or insect, that is involved in the indirect transmission of an agent by carrying the agent from a reservoir to a susceptible host.

Vehicle. An inanimate intermediary that is involved in the indirect transmission of an agent by carrying the agent from a reservoir to a susceptible host.

Virulence. The degree of pathogenicity of an infectious agent.

Zoonoses. An infectious disease that is transmissible under normal conditions from animals to humans.

Index